NURSING HISTORY REVIEW

OFFICIAL JOURNAL OF THE
AMERICAN ASSOCIATION FOR THE HISTORY OF NURSING

ISSN 1062–8061
ISBN 978-0-8261-0788-6

2011—Volume 19

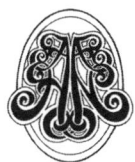

CONTENTS

11   GUEST EDITOR'S NOTE

       Historians and Health Care Reform:
       Avoiding the "Ash Heap"
       CYNTHIA CONNOLLY

       ARTICLES

15   Hell in the Family: Married Women and Madness Before
       Institutionalization at the St-Jean-de-Dieu Asylum, 1890–1921
       MARIE-CLAUDE THIFAULT

29   Life and Death in Philadelphia's Black Belt:
       A Tale of an Urban Tuberculosis Campaign, 1900–1930
       J. MARGO BROOKS CARTHON

53   Sickening Nurses: Fever Nursing, Nurses' Illness, and the
       Anatomy of Blame, New Zealand 1903–1923
       PAMELA J. WOOD

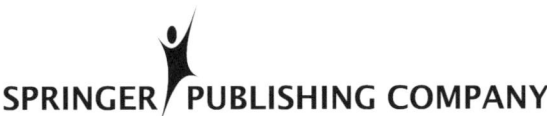

NEW YORK

78	Nurses Without Borders: The History of Nursing as U.S. International History JULIA F. IRWIN
103	Gender, Politics, and Regionalism: Factors in the Evolution of Registered Psychiatric Nursing in Manitoba, 1920–1960 BEVERLY HICKS
127	Political Dreams, Practical Boundaries: The Case of the Nursing Minimum Data Set, 1983–1990 JENNIFER HOBBS

REPORT FROM THE NURSING HISTORY SECTION AT THE 2009 INTERNATIONAL COUNCIL OF NURSES, DURBAN, SOUTH AFRICA

156	Guest Editors' Notes BARBRA MANN WALL SIOBAN NELSON
158	The History of Nursing in Ethiopia ABDURAHMAN ALI
161	The History of Nursing in Tanzania GUSTAV MOYO AND GREGORY MHAMELA
165	The History of Nursing in the Republic of Mauritius KRIST DHURMAH
168	The History of Nursing in the Togolese Republic BASSAN LAMBONI
171	The History of Nursing in the Islamic Republic of Iran MARYAM HAZRATI, G. MIRZABEIGY, AND AHMAD NEJATIAN
175	The History of Nursing in Romania ECATERINA GULIE
179	The History of Nursing in Turkey FUSUN TERZIOGLU

Notes and Documents

183   Networks of Identity: The Potential
      of Biographical Studies for Teaching Nursing Identity
      MARIA ITAYRA PADILHA
      AND SIOBAN NELSON

In Memoriam

194   Karen Buhler-Wilkerson,
      19 May 1944–13 February 2010:
      Spreading the Contagion of History
      SUSAN M. REVERBY

Media Reviews

198   *Cultures of Health: A Historical Anthology*
      REVIEWER: SONYA GRYPMA

200   *Brought to Life: Exploring the History of Medicine*
      REVIEWER: GERARD M. FEALY

202   *Canada's Role in Fighting Tuberculosis*
      REVIEWER: J. MARGO BROOKS CARTHON

204   *Classic Nursing Films 1927–1945*
      REVIEWER: MARILYN E. FLOOD

207   *Opening Doors: Contemporary African American
      Academic Surgeons*
      REVIEWER: ANNE Z. COCKERHAM

Review Essay: Women and War

210   *Mobilizing Minerva: American Women in the First World War*
      by Kimberly Jensen
      World War II Front Line Nurse
      by Mildred A. MacGregor
      REVIEWER: CHRISTINE E. HALLETT

REVIEW ESSAY:
NURSING IN NEWFOUNDLAND

214 *From the Voices of Nurses: An Oral History of
Newfoundland Nurses who Graduated Prior to 1950*
by Marilyn Beaton and Jeanette Walsh
A Life of Caring: 16 Newfoundland Nurses Tell Their Stories
by Marilyn Marsh, Jeanette Walsh,
and Marilyn Beaton
REVIEWERS: LYDIA WYTENBROEK
AND SONYA GRYPMA

REVIEW ESSAY:
PHARMACEUTICALS, HISTORY,
AND AMERICAN SOCIETY

217 *Prescribing by Numbers: Drugs and the Definition of Disease*
by Jeremy A. Greene
*Medical Research for Hire: The Political Economy of Pharmaceutical
Clinical Trials* by Jill A. Fisher
REVIEWER: CYNTHIA A. CONNOLLY

BOOK REVIEWS

220 *Mary Putnam Jacobi and the Politics of Medicine
in Nineteenth-Century America*
by Carla Bittel
REVIEWER: RIMA D. APPLE

221 *Health and Medicine in the circum-Caribbean, 1800–1968*,
edited by Juanita De Barros, Steven Palmer,
and David Wright
REVIEWER: KAROL K. WEAVER

223 *Rural District Nursing in Gloucestershire, 1880–1925*
by Carrie Howse
REVIEWER: JEANNINE URIBE

224 *Containing Trauma: Nursing Work in the First World War*
by Christine E. Hallett
REVIEWER: PATRICIA D'ANTONIO

226 *Place and Practice in Canadian Nursing History*
edited by Jayne Elliott, Meryn Stuart, and Cynthia Toman
REVIEWER: JULIA F. IRWIN

228 *Power, Politics and the History of Nursing in New Jersey*
by Frances Ward
REVIEWER: CARLA SCHISSEL

229 *When Sister Ruled: The Nursing Sister*
by Peter Arden
REVIEWER: TERESA M. O'NEILL

231 *Student Bodies: The Influence of Student Health Services in American Society and Medicine*
by Heather Munro Prescott
REVIEWER: BETH LINKER

232 *Caring and Curing: A History of the Indian Health Service*
by James P. Rife and Capt. Alan J. Dellapenna, Jr.
REVIEWER: CHRISTINE BREWER

234 *Examining Tuskegee: The Infamous Syphilis Study and Its Legacy*
by Susan M. Reverby
REVIEWER: JEAN C. WHELAN

236 *Make Room for Daddy: The Journey from Waiting Room to Birthing Room*
by Judith Walzer Leavitt
REVIEWER: SYLVIA RINKER

237 *Under the Radar: Cancer and the Cold War*
by Ellen Leopold
REVIEWER: BRIGID LUSK

239 *Officer, Nurse, Woman: The Army Nurse Corps in the Vietnam War*
by Kara Dixon Vuic
REVIEWER: MARY T. SARNECKY

241 *Moments of Truth in Genetic Medicine*
by Susan Lindee
REVIEWER: ELLEN D. BAER

242 *Observing Bioethics*
by Renée C. Fox and Judith P. Swazey
REVIEWER: CONNIE M. ULRICH

244 *The Adelaide Hospital School of Nursing 1859–2009: A Commemorative History*
by Gerard M. Fealy
REVIEWER: ANN MARIE WALSH BRENNAN

246 NEW DISSERTATIONS

Cover Photo: The original caption for this picture is "American Red Cross Nurses in Foreign Lands." It was first printed in the American Red Cross Courier in 1923. Reprinted courtesy of the American Red Cross; all rights reserved in all countries.

Nursing History Review is published annually for the American Association for the History of Nursing, Inc., by Springer Publishing Company, LLC, New York.

Business Office: All business correspondence, including subscriptions, renewals, advertising, and address changes, should be sent to Springer Publishing Company, LLC, 11 West 42nd Street, New York, NY 10036.

Editorial Office: Submissions and editorial correspondence should be directed to Patricia D'Antonio, Editor, *Nursing History Review,* University of Pennsylvania, 2017 Claire M. Fagin Hall, 418 Curie Boulevard, Philadelphia, PA 19104-4217. See Guidelines for contributors on page 8 for further details.

Members of the American Association for the History of Nursing, Inc. (AAHN) receive Nursing History Review on payment of annual membership dues. Applications and other correspondence relating to AAHN membership should be directed to: David L. Stumph, IOM, CAE, Executive Director, American Association for the History of Nursing, Inc., 10200 W. 44th Avenue #304, Wheat Ridge, CO 80033. Phone: 303 422.2685. E-mail: aahn@resourcenter.com

Subscription Rates (per Year): Volume 19, 2011. For institutions: $90. For individuals: $90. Outside the United States—for institutions: $90. For individuals: $90. Payment must be made in advance by check (in U.S. dollars drawn on a U.S. bank) or international money order, payable to Springer Publishing Company, LLC, or by MasterCard, Visa, or American Express.

Indexes/abstracts of articles appear in: CINAHL® print index & database, Current Contents/Social & Behavioral Science, Social Sciences Citation Index, Research Alert, RNdex, Index Medicus/MEDLINE, History Abstracts, America; History and Life.

Permission: All rights are reserved. No part of this volume may be reproduced or utilized in any form or by any means, electronic or mechanical, including photocopying (with the exception listed below), recording, or by any information storage and retrieval system, without permission in writing from the publisher. Permission is granted by the copyright owner for libraries and others registered with the Copyright Clearance Center (CCC) to photocopy any article herein for $5.00 per copy of the article. Payments should be sent directly to Copyright Clearance Center, Inc., 222 Rosewood Drive, Danvers, MA 01923, USA. This permission holds for copying done for personal or internal reference use only: it does not extend to other kinds of copying, such as copying for general distribution, advertising or promotional purposes, creating new collective works, or for resale. Requests for these permissions or further information should be addressed to Springer Publishing Company, LLC.

Postmaster: Send address change to Springer Publishing Company, LLC, 11 West 42nd Street, New York, NY 10036.

Copyright © 2011 by Springer Publishing Company, LLC, New York, for the American Association for the History of Nursing, Inc.

ISSN 1062–8061

ISBN 978-0-8261-0788-6

eBook ISBN 978-0-8261-0789-3

GUIDELINES FOR CONTRIBUTORS

The *Nursing History Review,* the official publication of the American Association for the History of Nursing, is a peer-reviewed journal, published annually for subscribers and members of the Association. Original research manuscripts are welcomed in broad areas related to the history of nursing, health care, health policy, and society. The *Review* prefers manuscripts of approximately 40 pages, inclusive of endnotes.

Submitted manuscripts must be prepared using the guidelines specified in the *Chicago Manual of Style,* 15th edition. Manuscripts must have a title page that contains the full title of the manuscript, the author(s) name(s) as they are meant to appear in print, institutional affiliations and preferred mailing addresses *for all authors,* and relevant contact information for the corresponding author. The title page must be followed with an abstract of approximately 150–200 words.

Manuscripts must be double-spaced and of letter-quality print. They must also use a type size of at least 12 characters per inch or 12 points. Please leave generous margins of at least 1 inch. All pages, including text, notes, and reference pages, must be numbered consecutively. All notes must be double-spaced and placed at the end of the manuscript as endnotes rather than footnotes.

Authors are responsible for securing permissions for all materials submitted. If more than 500 words of text are quoted from a book, or more than 250 words from an article, or if a table or figure has been previously published, the manuscript must be accompanied by written permission from the copyright owner.

Initial submissions of manuscripts may be sent by e-mail to *nhr@nursing.upenn.edu.* All submissions will be acknowledged when received. *Final versions of manuscripts accepted for publication* should be prepared in MS Word. The final packet must be submitted via e-mail to *nhr@nursing.upenn.edu.* Photographs or other figures accompanying the final manuscript must be attached as TIF files with resolutions of at least 600 dpi. All appropriate permissions and copyright releases must accompany the final submission.

All correspondence regarding manuscripts should be sent to: Patricia D'Antonio, PhD, RN, FAAN, Editor, *Nursing History Review,* University of Pennsylvania School of Nursing, 2017 Claire M. Fagin Hall, 418 Curie Boulevard, Philadelphia, PA 19104–4217. Phone: 215/746.8322. Fax: 215/573–2168. E-mail: *dantonio@nursing.upenn.edu* or *nhr@nursing.upenn.edu.*

AMERICAN ASSOCIATION FOR THE HISTORY OF NURSING, INC.

Sylvia Rinker
President

Carla Schissel
First Vice President and Chair,
Strategic Planning Committee

Arlene Keeling
Second Vice President and
Chair, Program Committee

Jean C. Whelan
Secretary

Jennifer Telford
Treasurer

Brigid Lusk
Director and Chair,
Publications Committee

Rima D. Apple
Director and Chair,
Awards Committee

Carol Daisy
Director and Chair,
By-Laws Committee

Barbra Mann Wall
Director and Member,
Finance Committee

Teresa M. O'Neil
Director, and Member,
Strategic Planning

Sandra Lewenson
Chair, Nominating Committee

Arlene Keeling
Past President

Gertrude Hutchinson
Archivist

NURSING HISTORY REVIEW

Patricia D'Antonio, Editor
Barbra Mann Wall, Book Review Editor
Jean Whelan, Media Editor
Elizabeth Weiss, Assistant Editor

Editorial Review Board

Ellen D. Baer
Florida

Nettie Birnbach
Florida

Eleanor Crowder Bjoring
Texas

Barbara Brodie
Virginia

Olga Maranjian Church
Connecticut

Julie Fairman
Pennsylvania

Marilyn Flood
California

Karen Flynn
Illinois

Janet Golden
New Jersey

Christine E. Hallett
Manchester, England

Diane Hamilton
Michigan

Carol Helmstadter
Ontario, Canada

Wanda C. Hiestand
New York

Arlene Keeling
Virginia

Joan Lynaugh
Pennsylvania

Lois Monteiro
Rhode Island

Sioban Nelson
Toronto, Canada

Anne-Marie Rafferty
London, England

Susan M. Reverby
Massachusetts

Naomi Rogers
Connecticut

Meryn Stuart
Ottawa, Canada

Nancy Tomes
New York

GUEST EDITOR'S NOTE

Historians and Health Care Reform: Avoiding the "Ash Heap"

Almost every president since Theodore Roosevelt in 1912 has tried to reform health care. Along the way, there have been major successes (Medicaid and Medicare in the 1960s) and spectacular failures (President Bill Clinton's Health Security Act in the 1990s).[1] As I write this editorial, many pundits are saying that President Barack Obama's health reform proposal is in serious jeopardy. Will this initiative be fated to end in history's ashheap, that place of failed ideas and philosophies so memorably named by both Leon Trotsky and Ronald Reagan, two men who held *widely* divergent beliefs about almost everything? At this point it is unclear, but many on all sides of the debate have been anxious to draw on the "lessons" of history to bolster their argument for, or against, this particular reform plan.[2] But what is the role of historians in informing this debate? The lives and careers of two prominent historians who died in the past year, John Hope Franklin (1915–2009) and Howard Zinn (1922–2010), provide one answer: the historian as activist.

Franklin, born in racially segregated Oklahoma, received his education at Fisk and Harvard universities. A prolific and meticulous scholar, he reshaped our understanding of United States history, particularly that of the American South.[3] The first African American to lead a major history department at Brooklyn College, he later held professorships at the University of Chicago and Duke University. But Franklin also pioneered the role of the historian as activist, marching in civil rights demonstrations in Selma, Alabama, and crafting a brief for *Brown v. Board of Education*, the landmark Supreme Court case in which the doctrine of racial separation was adjudicated unconstitutional. Franklin also served on a number of national commissions addressing issues of major importance to American society, among them President Clinton's One America: The President's Initiative on Race. The recipient of many honors, he received the United States' highest civilian award, the Presidential Medal of Freedom, in 1996.

The son of Jewish immigrants, Howard Zinn was born in Brooklyn. After military service in World War II, he attended New York and Columbia universities. Unabashedly radicalized by events roiling the nation in the 1950s and 1960s, Zinn's revisionist scholarship infuriated or inspired, depending on one's perspective. For example, Zinn challenged ideals cherished by many such as American exceptionalism, the notion that the United States has a unique, foreordained place at the center of the world's history. Again and again in his many articles and books, Zinn argued against what he saw as the celebratory impulse in historical thought, one that he believed ignored the genocide, racism, militarism, imperialism, and class exploitation nested within the American narrative. Zinn, like Franklin, believed that historians needed to insert themselves into history. For example, he, too, marched for civil rights and also traveled to North Vietnam with another radical, Father Daniel Berrigan, at the height of American involvement in Vietnam.[4]

Both Franklin and Zinn were also known as public intellectuals, a rather loosely defined phrase that can mean many things to many people. I use British geographer Kevin Ward's definition that what makes public intellectuals different from other scholars is that they write accessibly about matters of interest to the general public. "They are not just individuals who know things but people who shape the thoughts of a generation, through engagement, interaction, review, and synthesis."[5]

So, returning to the issue of health care reform: as nurse historians, do we have a role as public intellectuals in terms of shaping the debate surrounding the current proposal and if so, what is that role? Although each scholar needs to define notions of activism and involvement for himself or herself, I suggest a few strategies to better infuse nursing history into health care reform debates. First, I believe nurse historians must undertake scholarly inquiry that meets the standards of quality historical scholarship. Second, we need to situate our work clearly in the time stream of history while also translating it into narratives to that speak to issues that matter, not just to nurses, but to the broader American society as well as policymakers.

A few years ago I was lucky enough to spend time on Capitol Hill. Although it is a place where history is often cited, and ever present because of the museum-like structures in which the work takes place, as a tool for informing policy, history is not well used by lawmakers. The world of Washington tends to look at problems in a reactive, narrow, and often technical, manner. Staffers, the individuals who shape and write legislation, often have a weak understanding of their predecessors' attempts to address similar problems in the past. On Capitol Hill, knowing the history of a problem means reviewing materials from the previous Congress, not the last century.

Although historians of nursing in the past generation have generated a vibrant body of first-rate scholarship and forged innovative dissemination methods in an attempt to penetrate the consciousness of policy makers and the public, we need to do more. John Hope Franklin and Howard Zinn each challenged the traditional historical narratives governing their era. They positioned themselves as scholar-activists and so must we. In addition to actively seeking opportunities to communicate with the public, improving our reach not just through traditional venues such as newspaper editorials, we must also master the newer frontiers, such as social media. We need to insure that our students, whether at the undergraduate or graduate level, learn to think about the past in an integrated fashion. Nursing history is also American (or Canadian, South African, etc.) history, and nursing students' scholarship and thought processes need to reflect a broad understanding of our nation's history. We also must encourage more of our students to seek opportunities outside of clinical or academic settings and instead seek jobs with policymakers, advocacy groups, or think tanks. Health care reform, if it occurs, will be a process and involve a great deal of incrementalism. By positioning a new generation of nurses and nurse historians who understand the complexities and nuances of the past in the forums in which decisions are made, we can keep the embers of reform glowing and out of the ash heap of history.

CYNTHIA CONNOLLY
Associate Professor
University of Pennsylvania
School of Nursing
Claire M. Fagin Hall
418 Curie Boulevard
Philadelphia, PA 19104–6020

From the Editor: In Appreciation to our External Reviewers

On behalf of the Editorial Review Board, I thank the following colleagues who gave generously of their time and expertise in the review of manuscripts: Susan Brandt, Gertje Boschma, Winifred Connerton, Cynthia Connolly, Lynn Dunphy, Jayne Elliott, Judith Godden, Sonya Grypma, Rebecca Harmon, Sandra Lewenson, Dolly Macullen, Susan McGann, Kate Prebble, and Marie-Claude Thifault.

Erratum

Christoph Schweikardt corresponding address is:
Institute for History, Theory and Ethics in Medicine
University Hospital Aachen
RWTH Aachen University
Wendlingweg 2
D-52074 Aachen
Germany

Notes

1. Beatrix Hoffman, "Health Care Reform and Social Movements in the United States," *American Journal of Public Health* 93 (2003): 75–85.

2. See, for example, Robert Reich, "The Lessons from History on Health Care Reform," statement dated 8 September 2009, http://robertreich.blogspot.com/2009/09/lessons-from-history-on-health-care.html (accessed 10 February 2010).

3. John Hope Franklin, *Mirror to America: The Autobiography of John Hope Franklin* (New York: Farrar, Straus & Giroux, 2005).

4. Howard Zinn, *You Can't Be Neutral on a Moving Train: A Personal History of Our Times* (Boston: Beacon Press, 2002).

5. Kevin Ward, "'Public Intellectuals,' Geography, Its Representations and Its Publics," *Geoforum* 38 (2007): 1058–64.

ARTICLES

Hell in the Family: Married Women and Madness Before Institutionalization at the St-Jean-de-Dieu Asylum, 1890–1921

Marie-Claude Thifault
University of Ottawa

Abstract. Research in Montreal's St-Jean-de-Dieu Asylum archives has revealed a number of letters from family members and local physicians pleading for asylum care for married women between 1890 and 1921. When added to other admission documents in patients' medical files, these letters allow an intimate glimpse into private lives of families and highlight the pain and distress of dealing with mentally ill people in the home before the introduction of community mental health services. Far from easily abandoning a spouse or mother, close-knit French Canadian families struggled until they could no longer cope before seeking help. To comply with asylum regulations, family members (primarily husbands, who were often illiterate) and local physicians were required to justify their applications for admission, but they did so in different ways.

As historians of mental illness are now demonstrating, the link between the sex and social class of individual patients helps to refine our understandings of asylum populations of the nineteenth century. Patients (of either sex) who were deemed insane and who did not have family networks were vulnerable; being single had an impact on both the therapeutic plan and the duration of confinement of this class of patients.[1] Research has shown that these people often spent years longer than perhaps necessary in the asylum, primarily because asylum administrators were reluctant to send them out without community support. Scholars have also now shown that women were not overrepresented among those committed for insanity. Most scholars, however, have either studied institutionalized women as a group or focused on single women. As for married women, it was believed that they were admitted because their family had abandoned them.[2]

This paper examines a group of married women committed for insanity between 1890 and 1921 at the St-Jean-de-Dieu Asylum in Montreal. Opened in 1873, this hospital contained a population that was 90 percent French Canadian. Having had two centuries in Quebec to develop "solid networks to lighten the burden of a family in need," French Canadians typically resisted institutionalizing family members, and research on this specific group of women has already demonstrated that they were part of families who cared about them.[3] Although historian David Wright found that more married than single women were admitted to the asylums in Hamilton and Toronto in Ontario, single people of both sexes formed the majority of patients in Quebec asylums (see Figure 1). If single people without social networks in Quebec were more likely to be admitted to an asylum, what can we learn about the motivation of families to institutionalize a loved one who had family support, especially in such closely knit French Canadian families? What reasons did families have to admit their wives and mothers

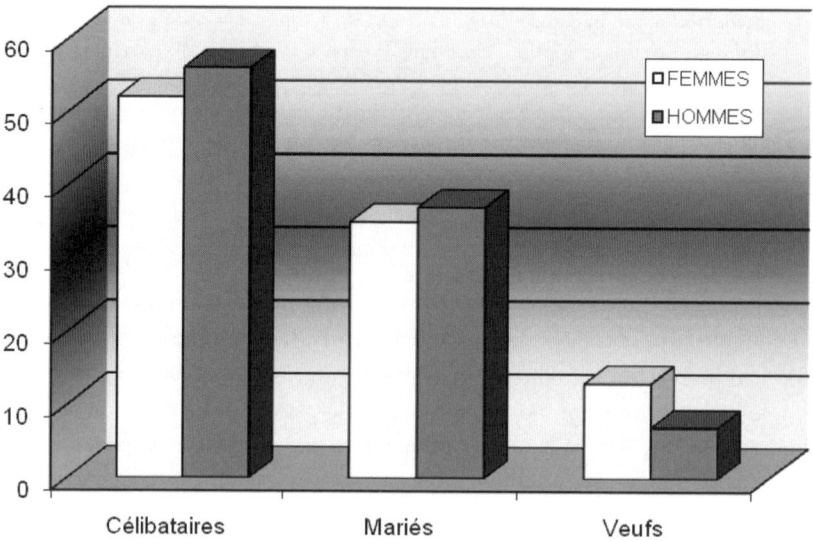

Figure 1. Civil status of the St-Jean-de-Dieu asylum population from a sample taken from admissions between 1879 and 1921. When the widowed and single categories are combined, single people outnumber married to an even greater extent. Femmes = women; hommes = men; célibataires = single; mariés = married; veufs = widowed.

to institutions, how did they explain their behavior, and how did they negotiate admission with asylum officials? Often needing help with putting their thoughts on paper, family members could only explain the extreme and threatening behavior of these women in terms of failure to carry out expected roles as wives and mothers. Local physicians, however, drew on their medical understandings of mental illness to convince the asylum's medical superintendent of the necessity for admission. This study suggests that, far from simply abandoning these women, families turned to institutional care only when they could no longer cope.

This study is based on records of patients admitted to St-Jean-de-Dieu between 1890 and 1921, and uses the official documentation on female patients along with, in some cases, correspondence addressed to institution authorities. There are 856 files on married women (37 percent of the women institutionalized during this period).[4] A sample of 284 files, 12.5 percent of married women admitted, were selected for this study because they contained enough explicit information justifying the need for commitment.

Commitment Procedure

Gaining admission to an insane asylum was complicated. An admission form, Form A, was usually filled out by a family member or friend of the patient. This form required the first and last name, profession, age, and residence of the person filling it out and the person for whom the placement was being requested. A medical certificate, Form B, filled out by a local physician, had to accompany the request for an admission. Following the rules established for admission procedures at English asylums,[5] this medical certificate could not be signed by a physician's relative, a distant relative of the patient, or the owner of the asylum. In cases deemed to be "idiotism" and "imbecility," the physician had to explicitly demonstrate that the sickness was dangerous or represented a cause of scandal, such as exposing themselves completely nude in public. Form C and its appendix gave the particulars of the illness and reasons why it was necessary to treat the sick person in an asylum. To complete the application for admission, Forms D, E, and K had to be signed by a priest and the mayor, attesting formally to the insanity of the patient and her place of residence. These last forms were used, among other things, to establish the ability of the applicant to pay the cost of care for the patient during her stay in the asylum.

Once these forms were completed (they were available in English and French), it was up to the medical superintendent of the institution to decide whether the patient was to be admitted and to advise the applicant of his decision.[6] Obtaining admission could be a frustrating procedure. If the medical superintendent found errors, he had to correspond with the applicant or official representatives to correct the anomalies detected. Georges Villeneuve, medical superintendent of St-Jean-de-Dieu hospital, had obviously made an exception for one local physician, but he made it clear he could only temporarily admit the patient if the forms were not completed correctly.

> I have the honor to send you the enclosed forms A. & B. which constitute the required medical certificate for the committal of patients. Would you please fill these in immediately and send them to me as soon as possible, because without this formality, it will be impossible for me to keep the patient in the asylum. I did you a favour because I received your letter. Please do not consider this case a precedent, because you have proceeded quite illegally, for, according to the text of the law, no person may be received at the asylum if the certificates required by law are not submitted beforehand to the medical superintendent.[7]

Some medical files that contained responses to these incomplete forms provided rich documentation on why families and local physicians wanted to admit women to the asylum. Families, helped sometimes by local physicians who examined the patients and recorded the information supplied by spouses or other family members, had to provide other details and facts about deviant behavior. Not only did both families and physicians have to correct the forms sent back to them, they were also provided with an opportunity to give more information on the trouble caused by the mentally ill wife or mother.

Trouble in the Family

The medical files demonstrate the severity of some family situations. Cruel mothers and violent wives were recognized as suffering from madness, and these symptoms were recurrent reasons for confinement in St-Jean-de-Dieu. Margaret[8] and Délia[9] broke everything around them, including clothing, furniture, and windows. Marie-Louise,[10] Azilda,[11] and Emma[12] attempted suicide. Céline[13] and Lucie[14] threatened to kill their husbands.

Some letters in the files added more explicit information about women's problematic behavior:

> There is an urgent need to admit this poor girl because she is a subject of scandal, and a continual threat to her old parents. Yesterday she took an ax to kill her brothers.[15]
>
> Sunday the 18th she suddenly took a nervous crisis, pulling her hair, crying, and calling herself damned etc. Every day since then brings more excitement, and despite administering sedatives, it takes 4 men to control her.[16]

According to information in their medical files, the married women caused disturbances, outrage, and exasperation. They kept those they lived with from sleeping. They tried to escape, they screamed, they howled, they made a racket. They seemed more or less unaware of the problems they caused to those around them. They ran away, slept very little, engaged in pitched battles with the neighbors, destroyed their clothes, and were a cause of scandal to their children. As Blanche explained to Villeneuve about her mother, "We are at the end of our rope, we can no longer keep her, we have problems."[17]

Family life was disrupted. The unexpected, the incredible, the unimaginable were part of daily life. The idea of a calm, quiet home became the stuff of fantasy. Living with Maria[18] was to fear the death threats that she shouted day and night; with Marie-Rose,[19] it meant accepting that she had to be shadowed every step to prevent serious injury from the blows she inflicted on herself; with Flora,[20] it meant protecting the children from her beatings; with Victorine,[21] it meant keeping her from destroying and burning everything around her. The forms suggest that the families of these women were constantly watching and listening for the slightest sign of danger. Their life was a perpetual struggle against the potential horror of an unfortunate action.

Exhaustion and discouragement built up within families living with these women. As years passed, unsettling experiences became difficult to manage, and misunderstandings became more frequent. Families became worn out by this life; those who experienced anxiety, fear, grief, and anguish on a daily basis were desperate for relief. Each family endured its share of problems, difficulties, and torments before it considered committing the patient to the asylum.

The powerlessness and shame provoked by a married woman's lewd acts, amoral words, and menacing gestures finally moved numerous spouses to take their ill wives to the St-Jean-de-Dieu Asylum. Very often, the request for the application forms was itself a call for help, a cry of desperation, and evidence of insurmountable discouragement. As Australian historian Bronwyn Labrum observed in her research on the Auckland Lunatic Asylum, the decision to confine an insane relative was often precipitated by the inability to control the sick person in the house: "Family members were admitted months and even years after the first signs of abnormal behaviour were perceived, often because events had taken a sudden turn for the worse."[22]

By the turn of the twentieth century, psychiatrists were beginning to offer hope for healing and a return to normal life through their confidence that patients who were admitted when the earliest symptoms appeared had a good chance to be cured.[23] Even French Canadian families were beginning to culturally integrate this institutional resource into their lives, wanting to share, in some way, the responsibilities of housing an insane woman.[24] They were evidently less reluctant to commit sick relatives to the asylum due to two factors. The first concerns all the efforts made to beautify the site of the asylum. Spaces in Montreal reserved for the insane were developed in exceptionally natural sites. Reading inspectors' reports, articles in the newspaper *La Patrie*, and A. Bellay's book *Histoire de l'hospice St-Jean-de-Dieu à Longue Pointe*,[25] one can imagine what St-Jean-de-Dieu was like at its beginnings and begin to understand the modifications made to it during the first decades of the twentieth century. These documents provide a wealth of detail highlighting a discourse based on the desire to "gild the image of the asylum." Adjectives and hyperbole followed one after the other, wiping out the memory of the legendary austerity of asylums, and the documents compare the asylums to houses of health with their charm and concern with aesthetics.

Second, the reputation of the asylum was based on the fact that the institution was becoming more and more "medicalized," with the implication that one could send sick relatives there without fear because they would be well treated. Developing the art of tending to the insane at St-Jean-de-Dieu, the community of the Sisters of Providence (Sœurs de la Providence), who headed the psychiatric institution, opened a nursing school in 1912 with a program that was accredited with the University of Montreal and fulfilled the requirements of the Association of Registered Nurses of the Province of Quebec. The nuns therefore contributed to the transformation from asylum to true hospital.[26] This school of nursing was created at first to improve the caring skills of the nuns for patients with mental illness. In 1917, lay students were admitted in a program to study to become graduate nurses with a specialization in psychiatric care.

The first goal of the nursing school was to develop a core of professional nurse-nuns to head each hospital department. The desire was to create a group of professional nurses who performed administrative or educational work, in contrast to what historian Cynthia Toman has called the "body work" at the bedside.[27] This latter work was done principally by the students in the school of nursing, who at that time were used as cheap labor in the same way as student nurses in general hospitals.[28] The community of nuns was thus able to have control over a cheaper staff of well-educated personnel. The nuns responsible for hospital service made sure that the old image of a residential facility for the deprived of spirit was banished by maintaining professional nursing standards in the care of those with nervous and mental illnesses.

Family Discourses

An exploration of the forms in the medical files permits us to see how families and local physicians seeking admission for these women described the behaviors of what they perceived to be mental illness. Investigating discourses in the medical files entails picking up traces of language from all the forms required for admission and the letters that sometimes accompanied them. Form C, for example, was filled out by family members applying to commit a spouse or mother; in some cases, someone in the hospital admission department helped them fill out their answers. This form was an official document found in the files of all patients admitted to St-Jean-de-Dieu. Applicants had to answer twenty-six questions to clarify the reasons why they thought their wives or mothers had to be admitted. Form B (also with some other correspondence) highlighted the discourse of local physicians who were obliged to fill out this form for the commitment procedure.

Recurrent problems justifying the need for commitment were related mainly to the difficulty in maintaining continual surveillance of the insane woman, who appeared to be dangerous to herself and to those around her. Often, the litany of concerns signaled that husbands and children were no longer able to cope. Rose-de-Lima's husband reported that she had ideas of persecution, which made her angry, sad, impatient, and irritable, but the primary problem was that she was highly suspicious. She complained and stormed against her neighbors. She slept little and was constantly criticizing her husband, accusing him of having an affair with a neighbor lady. She also accused him of being complicit with her persecutors and with the "electricity." The ideas of persecution made her suffer, and she was sure her husband was hiding the object of her suffering. She had had these ideas for about ten years, and they were accompanied by hallucinations of hearing and sight. The husband gave Dr. Villeneuve the sad story of his wife, who had "poisoned" his days and nights. "How many times . . . have I got home and found my woman and my poor dear little children each with a wide band around the head and all windows and doors closed because she was pretending that there was too much electricity, and she accused me of hurting our small children."[29] On 24 August 1897, Rose-de-Lima deserted his home, leaving her children behind. The next day, he was authorized to have her interned at St-Jean-de-Dieu.

The specific expressions husbands used to describe symptoms of madness were undoubtedly influenced by the questions on the admission forms. This helps explain the large number of similar expressions, such as women having auditory, visual, or "genital" hallucinations; attempting murder; refusing food; sleeping little or not at all; tearing clothes; breaking windows and furniture; or trying to set fires, as suggested in questions 16 to 20 of Form C. Such behaviors are not uncommon in the mentally ill, but it is unclear whether the husbands would have recognized them as manifestations of illness without being asked the questions on Form C. It is practically impossible to judge the frequency and intensity of these actions, and even more difficult to evaluate the capacity of these women, consciously or not, to hit, burn, or kill.

There is no doubt that the medical superintendent's opinion was influential when he asked applicants for the formalities necessary to make admission completely legal. When the information contained was not as explicit as he thought necessary and did not fulfill the criteria required by law to admit a person to the asylum, he so advised the applicants, who had to add more convincing details. For example, Villeneuve wrote to ask for explicit facts about Catherine's behavior.

> It is my duty to return to you the file of the above-mentioned Catherine and point out the few irregularities that it contains while expressing the hope that you will want them expunged. In Form C of your medical certificate, you mention none of the facts and symptoms that constitute proof of madness, and I find no technical information that enables me to conclude and observe with you that the ill person must in fact be committed. I therefore ask you to add to your testimonial everything that will seem to you of a nature to persuade me.[30]

It is clear upon reading this correspondence that the forms had to prove convincingly that patients required admission. The vigilance the medical superintendent demonstrated in the letters shows that it was not enough simply to place the words "dangerous" and "scandalous" (which reads as sexual) behavior on Forms B and C. To obtain the admission of an insane woman, it was necessary to convince the administrator of the extreme situations families experienced and the acts of indecency they observed. It is at this point, when we move away from the leading questions on Form C, that we can see families struggling to find language in order to add more details, so that the answers to the later sections of Form C reveal more about the families' situations.

The behaviors reported by husbands and family members in these instances reveal mainly their lack of knowledge about mental illness; to them, their mothers and wives seemed to be totally bizarre, distinctly unusual, or beyond comprehension. At first glance, the characteristics they identified seemed inoffensive—having a tic of the head, refusing to eat meat, having nightmares and suddenly waking, having dry tongue and lips, feeling sorrow, having changing moods, saying obscene words in the presence of children, or exposing the body. Families saw these symptoms as signs of madness, and inevitably commented that they made it impossible for the wife and mother to successfully carry out her role within the domestic sphere, and that she sought to flee elsewhere. It is therefore not surprising that they saw signs of madness in a woman who spent her day out shopping, left her house without closing the doors, refused to do her chores, detested her husband's children, hit her children, or took no care of her husband—with whom, on top of it all, she no longer wanted to live.

Families added to these observations worries about acts that they considered immoral, indecent, and scandalous. Women who admitted loving men other than their husbands, who either criticized or admired the physical attributes of the vicar, who masturbated, who had sexual impulses, or who walked around half-dressed, demonstrated actions that gave many family members reason to suspect madness and fill out applications for commitment.

Physicians' Discourse

Comparing the local physicians vocabulary on these forms with the families' vocabulary demonstrates the different levels of perception about symptoms of madness that required institutionalization. Family physicians were required to fill out Form B for these women to be admitted to the asylum, and the medical superintendent was required to return incomplete forms for the physician to provide more specific details of a women's madness, permitting additional qualitative information on how doctors understood mental illness at that time. This correspondence between the administrator and local physicians is a particularly rich source, since it helps reveal what doctors who were not specialists in mental health believed to be insane behavior in women. These men were being asked to pronounce themselves in a field of expertise that was not theirs, as they tried to make connections between their patients' physical and mental states.

Local physicians were well aware of the family's dramatic home situation as they attempted to respond to the request by the medical superintendent for clearer proof of a woman's insanity. They confirmed by examination that the woman was indeed dangerous or scandalous, legal stipulations for confinement to the asylum. Other signs and symptoms, which would have been insufficient confirmation for commitment on their own, were accompanied by various medical terms on the certificate to further define a particular woman's illness. This specialized vocabulary tagged female patients, for example, with hysteria, a taciturn character, ideas of grandeur, weakening of the intellectual faculties, motor excitation, nymphomania, and fits of mania.

One doctor provided this explanation of "scandalous" behavior: "If she goes to the Church office, it seems she amuses herself by criticizing the physical qualities of her pastor and admires the extreme beauty of the vicar or publicly mocks his education."[31] Another claimed that his patient was hysterical: "This young woman of 32 years has been married for just 3 months. Before her marriage she had a tendency to stop talking and be very unhappy in her surroundings. One time, she stopped talking because someone tracked mud into her house even though it was raining."[32] Another reported the fits of mania in one woman following the birth of her child: "For the first time [I saw her] after her delivery, I found her, though changed, emaciated and with shadows under her eyes, but nothing unusual in her language, for the quarter of an hour I spent with her. . . . Today, I went to see her again, I stayed long enough with her, and she gave me evidence that she was out of her mind. She was sure that her child was a stranger to her and her brother-in-law was a stranger too. Many here say she is mad, that she is dangerous and out-of-control."[33]

The B forms also caught the attention of historian Mary Glennon Okin, who studied the reasons women were confined over a fifty-year period at the Asile de St-Michel-Archange de Beauport. These forms were apparently more numerous in the medical files of the women at Beauport, and permitted Okin to suggest that physicians may have seen asylum admission as a means for women to flee tasks and responsibilities in the private sphere that had become too unwieldy, difficult, and demanding for the "fair sex."[34] My data suggest that this reading of female madness, which has also been proposed in the feminist studies of Yannick Ripa and Phyllis Chesler, for example, tends to ignore the reality of mental illness itself.[35] As many of the symptoms catalogued in the women at St-Jean-de-Dieu hospital suggest, some women truly appeared to be in real danger of harming themselves or their families.

Although only 2.3 percent of the quantitative data collected at St-Jean-de-Dieu in 1890 and 1898 linked the administrator's official diagnosis of madness to the pathology of female sexual organs, local physicians in the past commonly believed that women's madness was associated with their biology and biological differentiation from men. The Victorian period, which generated extraordinary change in the medical world, saw the development of new specialties such as gynecology and obstetrics. The marked interest in female biology was concentrated, more specifically, on the complexity of the uterus; this organ, seated in the woman's pelvic cavity, came to be seen as responsible for many "female troubles." For instance, physicians observed that symptoms of madness appeared after a difficult childbirth, a bout of puerperal fever, amenorrhea, or pregnancy. This was relevant information to be communicated to the medical supervisor, as it would assuredly help in making a diagnosis. Marie-Rose's physician noted, "What I wish to draw your attention to is the primary illness. I cannot tell you the current state of the womb and the appendices as I have not performed an examination since she discontinued treatment (July), but if there has been a change, it has been for the worse. A cure on this front may influence her cerebral state."[36]

Conclusion

The variety of documents found in these medical files at St-Jean-de-Dieu facilitated an analysis of how families and local physicians perceived mental illness in married women at the turn of the last century. Letters written to the medical superintendent of the asylum that further explained why a woman should be admitted added to the official documents and are crucial because they provide more detail about the range of abnormal behavior.

Explanations of a woman's illness resulted from two ways of understanding mental illness. The language used by husbands and other family members implies an emotional perspective—they could only communicate their distress at the women's behavior in terms of how it affected them personally. Lacking a medical understanding of mental illness, husbands could only express themselves in terms of the abnormal behavior of their wives that seemed to them to deviate from the expected roles and norms for spouses and mothers. From the perspective of husbands and other family members, women whose bizarre behavior prevented them from carrying out "normal" household duties demonstrated evidence of mental illness. Physicians applied medical terminology of the day to these same behaviors in order to convince the medical superintendent that these women needed admission. As evidenced by this language, their comprehension of mental illness was based on a contemporary understanding of "scientific" and "rational" connections between mind and body.

The upsetting, critical, and often dangerous situations for which families sought commitment highlighted the urgency of the situation. The fact that admission forms were often completed in haste, throwing formalities to the wind, illustrates that husbands and physicians thought they had indisputable, fully justified proof that commitment procedures should be undertaken for women who were causing so much trouble for their families. To them, the paperwork to be filled out may have been superfluous and secondary, because they had to move quickly—this woman, a wife and mother, had to be admitted immediately—and they believed that admission forms could be filled out later to meet the requirements of the medical superintendent for hospitalization.

This brief incursion into the pre-commitment world of families in crisis sheds light on private lives overwhelmed by the responsibilities involved with keeping an insane woman at home. The trouble, fear, and danger created by the actions of their spouses and mothers led husbands and other family members to seek and to justify admission for these women. The inability to always make themselves clear to officials points to the vulnerability of husbands "unqualified" to fill out the admission forms. Men who often could neither read nor write struggled to describe what they recognized was not normal. Although these admission procedures were complicated to complete, they nevertheless did not appear to discourage families from asking for admission of their loved ones. Increasing numbers of the asylum population, which included married women, show us that families became more successful in their efforts to find help for their wives and mothers to recover their health.

Marie-Claude Thifault
History Professor at the School of Nursing
Faculty of Health Sciences
University of Ottawa
451 Smyth Rd. (3245D)
Ottawa, ON, K1H 8M5, Canada

Acknowledgments

The author would like to thank Käthe Roth for the English translation of an earlier version of this article. She also thanks Jayne Elliott and Patricia D'Antonio for their comments, support, and help in writing the final version.

Notes

1. André Cellard and Marie-Claude Thifault, *Une toupie sur la tête: Visages de la folie à Saint-Jean-de-Dieu* (Montreal: Boréal, 2007).
2. David Wright, James E. Moran, and Sean Gouglas, "The Confinement of the Insane in Victorian Canada: The Hamilton and Toronto Asylums, c. 1861–1891," in *The Confinement of the Insane*, ed. Roy Porter and David Wright (Cambridge: Cambridge University Press, 2003), 100–28; Jonathan Andrews and Anne Digby, eds., *Sex and Seclusion, Class and Custody: Perspectives on Gender and Class in the History of British and Irish Psychiatry*, Clio Medica 73 (New York: Rodopi, 2004); Marie-Claude Thifault, "L'enfermement asilaire des femmes au Québec: 1873–1921" (PhD diss., University of Ottawa, 2003); Mary Glennon Okin, "'Madwomen' in Quebec: An Analysis of the Recurring Themes in the Reasons for Women's Committal to Beauport, 1894–1940" (PhD diss., University of Maine, 2008).
3. André Cellard and Marie-Claude Thifault, "The Uses of Asylums: Resistance, Asylum Propaganda, and Institutionalization Strategies in Turn-of-the-Century Quebec," in *Mental Health and Canadian Society*, ed. James E. Moran and David Wright (Montreal and Kingston: McGill-Queen's University Press, 2006), 100; Marie-Claude Thifault, "Sentiments et correspondances dans les dossiers des femmes internées à l'Hôpital Saint-Jean-de-Dieu, fin 19e siècle, début 20e," *Recherches féministes* 21, no. 2 (2008): 127–42.
4. For the nineteenth century, the sample included admissions of women from 1890 to 1898; for the twentieth century, the sample was collected every three years from 1900 to 1921.
5. David Wright, "Delusions of Gender?: Lay Identification and Clinical Diagnosis of Insanity in Victorian England," in *Sex and Seclusion, Class and Custody: Perspectives on Gender and Class in the History of British and Irish Psychiatry*, Clio Medica 73, eds. Jonathan Andrews and Anne Digby. (New York, Rodopi, 2004), 155. See also David Wright, "The Certification of Insanity in Nineteenth-Century England," *History of Psychiatry* 9 (1998): 267–90.
6. Statuts de la Province de Québec, 1880, chap. XXX: 117–20.
7. Letter from the medical superintendent to the local physician of Saint-Dominique, co. Bagot, Archives Hôpital Louis-H. Lafontaine (hereafter AHL-HL), correspondence, medical file 13839, 16 March 1910.
8. AHL-HL, medical file 3911, June 1890.
9. AHL-HL, medical file 4804, March 1893.
10. AHL-HL, medical file 4816, April 1893.
11. AHL-HL, medical file 9279, February 1909.
12. AHL-HL, medical file 4823, April 1893.
13. AHL-HL, medical file 3926, July 1890.
14. AHL-HL, medical file 4836, May 1893.
15. AHL-HL, correspondence, medical file 6048, 30 June 1898 (translated).
16. AHL-HL, correspondence, medical file 7243, 27 January 1903.
17. AHL-HL, correspondence, medical file 6770, 1904 (translated).
18. AHL-HL, correspondence, medical file 8358, 1906.
19. AHL-HL, correspondence, medical file 7243, 27 January 1903.
20. AHL-HL, correspondence, medical file 13377, undated.

21. AHL-HL, correspondence, medical file 7307, 8 April 1903.

22. Bronwyn Labrum, "Looking Beyond the Asylum: Gender and the Process of Committal in Auckland, 1870–1910," *New Zealand Journal of History* 26, no. 2 (1992): 141.

23. Trente-quatrième rapport des inspecteurs d'asiles pour l'année 1903, Session documents 38, *Parlementary publication of the province of Quebec*, no. 2 (1905): 211.

24. Cellard and Thifault, "The Uses of Asylums," 103.

25. Rapport des inspecteurs d'asiles, Session documents 21, no. 3 (1888): 140–43; Rapport annuel des inspecteurs d'asiles (1901): 188; (1908): 57; *La Patrie*, 24 July (1905): 5; 4 June (1903): 3; 19 July (1902): 8; 13 April (1901):1; A. Bellay, *Histoire de l'hospice de St-Jean-de-Dieu à la Longue-Pointe* (Montreal: Arbour/Laperle, 1892).

26. *École des infirmières de l'hôpital Saint-Jean-de-Dieu de Montréal*, Archives des Sœurs de la Providence de Montréal, 4.

27. Cynthia Toman, "'Body Work,' Medical Technology, and Hospital Nursing Practice," in *On All Frontiers: Four Centuries of Canadian Nursing*, eds. Christina Bates, Dianne Dodd, and Nicole Rousseau (Ottawa: University of Ottawa Press and Museum of Civilization, 2005), 89.

28. Yolande Cohen, Jacinthe Pepin, Esther Lamontagne, and André Duquette, *Les sciences infirmières: Genèse d'une discipline* (Montréal: Presses de l'Université de Montréal, 2002), 86–87.

29. AHL-HL, correspondence, medical file 5751, 22 April 1899 (translated).

30. AHL-HL, correspondence, medical file 8264, 18 May 1906 (translated).

31. AHL-HL, medical file 7345, Formule B, 9 April 1903 (translated).

32. AHL-HL, correspondence, medical file 7295, 27 May 1903 (translated).

33. AHL-HL, correspondence, medical file 9421, 31 May 1904 (translated).

34. Ibid., 248.

35. Phyllis Chesler, *Les femmes et la folie* (Paris: Payot, 1979); Marcel Gauchet and Gladys Swain, *La pratique de l'esprit humain: L'institution asilaire et la révolution démocratique* (Mayenne: Gallimard, 1980); Yannick Ripa, *La ronde des folles: Femmes, folie et enfermement au XIXe siècle (1838–1870)* (Paris: Aubier, 1986).

36. AHL-HL, correspondence, medical file 7243, 27 January 1903 (translated).

Life and Death in Philadelphia's Black Belt: A Tale of an Urban Tuberculosis Campaign, 1900–1930

J. MARGO BROOKS CARTHON
University of Pennsylvania School of Nursing

Abstract. The poor health status of black Americans was a widely recognized fact during the first third of the twentieth century. Excess mortality in black communities was frequently linked to the infectious disease tuberculosis, which was particularly menacing in densely populated urban settings. As health authorities in large cities struggled to keep pace with the needs of citizens, private charities worked to launch community-oriented attacks against the deadly disease. In 1914 a novel experiment to address excess mortality among blacks was launched in Philadelphia. The success of the health promotion campaign initiated by the Henry Phipps Institute and the Whittier Centre, two private charitable associations, has been attributed primarily to the presence of black clinicians, in particular public health nurse Elizabeth Tyler. This study suggests that community health efforts also rest on partnerships between like-minded organizations and coalition building.

Tuberculosis (TB) is an infectious disease with deep historical roots. For many centuries, "the white plague," known also as "phthisis" or "consumption," had wrought havoc both in the United States and in Europe, striking its victims during the most productive years of life, leaving them with little hope for cure.[1] During this period, TB was viewed primarily as a disease of heredity, preying on those of susceptible predisposition. By 1882, the pathogen responsible for TB, *Mycobacterium tuberculosis*, was isolated by bacteriologist Robert Koch, who established the disease as communicable, passed from person to person through respiratory secretions.[2] During the decades following Koch's discovery clinicians slowly acknowledged that TB was spread through close contact and prolonged intimate exposure. This concession came despite early resistance to the veracity of the germ theory and its less than auspicious reception.

By the turn of the twentieth century, ideas about TB had further evolved so that the disease once regarded as "the captain of death" was also recognized as a "social problem" brought on by environmental conditions.[3] This shift in scientific understanding helped shape the campaign for disease prevention, placing greater emphasis on environmental reform and personal responsibility.[4] According to one early twentieth-century writer, "the part played by social conditions in the propagation of the disease is twofold. First, the presence of the specific cause depends on . . . the duties of the *individual* [emphasis mine]. In the second place, the individual organism exposed to the danger of infection resists or succumbs to the invasion of the *bacillus tuberculosis* . . . as it has been predisposed by inheritance and environment."[5] In other words, though inheritance continued to be considered a factor in the development of the, individuals were increasingly expected to play a role in lowering their risks by increasing their health awareness and changing their lifestyles. Disease outcomes were now viewed as modifiable if environmental changes such as improved sanitation and ventilation were employed.

Turn-of-the-century Philadelphia was no stranger to TB or to this evolving discourse.[6] As in other northern cities such as New York, Baltimore, and Boston, Philadelphia's tenement housing, dense overcrowding, and poor sanitation served as breeding grounds for infectious illnesses like consumption.[7] Records of the Department of Public Health and Charities reveal elevated TB rates among all Philadelphian residents in the late nineteenth and early twentieth centuries, though blacks were hit especially hard. In 1900, TB mortality for black Philadelphians was two-and-a-half to three times that for native whites.[8]

The persistent high rate of TB among blacks, coupled with the risk of contagion to the city at large, prompted several civic groups to consider alternative methods to prevent the disease and attract black patients to clinics for treatment. The most familiar example of antituberculosis work among black Philadelphians is the work of the Henry Phipps Institute (HPI), which in 1914 hired a black nurse, Elizabeth Tyler, and a black physician, Henry Minton, to initiate antituberculosis efforts among black community residents. The HPI, established in 1903 by Lawrence Flick, was one of the nation's premier institutions for the prevention, research, and treatment of TB. Despite its prominence and its proximity to the black community, in its first eleven years, the institute largely failed to attract black patients. After the introduction of black clinicians this trend reversed and the numbers of black patients grew.

The HPI TB campaign in Philadelphia's black community was the subject of the early research of Sadie Mossell in 1923, and later twentieth-century historians David McBride and Barbara Bates.[9] These studies describe the work of the HPI among blacks as roughly involving three phases. During its first eleven years, the institute saw little participation from blacks; in 1914, the introduction of a black nurse and physician attracted blacks to the institute; and from 1914 to the 1930s black patient participation increased. This chronological summary largely attributes the efficacy of the HPI's antituberculosis campaign to the inclusion of racially concordant nursing and medical professionals.

While this assertion has much to recommend it as a plausible explanation for the increase in black patient attendance at the HPI, an alternative argument suggests that the accomplishment of the HPI antituberculosis efforts was more complex and involved the involvement of influential neighborhood civic associations within the black community. Looking toward other community institutions and key stakeholders adds important details to our understanding of the successful TB campaign. This level of inquiry is particularly relevant because the campaign was in reality a joint effort between the HPI and the Whittier Centre, an influential civic association. Scholars have generally recognized the Whittier Centre's role in providing the salary of the HPI's first black nurse, but little substantive consideration has been afforded to its function as a mediator between the black community and the HPI.

The Whittier Centre was established in 1912 with the mission to address the social, health, and housing needs of the black community. Its early work focused on members of two predominately black benevolent societies, the Co-operative Coal Club and the Rainy Day Society, both with roots dating to the preceding century. For many years Whittier Centre leaders worked closely with Co-operative Coal Club and Rainy Day Society members, and over time the strength of these contacts grew. Concerned with the pervasive threat of TB, Whittier Centre organizers partnered with the HPI to address TB in the black community. The hiring of a black nurse was the byproduct of this venture. While Elizabeth Tyler's addition to the HPI staff was of tremendous value, equally critical to the joint effort was the Whittier Centre's long-standing presence in the black community; its ability to leverage its relationship with black community members led to increased buy-in when antituberculosis measures were introduced.

The role of the Whittier Centre, while acknowledged by earlier scholars, has not previously been explored. Examining its mediating function between the black community and the HPI becomes increasingly important as we explore private sector organizations and their role in providing community level health resources. This study reexamines the renowned HPI TB campaign and the influence of collaborative partnerships between HPI and the Whittier Centre. The article begins with an overview of TB mortality among blacks in

Philadelphia during the first three decades of the twentieth century, a synopsis of ideologies by scholars of the time to explain elevated mortality rates in blacks, and the available treatment options. The efforts of the Whittier Centre and HPI and the response of black residents are explored in detail.

Death by Numbers: The Rise and Fall of TB in Blacks in Philadelphia

At the opening of the twentieth century, TB had long been recognized as a deadly menace in the city of Philadelphia. Efforts to eradicate the disease were taken up by the public and private sectors and included educating city residents on the importance of prevention and isolation to avert the spread of the disease. Whether due to the activities of the antituberculosis campaign, or to other factors such as improvements in nutrition or increases in per capita income, in the first decade of the twentieth century, TB rates started to decline precipitously.[10] The notable exception was the case of black Philadelphians, who experienced an overall but much slower decrease in mortality.[11]

Vital statistical records for 1900 show the death rate in Philadelphia due to TB as 197.3 per 100,000 for whites versus 447.0 per 100,000 for blacks.[12] Census records reveal continued elevated mortality for the next decade, so that by 1910 deaths due to TB in blacks were 57 percent greater than for native-born whites, and 44 percent higher than for foreign-born whites.[13] In 1908, TB mortality in blacks dipped significantly, but spiked in 1914 and continued to climb until 1918 (see Figure 1).[14]

Numerous factors may contribute to the variation in these death rates. Sharp elevations of TB among blacks at the opening of the century may have resulted from newly arriving blacks during the decades after the Civil War. Some scholars have argued that upon entering the city these blacks may have lacked acquired immunity, increasing their susceptibility to the disease.[15] So the higher TB mortality among blacks at the opening of the century might reflect more recently infected individuals. The drop in 1908–1913 is more difficult to explain; it may be attributed to city-wide improvements in sanitation or the natural peaks and troughs of the disease.

During the next seven years, TB rates again began to climb steadily, peaking in 1918. The elevation in mortality during this period has been attributed to the arrival of rural migrants between 1916 and 1920.[16] As newcomers entered the city, the combined effects of lack of acquired immunity, poverty, poor housing, and overcrowding likely led to increased susceptibility

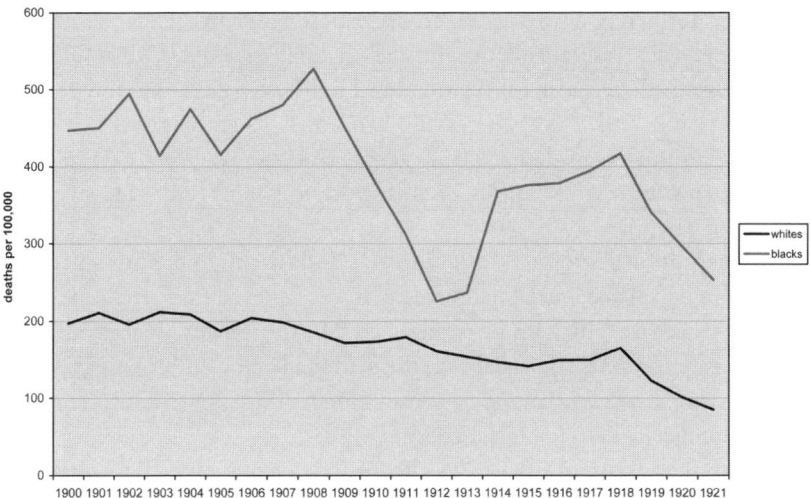

Figure 1. Death rate from pulmonary TB in Philadelphia, 1900–1921.
Note. Graph adapted from figures provided in Henry R. M. Landis, *A Report of the Tuberculosis Problem and the Negro* (Philadelphia: Henry Phipps Institute, 1923).

to the disease.[17] Other factors might include the 1918 influenza outbreak and the transient city population due to the upheavals of World War I.[18] Between 1912 and 1922, the rates of TB steadily declined in whites. Rates for blacks began to decrease between 1919 and 1921, though more slowly, and continued to fall throughout the remainder of the 1920s.[19]

Theoretical Considerations

Several theories have been proposed to explain why blacks incurred higher rates of TB. Many early twentieth-century scientists and reformers linked elevated TB rates to specific occupations such as domestic service, which required long, taxing hours; and jobs with high exposure to dust, such as marble, stone, plaster, wood, and textile work.[20] The nature of these jobs and the low wages connected with them suggest a relationship between income limitations and higher rates of TB. While there is limited empirical data for the early decades of the twentieth century to link actual income to TB mortality, occupation undoubtedly served as a reasonable proxy for economic status. Accordingly, individuals with better jobs were believed less likely to contract the infectious disease.

In a 1906 report of the HPI, TB expert Lawrence Flick noted that middle-class city residents with jobs such as teachers, bookkeepers, or saleswomen were at lower risk for contracting TB. These people typically lived in modern homes and if they did get ill, had access to the comforts necessary to insure improvement.[21] For blacks trapped at the lower end of the occupational spectrum, the hazards of their vocations and low wages weighed heavily on their health.

Other rationales for excessive rates of TB in blacks pointed to what were referred to as so-called racial handicaps.[22] It was believed that blacks inherited racial defects that left them physically and constitutionally weaker. Theories of racial inferiority relied partially on the field of physical anthropology, which used measurements of anatomical features in an effort to explain variances in disease frequency between racial groups.[23]

With the passage of years, other theories emerged, such as the "virgin soil" theory, which proposed that blacks were more prone to consumption due to their lack of exposure to infectious diseases while living in African villages, and led to a lack of inherited or acquired immunity.[24] Other members of the scientific community countered that "the Negroes as a race in the United States have long been in contact with the virus of TB. They are probably as well or nearly as well tuberculized as the white race."[25] These scholars contended that racial (inherited) differences in TB did not exist and that any increase in susceptibility was attributed to the same factors which caused increased rates among whites—"unwholesome" living conditions.[26] By the mid-1930s, most clinicians conceded that both racial and environmental factors played roles in the TB death rate among blacks; little could be done about racial differences, hence concerted efforts needed to focus on correction of the physical environment.[27]

Treatment Options: Fears and Limits

During the pre-antibiotic era, options to treat TB included isolation, bed rest, fresh air, and nutritious food, including milk in plentiful amounts. Many of these treatments were initiated in the home or dispensaries for incipient TB patients, or in hospitals or sanitariums for more advanced cases. The existence of treatment options did not, however, ensure accessibility to blacks. Several studies pointed to the lack of treatment facilities and hospital beds reserved for black patients.[28] In her 1923 study of TB in Philadelphia, Sadie Mossell reported that blacks were able to receive care for TB at only six facilities in the city.²⁹ Philadelphia General Hospital saw 96 percent of the total number of black TB patients, though the facility suffered from poor accommodations, overcrowding, and long waiting lists.³⁰ The two black hospitals in the city did not have beds for tubercular patients due to lack of funds.³¹ Mossell ended her study with recommendations for more beds and dispensaries for black residents because the number of facilities at which blacks could receive care was inadequate.³²

Options for blacks to enter sanitariums for treatment were also limited due to admission restrictions at both private and state sanitariums.³³ Some black residents refused removal from their homes for fear of the treatment they would receive on arriving at the sanatorium and placing themselves under the care of strangers. One black physician discussed these concerns, "the question for travel for the negro of some means and intelligence, seeking health in a sanatoria, is not worth consideration at this time; for a sick man traveling without civil rights, not knowing where he will be permitted to shelter his weakened body and quench his parching tongue, had better, yes far better, remain at home with his family and trust God for the rest."³⁴ Fear of mistreatment and the unknown left many blacks with the belief that they were indeed better off at home.

Low black patient utilization of the services that were available added to the problem of limited facilities. The HPI, established in 1903, was a well-regarded dispensary for TB treatment. Located for many years at 238 Pine Street, the institute was in the heart of the city's historic black district. Yet, despite its close proximity to black residents, "colored people did not avail themselves of the benefits of dispensaries, or if they did, made but a few visits, often but one, and then ceased coming."³⁵

HPI and Black Patient Attendance

Named after its benefactor, steel magnate Henry Phipps, the Henry Phipps Institute for the Treatment and Prevention of Tuberculosis was the nation's first endowed center aimed at curtailing the infectious disease.³⁶ Dr. Lawrence Flick, a nationally recognized authority on consumption and founder of the nation's first TB society, the Pennsylvania Society for the Prevention of Tuberculosis (1892), was the institute's first medical director, serving in this capacity for seven years.³⁷

In 1910, the University of Pennsylvania took charge of HPI, and the Institute's mission shifted largely from clinical services to research.³⁸ After the turnover, founder Lawrence Flick departed and soon after, Charles Hatfield was appointed executive director.[39] In 1913, HPI moved to Seventh and Lombard Streets.[40]

HPI originally inhabited a modest space in the midst of one of the city's poorest ethnically and racially mixed communities. Bare floors and walls, a few chairs, a clerk, and three physicians constituted the staff and equipment.[41] The dispensary was located on the first floor, with wards on the second, third, and fourth floors. The front room was divided into a consultation room and office, and the back room into a consultation room, waiting room, and drug store.[42]

Dispensary services grew rapidly, quickly outpacing the number of physicians and nurses available. At the end of the first year, the nursing staff consisted of five trained nurses and five student nurses; clinical staff increased as more patients entered the dispensary and wards.[43] During the first year, 1,903 patients were seen at the dispensary; of these, 904 made one visit only. Several reasons account for the low number of returning patients: some entered the hospital, some were deemed "unsuitable," some did not have TB, and others merely came for an opinion.[44] The racial composition of HPI patients during the opening year is particularly telling: 1,846 were white and 131 black.[45] These numbers are especially striking given the high TB mortality in the black community and the large number of blacks who lived near the clinic.

Flick recognized that the low number of blacks seeking treatment at the clinic did not reflect the rate of TB in the black community. He noted, "the vast preponderance of white people over colored people among the patients registered is no indication of the relative amount of tuberculosis in the races, nor of their relative poverty. The colored people are more prone to tuberculosis than white people. There probably is as much poverty among colored as there is among whites." Blacks, however, were "loath to become a public charge and are more disposed to help themselves. They will not go into a public institution if they can manage to crawl around."[46] Flick's observations held true: the number of patients grew steadily over first eleven years, but the number of black patients did not.

Clinic attendance patterns for HPI patients reveal interesting differences between blacks and whites. Henry Robert Murray Landis's 1923 study of TB in blacks compared individuals in the district of the HPI and those attending the dispensary. In 1903, there were 46 black patients; the numbers dropped to 11 in 1908 and 27 in 1913, then rose to 96 in 1918 and 427 in 1922.[47] There were 587 white patients in 1903, 566 in 1908, 1,253 in 1913, 1,408 in 1918, and 1,541 in 1922. Thus, from the clinic's opening whites tended to seek treatment there more frequently.[48] The figures also reflect a shift in black clinic attendance; blacks were a small fraction of the patients seen in 1903, but by 1921 they were nearly 30 percent of new patients.[49]

These numbers, while reflecting only a sample of those patients attending the clinic and living near the institute, are telling as they reflect trends in black and white patient clinic attendance over a span of time. The low turnout of black patients in the early years is striking, while the increase in attendance in 1918 and 1922 certainly reflects the purposeful outreach into the black community.

Other demographic information pertains to gender differences between racial groups. In 1903, black patients were 65 percent male and 35 percent female; in 1908, 55 percent male and 45 percent female; in 1913, 52 percent male and 48 percent female; in 1918, 47 percent male and 53 percent female; in 1922, 39 percent male and 61 percent female.[50] Clinic attendance according to gender in whites reflected a different pattern: in 1903, white patients were 60 percent male and 40 percent female; in 1908, 48 percent male and 51 percent female; in 1913, 54 percent male and 46 percent female; in 1918, 49 percent male and 51 percent female.[51]

These results taken together reflect interesting racial and gender differences in clinic attendance. In 1903 more black men attended the HPI clinic than did white and black women. Male/female patterns of attendance remained fairly even among blacks in 1913 and 1918, but the number of black men dropped significantly in 1922. After 1903, there appeared to be little gender difference in white attendance, while in 1922 the downward shift in black male attendance and increase in female attendance is quite notable.

It is difficult to attribute the dramatic shift in black male/female attendance in 1922 to any particular factor; several causes may have produced it. Possible shifts in work obligations during the war years may have made clinic attendance more difficult. A plausible rationale for the increase in black female clinic attendance may have been the types of outreach efforts, which, often occurring in the home, may have focused more on women than men. Landis's results take on more value when considered in connection with the health work among blacks beginning with the efforts of the Whittier Centre and the hiring of nurse Tyler.

The Whittier Centre–HPI Plan

Named after nineteenth-century poet and abolitionist John Greenleaf Whittier, the Whittier Centre's mission was to create solutions to the social and health problems plaguing black Philadelphia residents. The association's leadership were from the local community, including social progressive Susan Parrish Wharton, who served as the organization's first secretary, and physician Henry Landis, its first president. The other members of the board were a diverse group of black and white civic activists, including five physicians, five female volunteers, and a member of the clergy. Another group of eighteen individuals made up the Whittier Centre Advisory Board. Situated at 712 South Eighteenth Street and 510 South Seventh Streets, its geographical location placed it within the heart of the growing black community.

In its first year, the association focused its efforts toward the members of two black benevolent societies located in South Philadelphia, the Co-operative Coal Club and the Rainy Day Society. They had deep historical roots in the black community and together boasted a membership of over 1,000 individuals.[52] The Co-operative Coal Club (see Figure 2) was formed in 1893 and served as a way for blacks to work collectively to buy coal, which was then used as a fuel source for cooking and heating homes.[53] The Rainy Day Society, established in 1905, was similar to many other sick benefit societies operating in cities across the country; it served as a safety net to its members by providing financial assistance in the event of unexpected illness.

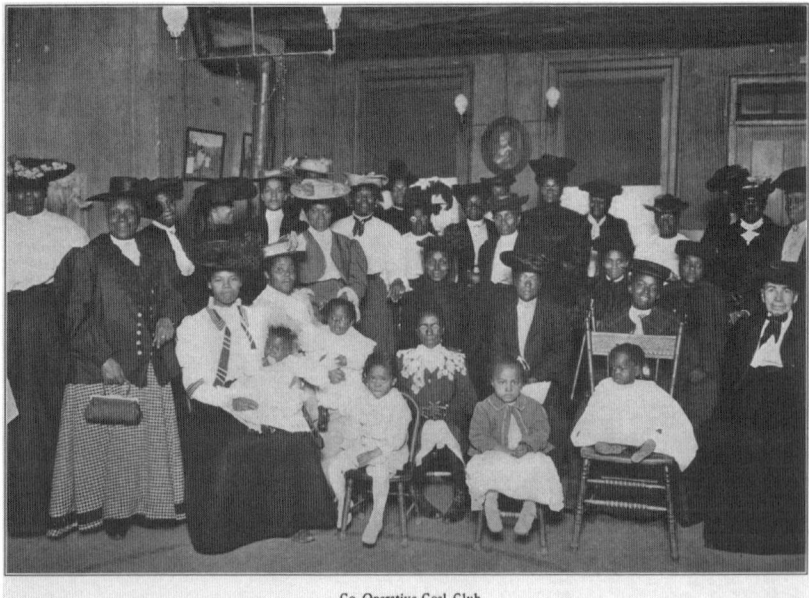

Figure 2. Co-operative Coal Club.

Members paid annual dues that they were able to withdraw in times of illness, or the total savings could be pulled at the beginning of each year for other purchases. By 1913, both groups were well-recognized entities within the black community. Though the Whittier Centre itself was new, many of its board members had served in the community for decades and brought to the Whittier Centre long-standing relationships with black club members.

These relationships prompted Whittier Centre organizers to discuss means to address poor health among black community residents, primarily through combating the excessive TB rates.[54] One early annual Whittier Centre report summarized the organization's goal, stating that: "No movement for the betterment . . . of the Negro, from a social as well as health standpoint, demands more attention than the one having as its object the prevention and arrest of tuberculosis."[55] Drawing on its knowledge of specific black neighborhoods, and by now having intimate acquaintance with members of the black community, the Whittier Centre thought it wise to provide funding for a black nurse to work in the community. It planned to carry out its mission by working cooperatively with the HPI. This partnership was solidified through Henry Landis.

With his dual affiliations with the Whittier Centre and the HPI, Landis was perfectly suited for oversight of the new program to reduce the high rate of TB in the black community. Born in 1872, Landis was a leading clinician and researcher in the field of TB. After graduating with an AB from Amherst College in 1894, and completing medical school at Jefferson Medical College in Philadelphia in 1897, he launched a career specializing in the treatment of TB; he later founded the National Tuberculosis Association and presided over the Pennsylvania Tuberculosis Society in 1928–1932. In addition, Landis was one of the original HPI clinicians, beginning his work there in 1903; he was assistant professor of medicine and director of clinical and sociological services, and served as visiting physician to the Commonwealth of Pennsylvania White Haven Sanatorium.[56] Landis's affiliations extended to civic organizations, including the presidency of the Whittier Centre, a position he held for more than 15 years. As such, he was influential in setting the center's organizational agenda toward consistent commitment to prevention and treating of TB.[57]

Under Landis's direction, the Whittier Centre executive board met in May 1913 to discuss the ongoing dilemma of TB plaguing the black community. Members resolved to provide funding for the salary of a black nurse, who would work on the HPI clinic staff to provide health services to members of the black community. Landis believed a black nurse could more easily gain access to the homes of other blacks, that she could "go with immunity, day or night, into districts in which it would not be safe for a white woman."

Moreover, she could establish a "greater degree of confidence with the residents in the community."[58] In a notice outlining the center's plan for public health reform, Landis explained the tripartite role of the nurse: visiting nurse, sanitary inspector, and social worker. To fill this auspicious position, the Whittier Centre board hired Elizabeth Tyler as nurse and "medical social worker."[59] See Figure 3. She would begin her work in a limited area (one or two blocks) at a salary of sixty-five dollars per month. She was also expected to live in the district and establish the beginning of a "neighborhood house."[60] As a community resident, she would work to strengthen bonds of racial and residential identification with hopes to increase her influence on the health practices of community residents.

Tyler's educational and past professional background had prepared her well for her new position. A graduate of the Freedmen's Hospital Training School in Washington, D.C., Tyler had a first-class education. After graduation, she worked as a private-duty nurse in Northampton, Massachusetts, caring primarily for students at Smith College. Hearing of employment opportunities in Alabama, Tyler traveled south, where she worked first at A&M

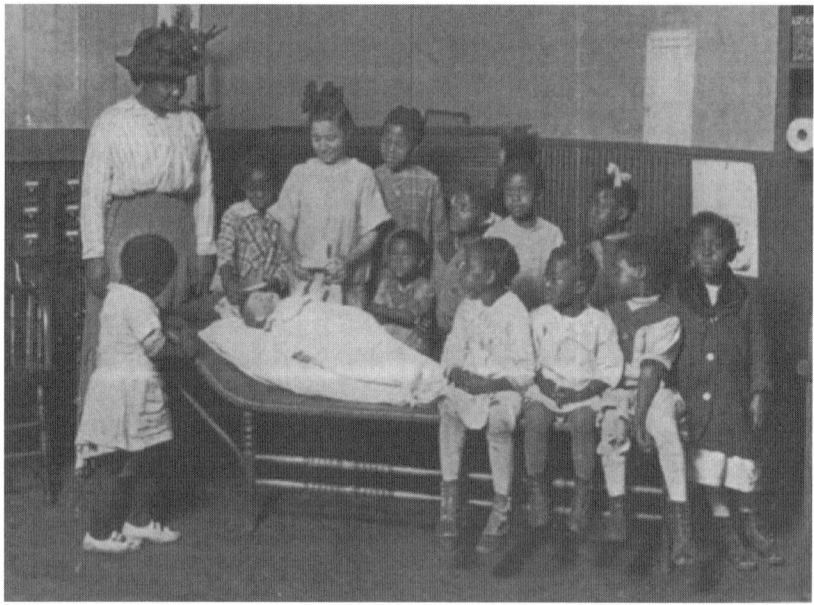

Figure 3. Elizabeth Tyler.
Note. Public health nurse Elizabeth Tyler with members of the "Little Mothers Club." *Whittier Centre Annual Report* (Philadelphia, 1915). Reprinted with permission of Temple University Urban Archives.

College in Normal, Alabama, as the resident nurse and then as an instructor teaching physiology and hygiene. In a move to further her nursing education, she moved to New York City and attended Lincoln School for Nurses for a postgraduate course. In 1906, she accepted a position as the first black public health nurse of the well-known Henry Street Settlement.[61]

TB Work in the Black Belt

Tyler began her new post on 1 February 1914, focusing her attention primarily on the area surrounding HPI, known as the "Black Belt" of Philadelphia. This area and its adjacent neighborhoods housed a large number of blacks, including more than 1,000 members of the Co-operative Coal Club and Rainy Day Society.[62] Club members had ties to the Whittier Centre, so many of Tyler's initial home visits were with families of which the center had "intimate knowledge."[63] In the Whittier Centre annual report for 1 November 1913 to 1 October 1914, Tyler provides a detailed report of her visits. The number of families visited totaled 327; families averaged 3 1/2 individuals; the total number of all individuals visited was 1,084.[64]

Tyler began her work by assessing the living conditions of each family, and found that about 62 percent required medical or social service. For Tyler, this meant offering advice, making referrals to other civic agencies, or recommending treatment at the HPI. Of the total number of families visited, 263 persons (24.5 percent) were ill "from one cause or another." About 12 percent of Tyler's visits found TB or symptoms of it.[65] For these individuals, Tyler recommended clinical treatment or hospital care; these suggestions were accepted voluntarily by nearly 75 percent.[66]

After Tyler's arrival, black patient visits increased rapidly at the HPI. In one of her early reports, Tyler noted that "it is gratifying to know that the number of colored people attending the Phipps Institute has been greatly increased as a direct result of these house-to-house investigations."[67] In the first year, more than twelve times as many black patients visited the clinic than during the first eleven years of the institute's history.[68] More advanced cases were referred to sanatoria, and sanitation measures were taught to remaining family members.[69]

Despite her overall success in attracting patients to the HPI clinic and increasing health awareness, some black patients did not take to receiving health advice from a nurse. Tyler recognized that she was "just scratching the surface," and that there were "gaps and leaks in the system which caused failure in too many cases."[70] Many cases refused to leave their unhygienic surroundings from fear or preference; others failed to improve under any circumstances. One of Tyler's early case notes reveals this paradox. During a routine investigation, Tyler came across a man, ill with a "bad cold." She persuaded him to go to the HPI for treatment, where his case was diagnosed as TB. Shortly thereafter, he became bedridden and hospital care was necessary. Despite his declining condition, he refused hospitalization until the woman with whom he was lodging could no longer provide food for him. After much coercion, the man was finally admitted to Philadelphia General Hospital, where he died three weeks later. The Bureau of Health fumigated the premises, but despite this action, the woman of the house soon became ill with TB; she was probably infected by the lodger. In homes such as these, Tyler believed that there was no protection for nontubercular members of the household. "Had the man been discovered earlier the woman might have been in good health today."[71]

Tyler pointed to early detection as the surest way of preventing further spread of the disease. This case, however, illustrates something else, perhaps more profound. As a visiting home nurse, Tyler surely recognized that understanding an individual's response to illness started with assessing the person's contextual reality. The woman in this case relied on this boarder to supplement her income, not realizing perhaps that there were risks involved—not only loss of family privacy, as some feared, but also threats to her own well-being. For many blacks, taking in boarders opened a de facto contractual relationship where economics and personal space overlapped. This exchange of living space for money, however, left both parties vulnerable to the health practices or non-practices, of one another. Pressing economic needs often forced blacks to think first of their livelihoods, but these choices often cost them their lives.

Tyler's health efforts were hugely successful, and while her work began with home visits, it quickly spread to a wider audience and included talks on sanitation, hygiene, and TB prevention to large crowds at local churches, "as it was the best way to reach the people en masse."[72] See Figure 4. An additional black nurse, Cora Johnson, was hired that same year, her salary provided for by the Whittier Centre and the Pennsylvania Society for the Study of Tuberculosis.[73] A black physician, Henry Minton, was added to the HPI staff in 1914, his salary provided by the Pennsylvania Department of Health.[74]

Minton, like Landis, served as both a staff member at the HPI and a board member of the Whittier Centre. His professional and civic background had much to recommend him for both. Minton is perhaps best known for his long-time affiliation with Mercy Hospital, the second of two black hospitals in Philadelphia. He was born in Columbus, South Carolina, on 25 December 1870. His father was head accountant in the office of South Carolina's state

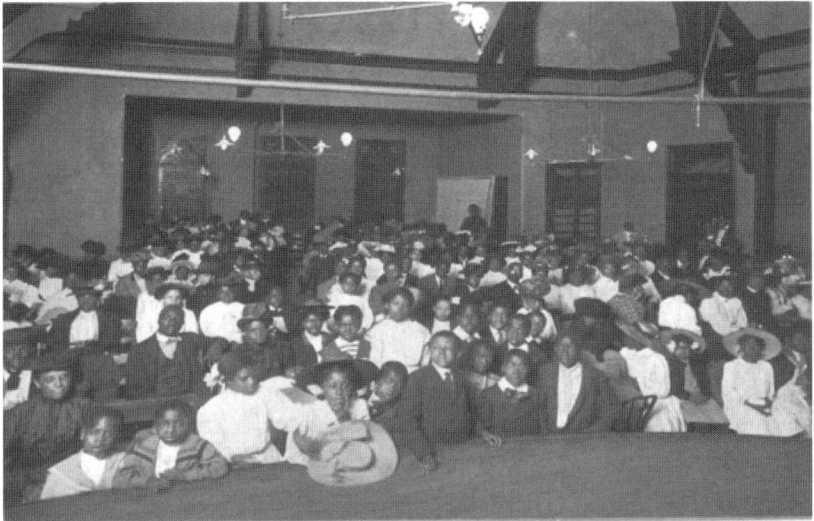

Figure 4. Coal Club "Ready for the Lecture to Begin."
Note. From *Starr Center Annual Report* (Philadelphia: 1906). Reprinted with the permission of the Barbara Bates Center for the Study of the History of Nursing.

treasurer at the time. Minton received his elementary education in the public schools of Washington, D.C., and an academy at Howard University before entering the prestigious Phillips Exeter Academy in New Hampshire, where he graduated in 1891. He briefly studied law at the University of Pennsylvania, but withdrew after his first year. Soon after, he entered the Philadelphia College of Pharmacy and Science, receiving his degree in 1895. Two years later, he opened what is believed to be the first black-owned pharmacy in Pennsylvania. In 1902 he entered Jefferson Medical College, where he received his MD in 1906. In 1904 he served as a charter member and founder of Sigma Pi Phi, the first black fraternity.[75]

Like many black physicians who graduated from white medical schools, Minton could not intern at the hospital associated with the school. To expand his clinical experience, Minton did his residency at Frederick Douglass Memorial Hospital and Training School. He left Douglass in the summer of 1907 to cofound Mercy Hospital, where he served as medical director until 1944.[76] Due to his professional standing, Minton was well respected throughout Philadelphia by both blacks and whites; he was also renowned as a TB expert, serving on the staff of HPI from 1914 until 1946.[77]

After working with the HPI and the Whittier Centre for more than seven years, in 1922 Minton was able to gather the fruits of his labor. In its formative years, the work of the institute was largely confined to black residents in South Philadelphia. By 1921, due to the large increase in patient volume, the number of black clinicians at the HPI had grown to six graduate nurses, one student nurse, and three physicians.[78] In March 1923, a new clinic was established at Ridge Avenue and Twentieth Street, allowing for expansion into northeast Philadelphia.[79]

During his musings, Minton reminisced on the many different collective strategies used by members of the nursing and medical staff to improve the health of the black community. First, he pointed to the work of black nurses, praising them for their hard work and noting that "the success of these clinics is largely dependent upon the efficiency and faithfulness of the nurse. Without proper follow up visits to the homes of the patients to see that they carry out the instructions of the physicians . . . the work of the clinic would scarcely be satisfactory."[80] Minton also recognized that information in the black community was disseminated in several ways: for example, through the church and word of mouth. In the winter of 1914, Minton and Tyler worked together on a church campaign, in which health information was provided for members of congregations.[81] Minton also solicited the support of other black physicians and ministers to aid in the health work. Of all the strategies used to attract blacks to TB clinics, probably none were more powerful than word-of mouth referrals through the social networks in the black community.

In a case note, Minton described Mrs. A., a twenty-three-year-old black woman who reported to the clinic with physical symptoms of incipient TB and a protracted cough. She was given medical treatment and instructed in proper methods of physical exercises, division of labor, rest, fresh air day and night, and nourishment. She diligently followed the instructions of both Minton and the medical social worker. The social worker made house visits to ensure that the instructions were followed. In subsequent visits, the young woman was free of her cough, she had gained twenty pounds, and her general condition was described as excellent. Mrs. A.'s progress prompted her to encourage her mother to visit the clinic for examination and treatment, along with a sister and two brothers. They all showed physical signs of incipient TB, were treated, and remained in close contact with the institute for three years.[82]

Revisiting the HPI "Experiment"

This article revisits a triumphant epoch in urban health history. Many health practitioners in the early part of the twentieth century did not understand why rates of TB in black American communities were much higher than in white American communities. This article reviews the many-faceted theories from that time, and more important, it revisits one of the better-known campaigns against TB in a black community and challenges previously held assertions that attribute the increase in HPI clinic attendance simply to the role of black clinicians. Rather, as is made clear here, the early success of HPI with blacks was due to a variety of different, though related, factors.

First, the Whittier Centre was not simply the benefactor providing "funding for the first black nurse." The center was the driving force and sustaining fire behind the initiative to combat TB in the black community. It had a longstanding commitment to the ideals of social justice and equality, and hoped to fight the burden of excessive illness in blacks through increasing access to health resources. The first effort toward this end was to hire a black nurse.

The success of this endeavor is undeniable. Tyler was skilled and adept, bringing with her years of experience in community nursing. Yet her early efforts were aided by the longstanding ties already established between the Whittier Centre organizers and black community residents. Due to the Whittier Centre connection with the community, they were able to leverage their ties with black families and introduce new health initiatives to an audience with whom they were already familiar. Hence, during the early and critical months of her employment, Tyler was exposed to an immediate pool of more than 1,000 actively engaged individuals. These families were familiar with the role of visitors and were apt to see Tyler as a "friend offering advice," making them less likely to reject her recommendations.

This examination does not deny that the presence of black clinicians contributed tremendously to the increase in black patient attendance at the HPI. The fact that the three early clinicians were members of the black community is critical. During this period, black medical professionals were few in number; thus, the increasing presence of black clinicians probably invoked a sense of racial pride among community residents, increased trust, and provided a sense of belonging.

The success of the Whittier Centre–HPI collaboration hinged, however, on the ability of health workers to extend their efforts beyond immediate TB prevention to include improvement of living conditions and provision of material relief to community residents. Working to meet both the material *and* health needs of black residents, the institute acknowledged the likely causes of excessive illness, such as poverty and joblessness, and appropriately addressed these factors as contributors to poor health in the black community.

These findings suggest that community health efforts rest on partnerships between like-minded organizations for the purposes of coalition building. The Whittier Centre partnership with the HPI is instructive in that it features the trajectory of two separate organizations that were able to collaborate to form a new shared vision. While the Whittier Centre explicitly began as an agency purposely organized to meet the social/welfare needs of black city residents, HPI had been unsuccessful for most of its early years in attracting blacks to its clinics. Together they were able to leverage their individual strengths and expertise to a positive end.

J. Margo Brooks Carthon
Barbara Bates Center for the Study of the History of Nursing
Center for Health Outcomes & Policy Research
University of Pennsylvania School of Nursing
Claire Fagin Hall, 3R, 392
Philadelphia, PA 19146

Acknowledgments

The author acknowledges that this research was supported by the Agency for Health Research Quality (Grant F-31 HS01029–02) and the National Institutes of Health, National Institute of Nursing Research T-32 NR0714. Special thanks to Drs. Julie Fairman, Joan Lynaugh, and Barbara Savage for their support and feedback on earlier drafts of this manuscript.

Notes

1. By the late nineteenth century, the infectious nature of TB had generated debate for years in the United States and Europe. Despite the discovery of the pathogen responsible for consumption, deeply rooted beliefs regarding "hereditary consumption" (transmittal of the disease from parent to child) prevailed. This belief gained traction as whole families succumbed to the disease. Lawrence Flick effectively argued, however, that consumption was indeed contagious and fully discussed the differences between heredity and predisposition in his journal article, "Contagiousness of Phthisis (Tubercular Pulmonitis)," *Transactions of the Medical Society of the State of Pennsylvania* 20 (June 1888): 164–82. Anticontagionists denied that consumption was spread between individuals—rather, they claimed that the disease was acquired when persons of a certain genetic predisposition came into contact with "miasmas" emanating from decaying garbage. For more on

anticontagionists see Barron H. Lerner, "New York City's Tuberculosis Control Efforts: The Historical Limitations of the 'War on Consumption,'" *American Journal of Public Health* 83, no. 5 (May 1993): 758–66.

    2. Lawrence F. Flick, Henry Phipps Institute Fifth Annual Report (Philadelphia, 1909) (hereafter HPI Annual Report). In his annual Clinical and Sociological Report, Flick explains the natural course of TB: "An individual inhales the dust carrying tubercle bacilli which is then implanted in the bronchial lymphatic glands or in the glands of the upper respiratory tract. The disease lies dormant in these glands or else slowly progresses during a period of years, until finally in the grown-up individual, under the stress and the vicissitudes of life and under the demands of labor and deprivation, the bacilli having gotten into the lungs or some other tissue by way of the lymphatic's or the circulation, it breaks out full force" (21).

    3. Lilian Brandt, "Social Aspects of Tuberculosis," *Annals of the American Academy of Political and Social Science* 21 (May 1903): 65. Brandt concluded that social conditions such as physical environment, poor ventilation, and lack of sanitation contributed the prevalence of TB.

    4. Bernard J. Newman, "The Relationship of Housing to Tuberculosis," in Pennsylvania Society for the Prevention of Tuberculosis, *Preventing Tuberculosis in Pennsylvania* (Philadelphia: The Society, 1914), 39.

    5. Brandt, "Social Aspects of Tuberculosis," 65. According to Brandt, physical predisposition to TB was not merely a function of heredity, but was also attributed to the "attendant evils of poverty, such as ignorance and carelessness, . . . all of which produce a physical condition predisposed to disease" (67).

    6. City of Philadelphia Bureau of Health, *Annual Report of the Director of the Department of Public Safety and Bureau of Health* (Philadelphia, 1901). In 1901, consumption caused 2,845 deaths. Due to the high death rates, "consumption of the lung" was placed on the list of reportable diseases on 12 March 1901. Physicians were then required to contact the Bureau of Health to report all cases of consumption.

    7. Henry R. M. Landis, *A Report of the Tuberculosis Problem and the Negro* (Philadelphia: Henry Phipps Institute, 1923), 10a, Table 7. Landis used the U.S. Mortality Statistics for 1920, which demonstrate that Philadelphia's TB was higher than that in any other region of Pennsylvania. It was also noted that not all cities shared Philadelphia's high mortality. Detroit, St. Louis, and Newark all reported death rates under 100 per 100,000 compared to Philadelphia's 137.3 per 100,000. Rates increased in the city in general and blacks specifically between 1916 and 1919 due to the combined effects of influenza, World War I, and increased occupational hazards.

    8. Bureau of Health Annual Report (1901), 80.

    9. Sadie T. Mossell, *A Study of the Negro Tuberculosis Problem in Philadelphia* (Philadelphia: Henry Phipps Institute, 1923); David McBride, "The Henry Phipps Institute, 1903–1937: Pioneering Tuberculosis Work with an Urban Minority," *Bulletin of the History of Medicine* 61 (1987): 78–97; David McBride, *From TB to AIDS: Epidemics Among Urban Blacks Since 1900* (New York: New York University Press, 1989); Barbara Bates, "P.S. I Am . . . Colored," in *Bargaining for Life: A Social History of Tuberculosis, 1876–1938* (Philadelphia: University of Pennsylvania Press, 1992), 288–310.

    10. It is worth noting that there is an ongoing debate regarding what factors contributed to the decrease in TB rates. While some historians argue that improved housing conditions, water filtration, and other environmental changes decreased disease rates, others

attribute the decline to the success of the antituberculosis campaign. In the 1916 Bureau of Health Annual Report, diminishing rates of TB were attributed to several factors, including increased health education of the lay public with an emphasis on how the disease was spread (by means of sputum) and how the disease can be destroyed; early diagnosis and immediate reporting of cases; and isolation and segregation of advanced consumptives. Last, decreased rates were attributed to the gradual establishing of "immunity against the disease" (279).

11. Bureau of Health Annual Report (1918).

12. First Annual Message of Mayor John E. Reyburn (Philadelphia, 1908), 96.

13. U.S. Department of Commerce, Bureau of the Census, *Negro Population in the United States, 1790–1915* (Washington, DC: GPO, 1918), 68, 350–51. It is also worth noting that while TB death rates were elevated in blacks, they were also elevated in some, though not all, European immigrants. Irish-born immigrants' TB rates were among those elevated in the early twentieth century, but trended downward rapidly as the decades progressed. While experiencing some elevation in TB mortality rates, European immigrant death rates were never as high as for blacks and dropped more quickly.

When considering mortality rates it was then and is now common practice to compare disease rates between racial and ethnic groups. While I make no specific attempt to make such comparisons, it is worth noting that a review of vital statistical records compiled by the Bureau of Health for 1900–1920 included comparative breakdowns of TB death rates by race and ethnicity. Categories such as "people of color" and "nativity" were used as broad taxonomic categories. The breakdown by race and ethnicity is helpful for stratifying disease, but it has limitations due to inconsistencies in the use of categories. For instance, a review of death rates due to TB in 1900–1918 shows that the term "people of color" generally referred to blacks except for in 1915, when "Chinese" were also grouped under this heading. It remains unclear why this change occurred in this singular year, given that every year before and after 1915 put Chinese under the subheading "nativity." Furthermore, when considering mortality rates that compared "colored" and "whites," it is not clear from the tables whether foreign-born whites were considered in the "white" mortality values.

14. Though death rates fell for both groups between 1908 and 1913, the rate for blacks reveals a remarkable 51 percent decline. Several plausible reasons may explain this drop. Blacks newly arrived in the city may have had low resistance. Some scholars have argued that, unlike native whites, some of whom had lived in the city for nearly a century, blacks may have been more susceptible to the disease once exposed to white society. As large numbers of black migrants arrived in Philadelphia after the Civil War, the high TB mortality at the opening of the twentieth century may reflect more recently infected blacks, whose rates were higher initially after arriving to the city, then fell off due to the natural progression (and the progressive development of resistance) of the disease. For further explanations for fluctuations in TB mortality in Philadelphia across racial and ethnic groups, see Landis, *A Report of the Tuberculosis Problem and the Negro*.

15. Bates, "P.S. I Am . . . Colored."

16. William D. Fuller, "The Negro Migrant in Philadelphia" (1924), Negro Migrant Study, 1923, Housing Association of the Delaware Valley, Records, 1923–1924, 5 folders and oversize worksheets, URB 31; Sadie T. Mossell, "The Standard of Living Among One Hundred Negro Migrant Families in Philadelphia," *Annals of the American Academy of Political and Social Science* 98 (November 1921): 173–218.

17. National Tuberculosis Association, *Report of the Committee on Tuberculosis Among Negroes: A Five-Year Study and What It Has Accomplished* (New York: The Association, 1937), 24. See also W.E.B. Du Bois, *The Philadelphia Negro: A Social Study* (Philadelphia: University of Pennsylvania Press, 1899), 147–63.

18. Landis, *A Report of the Tuberculosis Problem and the Negro*.

19. Bureau of Health Annual Report (1918), 343. While the mortality figures surrounding TB are helpful for capturing trends, the contextual background is equally important, and useful for those interested in "unpacking" the numbers. First, when considering the accuracy of available TB mortality rates during the early twentieth century, the reliability of TB reporting should be considered. A law adding TB to the list of reportable diseases was passed in 1901, but not formally put into practice until 1906. Thus mortality rates for TB before 1906 may have been influenced by underreporting in all groups (actual rates may have been higher).

20. Landis, *A Report of the Tuberculosis Problem and the Negro*, 12. Flick, "Work of the Year," HPI Annual Report (1906), 19. Differences in TB mortality between socio-economic class and occupational groups are discussed in Flick, "Clinical and Sociological Report," HPI Annual Report (1909), 31.

21. Flick, "Work of the Year," HPI Annual Report (1906), 19. Though few discussions in the primary sources discuss class differences in TB mortality rates, it is made clear that class distinctions existed and that it may be assumed that members of less affluent classes likely succumbed to the disease at higher rates.

22. National Tuberculosis Association, *Report of the Committee on Tuberculosis*, 6.

23. For further readings on early twentieth-century intellectual thoughts on heredity and race, see Edward A. Ross, "The Causes of Race Superiority," *Annals of the American Academy of Political and Social Science* 18 (July 1901): 67–89; William I. Thomas, "The Mind of Woman and the Lower Races," *American Journal of Sociology* 12, no. 4 (January 1907): 435–69.

24. See also C. R. Grandy, "Inherited Immunity in Tuberculosis," *American Review of Tuberculosis* 13, no. 373 (April 1926): 78; H. G. Carter, "Pulmonary Tuberculosis Among Negroes," *American Review of Tuberculosis* 6 (January 1923): 1002–7; C. R. Grandy, "The Control of Tuberculosis in the Negro," *Virginia Medical Monthly* 54 (December 1927): 566–71. Note that a similar debate was occurring regarding the high rate of TB in the Irish as compared to the English. Early twentieth-century writers continued to regard the Irish as a separate and inferior racial group, and as such, more inclined to develop TB.

25. George E. A. Bushnell, *A Study in the Epidemiology of Tuberculosis, with Special Reference to Tuberculosis of the Tropics and of the Negro Race* (New York: William Wood, 1920), 221.

26. National Tuberculosis Association, *Report of the Committee on Tuberculosis*, 21.

27. P. P. McCain, "Tuberculosis Among Negroes in the United States," *American Review of Tuberculosis* 35 (January 1937): 25–35.

28. David McBride, *Integrating the City of Medicine: Blacks in Philadelphia Healthcare, 1910–1965* (Philadelphia: Temple University Press, 1989).

29. Mossell, *A Study of The Negro Tuberculosis Problem*, 18. Mossell found that blacks could receive care for TB at Philadelphia General Hospital at Thirty-Fourth and Pine Streets, Rush Hospital and Clinic at Thirty-Third Street and Lancaster Avenue, Jefferson Chest at 238 Pine Street, State Clinic no. 21 at 1724 Cherry Street, State Clinic

no. 107 at Frankford Avenue and Palmer Streets, and the Henry Phipps Institute at Seventh and Lombard Streets.

30. Ibid. Philadelphia General Hospital's large number of black patients was likely due to its open admission policy, which did not bar them. It was also large and had 300 beds devoted to TB patients. Despite its size it was frequently overcrowded and accommodations were lacking. Several of the other facilities mentioned had limited bed availability on their inpatient wards.

31. Landis, *A Report of the Tuberculosis Problem and the Negro*, 3. Landis noted a lack of hospital beds at the two black hospitals, Douglass Memorial Hospital and Mercy Hospital, and attributed this to lack of funds. See also Barbara Bates, *Bargaining for Life: A Social History of Tuberculosis, 1876–1938* (Philadelphia: University of Pennsylvania Press, 1992), 220.

32. Mossell, *A Study of The Negro Tuberculosis Problem*.

33. Historian Barbara Bates attributes the prohibition of admitting blacks to private sanatoriums to open prejudice and the desire of white patients to limit social interaction with blacks. This was the case at White Haven Sanatorium, which enacted a policy prohibiting blacks in December 1914. In the early twentieth century, White Haven was among the institutions that accepted black patients, but white patients were angered when forced to share the same space as blacks and sent letters of protest and threats. The board of directors capitulated to the demands of white patients who threatened to leave. The fear of reprisal from private patients was of particular concern to proprietors who relied on these patients as their primary means for reimbursement for services. For more see Bates, *Bargaining for Life*, 294–95, 323.

34. John E. Hunter, "Tuberculosis in the Negro: Causes and Treatment," in *Germs Have No Color Lines. Blacks and American Medicine 1900–1940*, ed. Vanessa N. Gamble (New York: Garland Publishing, 1989), 12–19; quote on p. 18.

35. Landis, *A Report of the Tuberculosis Problem and the Negro*, 1. See also HPI Annual Report (1909), 10, 19. In his Clinical and Sociologic Report, Flick notes the low percentage of blacks treated at the institute from its beginning. During its first five years the percentage of black patients was low: in 1904, blacks represented 6.63 percent of HPI patients; in 1905, 5.65 percent; in 1906, 5.96 percent, in 1907, 9.83 percent; and in 1908, 7.68 percent. Blacks held nearly the highest rates of single visits with no return follow-up compared to other racial/ethnic groups.

36. *Who's Who in America* (1903), 1856; news clipping, "$5,000 Is Phipps Gift to University of Pennsylvania for Tuberculosis Fight," December 1909. Born in Philadelphia on 27 September 1839, son of an immigrant English shoemaker, Phipps moved to Allegheny City, close to Pittsburgh, in 1845. As a young boy, Phipps made the acquaintance of the Carnegie family, forming in particular a friendship with Carnegie sons Andrew and Tom. The boyhood friendship between Henry and Andrew turned into a profitable business partnership in the iron forge and manufacturing industry. In 1901, after four decades, Phipps sold his business interests to the United States Steel Corporation, netting $100 million. In his early sixties, Phipps increasingly focused his attention on humanitarian efforts.

37. Bates, *Bargaining for Life*, 99–100; Pennsylvania Society for the Prevention of Tuberculosis, *Preventing Tuberculosis in Pennsylvania* (Philadelphia: The Society, 1914), 55. The Pennsylvania Society for the Prevention of Tuberculosis was one of the first organizations in the United States to mount an organized campaign against TB. One of Flick's

early endeavors began with the founding of Rush Hospital for Consumption and Allied Diseases. The hospital opened in 1891 and accepted its first patients in 1892.

38. "The Phipps Gift," *Gazette*, 5 March 1926, University of Pennsylvania Archives Information Files Collection (UPF 8.51), Folder Henry Phipps Institute; news clipping, "Dedication of the Phipps Institute," December 1909. The HPI takeover was completed with the continued annual support of $50,000 per year from Phipps.

39. News clipping, "Dedication of the Phipps Institute."

40. News clipping, "$5,000 Is Phipps Gift."

41. Bates, *Bargaining for Life*, 101.

42. HPI Annual Report (1904), 4–5.

43. Ibid., 6. The early annual reports of the institute do not explicitly provide the racial makeup of its nursing staff. It may be surmised with a great deal of certainty that these nurses were white, since as indicated in subsequent Phipps records, the first black nurse, Elizabeth Tyler, is hired in 1914.

44. Ibid., 8.

45. Ibid., 12.

46. Ibid., 12.

47. Landis, *A Report of the Tuberculosis Problem and the Negro*, Table 1, "Analysis of Negro Patients Within Present District, in Attendance at Phipps Institute Tuberculosis Clinic in 1903, 1906, 1913, 1922, by Diagnosis, Prognosis, and Result."

48. Ibid., Table 3, "Analysis of White Patients Living Within Present District, in Attendence at Phipps Institute Tuberculosis Clinic in 1903, 1908, 1913, 1922, by Diagnosis, Prognosis, and Result."

49. Ibid., Table 9, "Attendance at Five Tuberculosis Clinics in Philadelphia in 1921, Showing the Number and Percent of White and Negro Patients Examined and the Number of Negro Patients Diagnosed."

50. Ibid., Table 3.

51. Ibid.

52. Whittier Centre Annual Report (Philadelphia, 1914), 4.

53. Starr Centre Association, Untitled Pamphlet (Philadelphia, 1907), Barbara Bates Center for the Study of the History of Nursing, Starr Centre Collection, Box 9, Folder 105.

54. Whittier Centre Executive Board Meeting Minutes, 1913.

55. Whittier Centre Annual Report (1914), 5.

56. "Who's Who, 1924–25 American Men of Science," University of Pennsylvania Archives, Information Files Collection (UPF 8.51) Folder Henry Phipps Institute; Bates, "P.S. I Am . . . Colored," 296.

57. Whittier Centre Annual Report (1914), 3–4.

58. Whittier Centre Annual Report (1915).

59. Ibid.

60. Whittier Centre Executive Board Meeting Minutes, 1913.

61. Marie O. Pitts Mosely, "Satisfied to Carry the Bag: Three Black Community Health Nurses; Contributions to Health Care Reform, 1900–1937," *Nursing History Review* 4 (1996): 65–82. Elizabeth Tyler's career as a public health nurse did not end in Philadelphia. In 1921 she left the HPI to take a position in Delaware for the State Health and Welfare Commission. Later she held positions in Newark and Essex County, New Jersey, for the New Jersey Tuberculosis and Essex County Tuberculosis

leagues, respectively. In each position Tyler maintained her community outreach efforts for education and disease prevention. In the current examination of Tyler's public health activities, I attempt to layer her nursing work alongside those of civically active community residents and thereby recontextualize her health promotion success within the larger scope of community-building initiatives already perculating in local black communities.

62. Whittier Centre Annual Report (1914), 4.
63. Ibid.
64. Ibid., 6. The total number of visits for each family is not provided.
65. Ibid., 4.
66. Ibid.
67. Ibid., 7.
68. Whittier Centre Annual Report (1916), 6.
69. Whittier Center Annual Report (1915), 5. In my examination, I saw no evidence of forcible removal of patients from their homes. Tyler could only encourage patients to go to hospitals or sanatoriums for treatment; ultimately black patients had the right to refuse.
70. Ibid., 6.
71. Whittier Centre Annual Report (1916), 6.
72. Whittier Centre Annual Report (1915), 6.
73. Whittier Centre Annual Report (1916), 2.
74. Whittier Centre Annual Report (1915), 6.
75. *Philadelphia Colored Business Dictionary* (Philadelphia, 1913), 81.
76. Russel F. Minton, "The History of Mercy-Douglas Hospital," *Journal of the National Medical Association* 43, no. 3 (1957): 153–59.
77. Ibid., 154.
78. Whittier Centre Annual Report (1924), 13.
79. This new clinic was established based on the Whittier Centre–sponsored research conducted by Sadie Mossell under the supervision of Landis. Mossell's study indicated the need for increased treatment facilities due to persistently high rates of TB. Mossell, *A Study of The Negro Tuberculosis Problem*.
80. Whittier Centre Annual Report (1924), 13–14.
81. Whittier Centre Annual Report (1915), 6. The names of the churches are not provided.
82. Whittier Centre Annual Report (1919), 11.

Sickening Nurses: Fever Nursing, Nurses' Illness, and the Anatomy of Blame, New Zealand 1903–1923

PAMELA J. WOOD
Victoria University of Wellington, New Zealand

Abstract. In the early twentieth century, patients with infectious fevers represented a danger to the health of others including their nurses. This research describes the training New Zealand nurses received in fever nursing during the period 1903–1923, and considers how they applied hospital cross-infection principles in emergency tent fever camps in remote rural areas. It examines the reaction of nurses, hospital boards, and physicians to nurses who succumbed with their patients' fevers. It therefore reveals attitudes to nurses, prevailing ideas about responsibility for nurses' health, and elements in the emerging professional culture of nursing. Although some measures protected them against epidemic fevers, nurses were held responsible for their own health. A complex anatomy of blame is evident against those who sickened; the nature of the blame shifted, depending on the observer, disease, and practice setting. Physicians blamed nurses, especially when they sickened with typhoid fever. The country's chief nurse and other nurses blamed those who jeopardized their health through ill-spent leisure time. Sick nurses could be absolved from blame for the lax discipline evident through their failure to observe cross-infection principles if their practice setting was the fever camp. Willingness to work in difficult circumstances showed they embodied the ideal of sacrifice that, like discipline, was part of the emerging nursing culture.

Agnes Maud Snell, a carpenter's daughter, was born in August 1880 in New Zealand, the British Empire's farthest colony that had been established just forty years before. She began her nursing training at Wellington Hospital during 1904 but in January 1908, Snell died at the age of twenty-seven. Her cardiac failure followed a year of chronic endocarditis, the result of contracting scarlet fever.[1] It is likely that Snell caught the disease from a patient while she was training at the hospital. Nearly all hospital care in the country was provided in public (government-funded) hospitals where nurses were required to train. The Nurses Registration Act of 1901 had instituted a three-year program for the country with a state examination system leading to state registration as a nurse. The year before Snell started her training, legislation had shifted responsibility for the care of patients with infectious diseases from municipal authorities, such as town boards, to the boards responsible for the hospitals in their regions. This added a new dimension to nurse training and increased nurses' exposure to the health risks of infectious fevers.

This research examines New Zealand nurses' training and practice in fever nursing, particularly in preventing the spread of disease to others and themselves. It considers the difficulties in implementing this, especially in the challenging practice setting of rural fever camps, and the issue of fever sickness among nurses. An indicator of nurses' proficiency, even if not a formal measure, would have been their ability to avoid contracting a patient's disease. Such a failure of preventive principles could have carried a powerful message within the professional culture. This research therefore considers the reaction of nurses, hospital boards, and physicians to nurses who succumbed to their patients' fevers. It reveals attitudes toward nurses, elements in the emerging professional culture of nursing, and prevailing ideas about responsibility for nurses' health in the time when New Zealand hospital boards first became responsible for the care of patients with infectious fevers. Only a little attention has been paid to the history of epidemic infectious fevers among nurses in the early decades of the twentieth century.[2] Yet studying the history can reveal much about attitudes toward nurses, elements in the emerging professional culture of nursing, and ideas about responsibility for nurses' health.

This study focuses on New Zealand from 1903 to 1923, a twenty-year span from the point when the Public Health Amendment Act of 1903 transferred responsibility for fever patients to hospital boards. Nurses were required for staffing the new isolation wards and hospitals for infectious patients and were therefore more exposed to the risk of contracting fevers than in their previous general hospital work. It also covers the period when the Department of Health was most active in responding rapidly to rural epidemics. The research therefore allows an exploration of the realities of protecting nurses' health when caring for patients with infectious fevers, not only in urban hospitals (as in many other countries) but in emergency fever camps. The research concentrates on typhoid fever and scarlet fever as these were two of the epidemic infectious diseases nurses encountered most often. Smallpox also warrants inclusion. Although fourteen mild cases of smallpox occurred in Christchurch in 1904, there is no documentation that nurses encountered the disease elsewhere in New Zealand.[3] As Dr. William Irving remarked in a lecture to a meeting of the local branch of the New Zealand Trained Nurses' Association there in 1909, many nurses would "probably have never seen anyone vaccinated, and still fewer have seen a case of smallpox."[4] The 1913 smallpox epidemic therefore taxed nurses' skills and offers a significant example of guarding against cross-infection in fever camp nursing. In particular, the research examines the different responses to nurses who became ill with an infectious fever. Was the idea of a nurse sickening with her patient's fever "sickening" to others? If so, did they hold the nurse or others responsible? And what does this tell us about attitudes toward nurses, aspects of nursing culture, and the protection of nurses' health in this time period before authorities internationally acknowledged responsibility in response to concern over tuberculosis?

Response to Epidemics

The prevalence of epidemic infectious diseases in general had been declining in the late nineteenth century among the European (mostly British) colonial settler population in New Zealand. For example, the mortality rate for typhoid fever had fallen steadily from 50.9 per 100,000 in the 1872–1876 quinquennium, to 24.4 in 1882–1886, 16.7 in 1892–1896, and 6.6 in 1902–1906, and continued to fall. The mortality rate for scarlet fever fell steadily from 30.0 per 100,000 in 1882, 5.0 in 1890, and 0.3 in 1898, but rose dramatically to 4.9 in 1902 and 16.0 in 1903. This sharp and worrisome reversal spurred the Public Health Amendment Act's addition to hospital boards' responsibilities that year. Between 1872 and 1900, only nine deaths from smallpox were recorded. Although legislation in 1872, 1876, and 1900 had made vaccinating children against smallpox compulsory, it was ineffectual. Even the fourteen mild cases reported in Christchurch in 1904 did little to change public attitudes. Of all children born that year only 10 percent were vaccinated. From 1920 on, infant vaccination was no longer compulsory.[5]

In contrast to the decline in the prevalence of infectious diseases among settlers, typhoid fever was increasingly affecting the indigenous Maori population, who lived mostly in remote rural areas. When epidemics broke out in these regions, the Department of Health quickly sent nurses to care for people in tent hospitals or the meeting-houses in Maori *kainga* (villages). The response to a 1913 smallpox epidemic in the same remote rural areas, in which 55 Maori died, was equally rapid but larger in scale, perhaps because of the fear the disease generated. Fever camp nursing challenged nurses in unexpected ways, not least in applying hospital-based nursing principles, including measures to prevent cross-infection, in a far different and more demanding environment.

Hospital Training for Fever Nursing

Probationers learning to care for fever patients had to become proficient in preventing cross-infection. The two central principles in preventing the spread of fevers were cordoning off patients' capacity to infect others by isolating them and quarantining their contacts, and killing infective organisms by thorough disinfection. In the first years of the twentieth century, how to put these principles into action was a contentious subject discussed in medical literature. Journals like *Lancet* debated the value of isolation hospitals for large population groups such as those in London, but many isolation hospitals did exist.[6] In smaller British hospitals, an outbuilding for isolating infectious patients often stood empty and lacked experienced staff when needed.[7]

In New Zealand, patients with infectious diseases could be quarantined and nursed at home. Some households could afford a private nurse; others relied on family members. Severely affected patients could seek admission to the local hospital. This was not guaranteed as physicians could refuse to admit patients and often did during an epidemic, especially if the hospital did not have a separate isolation ward or if they felt the admission would endanger patients already there, perhaps by introducing an additional fever. The Public Health Amendment Act of 1903 did not resolve this issue as it addressed the matter at the level of hospital boards rather than hospitals. With the possibility that physicians could refuse admission, the boards had to meet their responsibility for infectious fever patients in other ways.

New Zealand's main hospital boards followed the international trend and gradually built separate isolation wards or fever hospitals either at the edge of the main hospital grounds or at the margins of the town. Nurses in towns could also find themselves caring for infectious patients in tents while more permanent buildings were being planned and constructed. This was the case in 1908 when the resident medical officer of the Dunedin Hospital, A. R. Falconer, refused to admit scarlet fever patients during an epidemic and wanted others who had caught the disease after admission to the hospital to be sent elsewhere. The hospital board had been slow in setting up a separate infectious diseases hospital. There were delays in finding a site, approving plans, and gaining agreement with town and rural local authorities for their contribution to costs, as allowed by the 1903 legislation.[8] The scarlet fever epidemic overtook this process. Faced with the urgent need for alternative accommodation, the board erected a separate, temporary fever hospital for the district. Known informally as "The Camp," it consisted of three bell tents and two large marquees, one with a wooden floor, erected on a rather cold, dank, swampy edge of Pelichet Bay in Dunedin's inner harbor. A woman, six children, and three sick nurses were transferred there on 25 January 1908 as soon as the camp was ready. Two nurses (one designated matron) managed all the care, one during the day and the other at night. At the beginning of March, the matron, a Miss Stronach, reported that two of the nurse patients were by then convalescent and had taken on the duties of night nursing so the night nurse was no longer needed.[9]

In Britain, nurses could train solely as fever nurses and could take an examination to have their names recorded by the Fever Nurses' Association. From 1919 they could register as fever nurses with the General Nursing Council.[10] This did not give them reciprocal registration in New Zealand. No separate training or registration as a fever nurse existed, as the country's comparatively small population did not warrant such a specialty. Instead, New Zealand needed nurses with a broad general training. Each year registered nurses were asked to supply information on their clinical experience and professional appointments following registration, for publication with the nursing register. By 1910 only two New Zealand trained nurses had recorded post-registration experience in New Zealand fever hospitals. One of them, Barbara Smith, was the matron of the permanent fever hospital finally built in Dunedin on the site used in 1908 for the tent hospital. Eleven nurses from Britain and Australia registering in New Zealand by 1910 had recorded training or experience in special fever hospitals, and another had a certificate in fever nursing.[11] At the end of the time period, an additional six New Zealand–trained and eleven overseas-trained nurses who were registered in the country had recorded fever nursing experience. These 31 nurses were only a fraction of the approximately 3,400 nurses on the register in 1923.[12] This would not have been an accurate portrayal, however, of the extent of registered nurses' experience in caring for patients with fever. A nurse would only note this if she had worked for a significant period of time in a ward or hospital dedicated to isolating infectious patients. If infectious patients were nursed in general wards, a nurse who had worked there would not record fever nursing as a separate item in the information she sent for the register. Nevertheless, few nurses in the country had special training or intensive experience in fever nursing. In 1910 only two boards were sending probationers to the fever hospital in their districts for part of their training.[13] This changed as more boards built fever wards and hospitals and required probationers to staff them, particularly during epidemics. Nurses' preparation for caring for fever patients was therefore undertaken where infectious patients were nursed in the same wards as non-infectious patients or in separate isolation areas.

The principles of preventing cross-infection that probationers learned were debated internationally among the medical profession. Medical journals such as the *Lancet* discussed the various ways to separate patients with different infectious diseases within an isolation ward, or infectious patients within a general ward. The two commonly accepted methods were "cubicle" and "barrier" (or "bed") isolation. The first method relied on a partition between patients, the other on nurses' actions to create a "barrier" between the patient and others.[14] One British physician in 1910 disliked the cubicle method because of the cost of partitions and the fact that the nurse's attention became fixed on the partition as the safeguard. He believed patients should be separated by a barrier of "ritual observance only" to overcome the nurse's misplaced reliance on a physical barrier. This ritual included wearing overalls, donning gloves for certain procedures, and disinfecting all articles as well as the nurse's hands. Its success also required that the matron have "the fullest control of her staff and the keenest appreciation of the ideas."[15]

The techniques involved in barrier nursing were described in detail in nursing journals and textbooks. Method was everything. Precautions were likened to those in an operating theater except that they were observed continuously throughout the patient's stay in the hospital.[16] One nursing textbook reported research at a Liverpool isolation hospital in a ward run by a "highly trained sister possessing surgical and fever experience." Strict cleanliness and "the loyal and intelligent observation of all concerned" meant that of the 741 cases admitted over two years, only two had contracted an additional disease through cross-infection.[17] A question on barrier and cubicle nursing included in the Fever Nurses' Association examination in October 1919 was used by the *British Journal of Nursing* in November as the subject for its monthly essay competition.[18] Details in the prize-winning essay, published in December, were consistent with those conveyed in textbooks and journal articles but also reflected the practice in the particular fever hospital where the nurse worked.[19] The importance of proficiency in barrier nursing was emphasized whenever possible, for example, in lectures physicians gave nurses outside their training courses.[20]

While the international medical profession debated the benefits of these different practices, nurses grappled with the intricacies of the regimented cross-infection prevention routines for that had been decided for their locality. Emily O'Callaghan, who trained at Wellington Hospital in New Zealand between 1915 and 1918, remembered the tedious and somewhat arbitrary nature of precautions there. Probationers went to the separate fever hospital inside the grounds for six weeks during their training and, as she noted, did not leave the place *at all*. It had its own Nurses' Home, and the nurses walked to the hospital in a different uniform than the one they worked duty in (even shoes). After work, on the way out the nurses bathed in disinfectant and put on their "walking" uniform again. The doctors didn't do all that![21]

Nurses were trained to prevent cross-infection whether nursing patients in hospital or home. New Zealand probationers were taught that scarlet fever, for example, could be spread by direct contact with the patient, droplet infection, or fomites (items such as clothing, brushes, bed linen, or books). Patients were isolated for six weeks once diagnosed, as they were considered infectious until their skin had finished desquamating. Even this bodily detritus was capable of spreading infection. Giving the twice-daily bath and lubricating patients' desquamating skin with Vaseline or carbolized oil required careful handling. Nurses learned to take particular care when brushing or syringing patients' throats with an antiseptic lotion to destroy the hemolytic streptococci. Disinfecting patients' excreta in carbolic 1–20 solution, and soaking clothes and soiled linen in disinfectant or fumigating them with formaldehyde or sulfur, established a chemical barrier between the infective power of the patient and susceptible others.

Nurses' grasp of precautionary principles was often tested in the state examination for nursing registration. One nurse, answering a question on scarlet fever in 1910, explained that she would protect her health by washing her hands and soaking them in disinfectant, by gargling frequently with antiseptic and, to the examiner's surprise, by turning her head away from the patient when attending to his or her throat—undoubtedly an ambitious and fraught maneuver when trying to aim a stream of antiseptic accurately from a syringe.[22]

By contrast, the examiner in 1921 clearly approved of a candidate's answer that the nurse caring for someone with scarlet fever in their home had a distinct responsibility to prevent the spread of the disease. She would hang a sheet wrung out with strong disinfectant across the outside of the sickroom door. Just inside the room she would have gowns, caps, masks, and shoes to be worn by herself and the doctor. Soaking soiled linen for two hours in a pan of disinfectant in the corner before laundering it, burning all excreta and bodily discharges, keeping the patient's eating utensils separate, allowing no visitors, and thoroughly disinfecting the room and its contents when the patient had recovered would all help prevent cross-infection. Turning to her own health, she added that she would always wash her hands and face before leaving the room or eating any food, and would endeavor to get as much sunshine and fresh air as possible.[23] In her perspective, at least, responsibility for her health rested with her.

As historian Alison Bashford has noted, hanging a disinfectant-soaked sheet across the door to prevent cross-infection was a literal translation of the older practice of using a carbolic spray during surgery "as an antiseptic shield or curtain" and technique for purifying the air.[24] The evidence from this research indicates, however, that its efficacy relied more on the visible, physical, and olfactory barrier it presented to people trying to enter the room than on any belief in its ability to screen out microbes. The sheet was a clear, visible sign that people should be cautious in entering the room. As an Australian matron noted, the sheet had little value as a disinfectant but acted as a "warning to forgetful members of the household."[25] Opening the door also required extra effort in managing the physical barrier of a wet, clinging sheet. And the smell of disinfectant carried a subliminal warning of infectious danger, as households were familiar with the distinctive odor of disinfectants and their use to destroy harmful microbes. As one 1922 article on this common practice commented, a weak solution of carbolic acid or Sanitas could be used to wet the sheet, but water was "equally effective, though perhaps less impressing."[26]

Examinations similarly tested nurses' understanding of precautions when nursing patients with typhoid (or enteric) fever. In 1913, an examiner was again amused and surprised by some of the nurse candidates' answers. One candidate wrote that she would wear a respirator; another would don rubber slippers. A third nurse caught the examiner's imagination by stating that "nurses should remove their clothes on leaving the room." He commented wryly that she "excelled in precautions."[27]

Amelia Bagley, the Department of Health's supervising nurse for fever camps in remote areas, worried about nurses' training. The reason so many nurses contracted typhoid fever needed to be investigated, especially as they were supposed to be trained in proper nursing precautions to minimize danger. Bagley was forced to conclude that precautions received insufficient emphasis. Teaching seemed to be too narrow as it only met the particular conditions in that hospital. Nurses should be taught to adapt and contrive safety measures so they would be equally effective in "widely different conditions" when nursing patients with typhoid fever, to ensure "safety to themselves as well as others." Bagley advocated training nurses not only in general and personal hygiene but also in domestic and rural sanitation and the care of drains, and the safe disposal of typhoid and other infectious excreta in places without drainage, including camp hospitals. State examination questions could embody these points.[28] Her recommendations were not enacted but she at least was one to recognize from firsthand experience the need for well-trained, adaptable, resourceful nurses who could care for themselves as well as patients while nursing in fever camps.

Fever Camps

The Department of Health responded rapidly to news of typhoid fever epidemics affecting Maori living in remote regions. Registered nurses were immediately dispatched to set up an emergency fever camp. Some nurses came from hospitals; others were drawn from those already in the department's district nursing schemes for settlers and Maori living in these remote "backblocks" areas. Traveling by coastal steamer, wagon, and horse, nurses arrived with rudimentary supplies and set about erecting tents or arranging for the use of the local Maori meeting-house. They enlisted help from the Maori and gathered patients into the temporary hospital. Once a fever hospital had been set up, usually two or three nurses and a local assistant worked alone and could sometimes be responsible for the twenty-four-hour care of twenty to sixty patients at a time.[29] They were supported by only occasional visits from Bagley, a sanitary inspector, or government doctor. Nurses stayed for two or three months before moving to the next epidemic site, bringing their camp equipment with them, often by packhorse.

In 1913 the nursing service was severely taxed by the additional challenge of running fever camps for more than 2,000 mostly Maori patients with smallpox.[30] Some were admitted to the isolation hospital at Point Chevalier, a suburb of the city of Auckland. The number of cases there increased daily until for some time it did not fall below sixty. Two trained nurses, one untrained nurse, two porters, and convalescent patients provided all the care for four months. At the tent fever camp in the most affected rural area in the far north, three nurses cared for more than fifty patients at its busiest time.

A nurse (probably Bagley) reported how cross-infection principles were applied to the camp as a whole. It was organized into two distinct areas—infected and clean—separated by a barrier. The infected side housed patients and those caring for them. It was equipped with the patients' tents, the nurses' marquee, and a disinfection tent used before patients were discharged. Convalescent patients did the domestic work. The clean side accommodated doctors, medical students, and sanitary inspectors attending to the public health aspects of the epidemic, including liaising closely with kainga committees. No one in the infected area crossed over the barrier, went to the clean linen tent, or handled anything after its final disinfection. No one from the clean side entered the infected area, except doctors who wore special clothing during any visit. Laundering patients' clothes was divided on the same lines. Convalescent patients washed them in the infected area. After the washing had been well boiled it was taken away in clean tubs, rinsed, and hung out by others from the clean area. Anything contaminated by infective matter from smallpox patients' pustules had to be disinfected or destroyed. The greatest risk was to nurses. As they were continually handling patients, they needed to find ways to manage bodily contaminants. When turning a smallpox patient whose body was covered in pustules, one nurse manipulated the patient with a drawsheet while the other supported the patient's shoulder and buttock, holding large swabs of wool wrung out with warm Lysol.[31] No nurses contracted smallpox.

Preventing cross-infection in typhoid camps was also demanding. Maintaining sanitary standards was awkward when nurses had to kneel on the rough ground to nurse patients lying on mats over bracken, when no camp stretchers were initially available. Keeping patients clean was particularly difficult when they were incontinent with pea-soup diarrhea and all water had to be brought from a creek. It was challenging to disinfect and dispose of patients' excrement without a sluice. Nurses had only old kerosene tins to use for containers for disinfecting the waste and boiling it over a camp fire before burying it.[32] In addition to the dangers of handling infective bodily material, nurses' health could be undermined when they had to try to sleep in the same tent as delirious patients, got little rest even when they had a separate tent, and had no respite from the heavy, demanding work in successive typhoid outbreaks. Inevitably some nurses became sick.

Sick Nurses

The task of replacing camp nurses who sickened rested with Hester Maclean, the person responsible between 1906 and 1923 for all nursing matters in the country. She initially held the post of Assistant Inspector of Hospitals, but in 1920, when the Department of Health restructured, her broader responsibility for nursing was recognized in the new position of Director, Division of Nursing. In her role as the country's chief nurse she received news of sick and convalescing fever camp nurses and promptly reported it in the country's only nursing journal, *Kai Tiaki,* which she owned and edited. Nurses were sent as quickly as practicable to replace any colleagues who became ill. Florence Gill was one who contracted typhoid after a long stint of camp nursing in 1911. Initially she and one other nurse had worked twelve-hour duties on their own without a day off, exchanging night and day duty at the end of a fortnight. After three weeks, when the number of patients had increased to thirteen, another nurse was sent to assist with the day work, which they "found the heaviest." After several weeks and despite taking every precaution, including boiling water and milk and washing any fruit, Gill contracted typhoid. Once convalescent, she was quick to assure Maclean that she would soon be "ready for action again."[33]

Two years later, at Pakaraka, it was Gill's turn to nurse a colleague who developed typhoid "very badly."[34] Another nurse became ill just as the last of her thirteen patients was nearly recovered. She was thankful to have seen the epidemic through before succumbing.[35] Some fever camp nurses died from typhoid. One of the first Maori registered nurses, Akenehi Hei, nursed in the epidemic among Maori living up the Wanganui River, then cared for affected members of her own family in Hawkes Bay before succumbing herself and dying in November 1910.[36] Two nurses died at Te Araroa in the remote East Cape: Rose Winfield in 1917 and Elizabeth Ensor in 1919.[37]

Maclean admired the fortitude of fever camp nurses who were undaunted by nursing under canvas and were willing to volunteer again and again, even after contracting the disease. As so many wrote saying they were nearly "ready again for the fray," she was moved to say "we shall not despair of the future of the profession."[38] The location of practice and a nurse's response following illness could therefore counteract any doubt about her professional worth that might have been generated by her succumbing to illness.

It was not only the rough and rugged conditions in fever camps that endangered nurses' health. In urban hospitals and patients' homes, other nurses sickened with scarlet fever and some, like Agnes Snell, died. When the temporary tent hospital opened in Dunedin in 1908, one of the three sick nurses admitted, Agnes Redwood, died.[39] The following year Helen Robinson, who had been nursing a Dunedin family with the disease, was admitted to the now permanent fever hospital there and died the same day as the family's youngest child.[40] Dunedin nurses could choose whether to work in the fever hospital and were paid a higher rate as compensation for the extra risk involved.[41] In the ten-year period from 1 April 1910 to 31 March 1920, thirty-one nurses were admitted to the Dunedin fever hospital as patients. Although their diagnoses were not recorded in the patient register, all but five stayed for the distinctive forty-two-day period of isolation for scarlet fever.[42]

Anatomy of Blame

A complex anatomy of blame is evident in relation to nurses who contracted disease from their patients. Nurses who sickened were vulnerable to blame for transgressing precautionary principles. The likelihood of blame depended on an intricate interplay of observer, disease, and setting. Embedded in this interplay were varying attitudes toward nurses, professional cultural values of discipline and sacrifice, and differing opinions regarding who should take responsibility for nurses' health. Evidence appears in textbooks and articles written by both nurses and physicians. The textbooks were mostly British but were used in training or known more generally in New Zealand (as reviews in the journal indicate).[43] Maclean also reprinted articles from overseas journals in *Kai Tiaki*. New Zealand physicians' views can also be found in the journal, in articles, published lectures, and reports on examinations. Maclean's own views are clearly voiced there and perhaps predominate. As editor, she also used the journal as a vehicle for voicing her opinion when it differed from the official department or government agenda. The views of other nurse leaders (like Bagley) and rank-and-file nurses, while appearing in the journal less frequently, show important variations within this complex and nuanced anatomy of blame.

Nurses' instruction in measures to prevent cross-infection generally focused on guarding others rather than themselves from the disease. Some textbooks made no mention of the risk to the nurse.[44] Nurses could be given advice on maintaining their general health as well as specific precautions to take, but this was usually presented not as concern for their welfare but in terms of their obligation to protect others.[45] They were a potential vehicle for spreading disease beyond the patients they nursed, either by carrying infective material outside the sickroom or by succumbing to the disease themselves, and were blamed for any failure in preventive measures. This message was delivered in a variety of ways, from a straightforward manner to a strongly emotive style. It could be a warning that needless exposure to danger was "always foolish," and it was the nurse's duty to safeguard herself just as it was the "duty of the soldier to take cover in battle."[46] It could be stated more strongly as a duty to the community. The nurse should "carry out faithfully the minutest details for isolation"; otherwise she was a "source of danger to the public." As this textbook noted, carelessness was the chief crime, as a single case could cause an epidemic in a town.[47] Their duty to guard themselves against infection did not mean they should put their own safety first; rather, they should realize that nurses who were careless about themselves were apt to be the same about other people and therefore more likely "to carry contagion away with them from the sick-room."[48] Two nurse-writers doubted nurses' diligence. One said that nurses were "constantly washing their hands and touching their faces, screens, door handles, etc., before disinfecting them."[49] The other conveyed the stronger message that, as success depended on conscientious care, nurses were to regard cross-infection "as a disaster" for which they were "individually responsible."[50] Perhaps the most vehement expression of this view had come earlier, in 1888 from Eva Lückes, matron of the London Hospital. She told probationers that in regard to contracting infection they should avoid two extremes: cowardly dread and careless disregard. The latter worried her more, as familiarity with disease made many experienced nurses careless, indifferent, lax, slovenly, and culpably negligent in failing to put their knowledge into practice. It arose from sheer laziness.[51] In nursing textbooks at least, nurses were not only responsible for their own health but accountable for protecting all others as well.

Physicians tended to blame sick nurses for poor technique, particularly when sickening with typhoid fever. Archibald J. Aspinall, the medical superintendent of Sydney Hospital in Australia, for example, gave detailed instructions for preventing cross-infection when nursing patients with this disease. He extended the potential for blame and guilt by pointing out the risk the nurse created for her colleagues. The nurse who was "careless in these matters" was "a danger to every other Nurse on the staff."[52] An article in the *British Journal of Nursing* in 1908 by Manchester physician Alec Knyvett Gordon, reprinted in an Australian nursing journal, castigated nurses in hospital and private practice for inadequate hand-washing. How many nurses, he said, would think that a surgeon whose hands were contaminated with pus from an abscess would really remove all traces by simply washing his hands in a basin in the ordinary way? Yet how many nurses did anything else when leaving a typhoid patient's sickroom? It was a wonder not that so many nurses caught typhoid fever, but that so few did. He reminded them that there was no chemical or soap that would "sterilise hands at sight." Nurses should rub their dry hands with soft soap, taking special care with crevices round the nails, then scrub them with a nailbrush and hot water, and finally rub them with methylated spirits. Yet however carefully hands were sterilized, he added, it was unwise to court infection by eating bread with the fingers, especially as there was no reason why a fork should not be used for the purpose.[53] As he applied these comments to nurses working in either hospitals or patients' homes, the location of the practice setting was not a factor in his criticism. He held nurses responsible for their own health, as he believed that it was their poor technique that led to their illness. This physician's views were conveyed as forcefully to New Zealand nurses as to their British and Australian counterparts, as Maclean made the most of it when reprinting the article in *Kai Tiaki* by positioning it immediately after the death notice for an Auckland nurse who had contracted typhoid fever from a patient. Maclean admonished that her death called attention to the great need for care in nursing such cases, especially as an epidemic was currently "raging" in the city.[54]

Physicians were most outspoken in relation to typhoid fever, perhaps because its transmission by fecal contamination added to their repugnance for the sickening nurse, but their readiness to blame them extended to other diseases. In 1917 another article, most likely by a New Zealand physician, gave a similar warning about scarlet fever. It was explicit in stating that in the "vast majority of cases, when a nurse contracts scarlet fever, the fault lies at her own door. Through ignorance or carelessness she has exposed herself to the risk of infection." If she disregarded "the many little rules set down to keep her physically fit," it was "small wonder if she succumbs and is nursed, instead of nursing."[55] Physicians were therefore ready to blame the nurse for succumbing to illness as well as endangering others.

Nurses showed a mixture of attitudes toward other nurses in relation to health and illness. They wrote articles chastising those who grumbled about conditions they felt were jeopardizing their health. Maclean insured these bracing articles reached a wide audience and contributed editorial comment.[56] In 1911 she complained that it appeared a habit for nurses to make the most of their troubles. "We seem to think that because we are working in the cause of sick humanity, we must not in our own bed have even a crumpled rose-leaf; we must not be subjected to the ordinary vicissitudes of life." Nothing made her more indignant than the "uncalled-for pity and commiseration" it was the fashion to give nurses, who were after all only doing the work they had chosen.[57] She was irked again in 1918 by Nurses' Homes that gave nurses "extreme consideration." Comfort a nurse should have, yes; restfulness and beauty surrounding her; but not to a higher degree than a patient or the standard the nurse had previously enjoyed in her own home. She was particularly irritated by the "bitterly waged" controversy over the provision of steam-heating in bedrooms, a luxury not available to nurses who were at that time "enduring with fortitude and cheerfulness" the hardships and biting cold of wartime service in France.[58]

Maclean also abhorred the eight-hour day. This had been instituted for nursing staff at some New Zealand hospitals in the 1880s and 1890s. Maclean sidestepped her official role as chief nurse and used her editorial position to rail against the government's 1909 legislation that consolidated a fifty-six-hour working week for all probationers in the country as a measure to improve their working conditions and health. Commonly called the "eight-hour day," it was a significant reduction from the twelve-hour day, although it remained the ideal rather than the reality in some hospitals. The wisdom of giving nurses a shorter working day was sometimes fiercely debated. Maclean took pleasure in reprinting a 1912 letter from a nurse to a Wellington newspaper, claiming nurses' extra freedom and time used up their strength "unprofitably." The system of pampering produced "feather-bed nurses."[59]

Maclean believed that training needed to be stringent enough to toughen the nurse for the rigors ahead, instilling discipline and backbone. In a 1917 editorial, she again veered from official policy to criticize the way hospital authorities were expected to guard probationers from any possible risk, to the extent that boards were forbidden by the department to place a first-year probationer in a ward where any infectious disease was treated. It hampered staffing and training. It also engendered a "fear of danger" that resulted in nurses later "picking and choosing cases" in private practice.[60] Not relinquishing her editorial campaign, in 1921 she repeated her belief that the eight-hour day was "responsible for much of the ill-health of our nurses." Nurses on afternoon duty spent the morning in town "shopping, having morning tea with friends, even lunching out," then rushed back "at the last moment to scramble into their uniforms" before hurrying onto their wards. They had already "spent their freshness," came on duty tired, and had to make an effort to carry out their duties.[61] A measure designed in part to bolster nurses' health was therefore held up as a danger to it.

Maclean's view that nurses had chosen their profession and should therefore endure its occasional hardships and not complain was matched by a speaker at a hospital board conference in 1911. The chairman of the Hawera board, Robert H. Nolan, delivered the strong message that with an eight-hour day and comfortable accommodation, better work could be expected of the probationer and less illness. After all, she worked in a large, bright, airy ward, was in and out to the ward veranda and balcony all day, and had the bustle of life around her. Moreover, the constant variation of her work was in itself a rest.[62] This put responsibility for nurses' health squarely on nurses, even suggesting that hospital boards were actually enhancing nurses' well-being through the apparent benefits of the ward environment and the variety inherent in nursing work. Maclean bolstered her case by publishing the speech in the journal.⁶³

Whatever board members thought, they could not ignore the economic impact of nurses' illness. Probationers in New Zealand received a salary throughout their three-year training, and boards also invested funds in providing accommodation for them in Nurses' Homes. Having a probationer's training disrupted by illness jeopardized these investments in training, salary, and accommodation. A nurse's illness also had an impact on available staffing and meant increased costs in addressing this. The Department of Health advised boards in 1918 that it would be reasonable to terminate a probationer's training during illness, including her pay, and allow her to resume her training later. On the other hand, boards could pay registered nurses while sick. The department suggested perhaps full pay for one month and half pay for two further months, with the provisions extended in time and amount for longer service.⁶⁴ This differentiation between probationers and trained nurses could perhaps be explained by the fact that most of the hospital care was delivered by probationers. As they represented a much greater proportion of hospital staffing than registered nurses, their illness had a greater impact on staffing costs. Once nurses were registered, boards would also have wanted a return on their training investment. In light of this, those who remained working in their hospitals once qualified were a valuable group who needed consideration.

The expectation that boards would pay part of a qualified nurse's salary when sick did not address the problem of sickness among the majority of registered nurses. Most worked outside hospitals, undertaking private practice caring for patients in their homes. Recognizing the reality of needing to provide for themselves when unable to work, they acted collectively to set up a fund in 1911 through the New Zealand Trained Nurses Association. The secretary put into the small starting sum "all the spare bawbees" she could "make out of anything."⁶⁵ It was then put on to a formal footing as a protection and savings fund that nurses could subscribe to, in order to counteract loss of income. The company managing it advertised the scheme as encouraging thrift, giving independence in the autumn of a nurse's life, and in the spring and summer of a career a feeling of security and contentment. It would enable a nurse to direct all her energies with pleasure to her work, free from anxiety for when her physical strength became impaired.⁶⁶

The company regularly reported recent claims, often including the nurse's initials, town, medical condition, and payment. In 1916, for example, besides accidents, operations, pleurisy, and infected fingers, seven received payments for loss of income from typhoid fever, four from diphtheria, four from measles, and two from scarlet fever.[67] Although including initials and town meant that in a small country like New Zealand with a small nursing population the nurses who had been ill could probably be identified, this does not seem to have carried with it any sense of blame. It appears to have been a way of showing prospective contributors the value of joining the scheme. As it was the professional nursing association that had established the fund and nurses themselves who contributed to it, they clearly had a sense of collective and individual responsibility for their own well-being when affected by illness. This suggests a counterpoint to others' readiness to blame nurses who sickened, or was perhaps simply a more pragmatic approach to the issue. Sickness was inevitable, wherever the fault lay, and needed to be addressed.

Another tension in dissecting a culture of blame was the mixed views even one individual could hold. This is seen most clearly in Maclean's attitudes. Despite her irritation at nurses' grumbling, she did advocate measures to protect their health. In 1913, for example, she reminded them that a dozen nurses had become ill in an Auckland typhoid fever epidemic five years earlier, with one dying. Three "valued lives" had been lost since then and many more nurses had been very seriously ill. At least a dozen were sick that year alone. She therefore drew their attention to the advised anti-typhoid inoculation.[68] Auckland Hospital made inoculation available to nurses but "no pressure" was used "to induce them" to have it. Maclean reported that a "good many nurses" had accepted.[69] This protection was also being offered to nurses in countries such as the United States, Canada, and Australia. At the Winnipeg General Hospital, a review of records for 1901–1910 had shown that on average seven cases of typhoid occurred each year, and 5 percent of these were nurses, usually probationers or juniors. A hospital nurse was eight times more likely to contract typhoid than anyone else in the community and cases were usually severe. Since inoculating nurses, no cases had occurred.[70] An Australian editor reported that at a large metropolitan hospital where patients with typhoid were continually admitted but all precautions taken, twenty-one nurses contracted typhoid in the 1904–1910 period and six died. This was a mortality rate far above the average for the disease. All nurses had been inoculated after that, and no cases had occurred.[71]

Maclean used excerpts from these reports in the journal to urge nurses to be inoculated. Her additional comment in 1913—that she hoped hospital and health authorities would afford nurses every possible facility for gaining immunity and that the Department of Health would discharge its duty—suggests she was struggling to achieve this in the department and using her editorial role to bolster her official efforts.[72] The following year, when two more nurses died from typhoid, she added the weight of opinion from "distinguished men of science" in repeating her argument, reprinting a letter by two physicians to the editor of the *British Journal of Nursing* on the question of inoculation.[73] By 1915 she had achieved partial success, as all nurses working among Maori in the rural areas of New Zealand had to be inoculated "for their own protection."[74]

Maclean's attitudes toward sick nurses could be mediated by their practice setting. Her irritation with feather-bed nurses who jeopardized their health in their extended leisure time was clear. In contrast, she clearly sympathized with those who succumbed to typhoid while working in fever camps and extolled their virtues. It was more the location of practice and nurses' willingness to cope with difficult circumstances that shaped her attitudes to those who became ill. Her position as the country's chief nurse and editor of its nursing journal would have carried considerable influence. Nurses who sickened in these difficult circumstances were not portrayed as sickening to others. Their illness was regarded as a regrettable outcome of their extraordinary and devoted service and self-sacrifice. Maclean's assistant, however, did not completely share this view. Amelia Bagley, the supervisor directly responsible for fever camp nurses' work, was clearly frustrated by so many nurses sickening with typhoid. She positioned her view as that of the "generally accepted opinion in medical and nursing circles" that proper nursing precautions would reduce danger to the nurse to a minimum.[75]

Location of practice is less evident in influencing attitudes among the nurses who became sick. They blamed themselves. They would not have done so unless they felt they had transgressed fundamental nursing principles and that others would be likely, and right, to blame them for the consequences. Nurses sickening with typhoid perhaps felt exposed as careless and inefficient. Even the trying conditions of a fever camp did not absolve them in their own eyes, but added to their faults, as by becoming ill they created additional work for their already burdened colleagues and let their patients down. One nurse was thankful to have become ill only at the end of an epidemic; she had already fulfilled her duty. The two nurses ill with scarlet fever in Dunedin in 1908 took over the night nurse's duties as soon as they were convalescent.

Nurses learned this subtext of responsibility and blame between the lines of their textbooks and lecture notes. This was illustrated by the length one nurse went to in 1911 to publicly disclaim Maclean's announcement that she had contracted typhoid from her fever camp patients. The nurse felt sufficiently concerned, even irritated, to write to *Kai Tiaki* to correct the report. "I have never had typhoid in my life," she said, "and I am happy to say that after ten weeks hard nursing I was as strong and well as when I began." She further quashed any speculation of her own nursing technique by turning the lamp toward others, commenting that "the other two nurses who were with me were both unfortunate enough to contract the disease."[76] This nurse was upset by being wrongly identified as having succumbed to fever, almost as though she felt wrongly *accused* or publicly shamed by it, regardless of Maclean's admiration and concern for those working in fever camps. There were clearly elements in the emerging professional culture of nursing that shaped their attitudes.

Chief among the cultural elements were the notions of discipline and sacrifice. Maclean's impatience with feather-bed nurses and her views of the need for stringent training to toughen nurses for the difficult work ahead reflect the values of discipline and sacrifice extending from nursing in the Victorian period. Respectable young women of good character were to be trained in strict codes of behavior and discipline of practice that ensured the smooth functioning of the hospital. Historians Alison Bashford and Susan Reverby have identified the rigid ordering of time, observation of detail, drill, discipline, hierarchy, duty, character, and service as hallmarks of nurse training that imparted idealism and sense of self-sacrifice.[77] Discipline in practice was certainly needed in observing the stringent measures to prevent cross-infection. Nurses had to realize "the necessity for absolute conformity to every rule" and that "the sternest antiseptic discipline must be enforced."[78] Personal discipline was also expected from nurses tempted by their expanded off-duty time. They were to conserve their energy for the benefit of their patients rather than squandering it in selfish frivolous pursuits before going on duty. Dedication to nursing meant a sacrifice of pleasure.

The extent to which nurses consistently embodied these ideals is another matter. Flouting the rules, however, could bring severe consequences. In 1926, for example, five probationers and a registered nurse were dismissed from Wellington Hospital for "the very disgraceful action" of returning after hours to the Nurses' Home by means of the fire escape.[79] And at least one nurse in Christchurch in 1913 ignored both fever nursing discipline and the need to sacrifice pleasure by leaving an isolation ward to attend a party, conveying scarlet fever to two other party-going nurses.[80] The willingness of nurses on wartime service and those who worked in fever camps to sacrifice their personal comfort and hospital environment, even their own safety, for the rigors of caring for patients in demanding circumstances engendered Maclean's deep admiration. When Elizabeth Ensor died from typhoid fever in the remote backblocks area of Te Araroa in 1919, Maclean described her death in terms more familiarly used for deaths on active wartime service. Nurse Ensor had "volunteered" to nurse in the epidemic and had "therefore given her life for her profession."[81] This was reminiscent of Lückes's call to probationers in 1888 that if they contracted their patient's illness and died "at their post," they would have used their "nurse's talent faithfully to the end." The highest things that were worth living for were "worth dying for too."[82] In Maclean's eyes, nurses who showed discipline and sacrifice, ideals of the new profession, in volunteering for fever camp nursing could not be blamed for any ensuing illness.

Conclusion

When hospital boards became responsible for the care of patients with infectious fevers beginning in 1903, hospital nurses and probationers in training were more exposed to the risk of illness than in previous general nursing. Nurses learned strict measures for preventing cross-infection, but some inevitably contracted their patients' diseases. Whether they were blamed for succumbing to fever depended on a complex interplay of observer, disease, and practice setting. The anatomy of blame when a nurse became ill therefore requires careful dissection.

Hospital nurses were reprimanded by Maclean, other nurses, and boards for unwarranted grumbling. The Department of Health advised boards that they could cease probationers' training and salary when they became sick, but guarded probationers from infectious patients, at least in their first year of training. On the other hand, they did not make typhoid fever inoculation or smallpox vaccination mandatory for all nurses. Physicians castigated hospital and private nurses careless enough to catch typhoid fever, a disease contracted through fecal contamination, and were clear that the fault for succumbing to scarlet fever lay at the nurse's own door. Textbooks warned that cross-infection was a disaster entirely attributable to the nurse's carelessness. The sense of impatience, disdain, and even repugnance for nurses who succumbed to fever suggests that they were "sickening" in two ways: disrupting both their own health and others' sensibilities. On the other hand, others did not blame nurses who became ill when working in a typhoid fever camp, although these nurses blamed themselves. Bagley blamed their training. Maclean greatly admired their willingness to relinquish a comfortable personal and working environment to take on the difficulties of fever camp nursing, and to volunteer again after succumbing to illness.

Within these attitudes to nurses who succumbed to patients' infectious fevers were the ideals of discipline and sacrifice, values embedded in the emerging professional culture of nursing. Nurses were inculcated with the notion of sacrifice, to put their patients' needs always before their own, and were trained to demonstrate discipline in their behavior and practice. Measures to prevent cross-infection when nursing patients with infectious diseases required extreme discipline, especially when barrier nursing depended on the nurse's visualization of an imaginary barrier and strict observance of precise rules. The sick nurse was one who could be blamed for laxity in discipline but could be absolved when the location of her practice—the fever camp—showed that she embodied the sense of sacrifice so valued within the emerging nursing culture.

PAMELA J. WOOD
Associate Professor and Director, Research Degrees
Graduate School of Nursing, Midwifery & Health
Victoria University of Wellington
New Zealand
Graduate School of Nursing, Midwifery & Health
Victoria University of Wellington
P.O. Box 600
Wellington 6140
New Zealand

Notes

1. Details written on the back of a photograph of Agnes Maud Snell, c. 1904, ABRR 7563 W4990/10f, Nursing Staff, Archives New Zealand, Wellington; details from death certificate.
2. The few studies of nurses' health tend to relate to tuberculosis, reflecting the international concern that arose particularly in the 1930s about nurses succumbing to this disease. For this historical concern, see, for example, Dominika A. Pietzcker, "The Maintenance of High Standards of Health in the Nursing Community," Section II, Session 3, *Congress Papers 1937* (London: International Council of Nurses, 1937), 56–66; Mary I. Lambie, "The Maintenance of High Standards of Health in the Nursing Community," Section II, Session 3, *Congress Papers 1937* (London: International Council of Nurses, 1937), 67–69. For New Zealand nursing, two studies have focused on tuberculosis, one covering the 1900–1950 time period and the other the 1940–1950 decade. Natali Allen and Eve Brewster, "Nurses with Tuberculosis: A Preliminary Study," *Women's Studies Journal* 5, no. 2 (December 1989): 38–60; Bronwyn Paterson, "Tuberculosis Amongst New Zealand Nurses, 1940–1950," *History of Nursing Society Journal* 3, no. 2 (1990): 46–59.

A study of nurse training at Auckland Hospital between 1913 and 1947 considered the issue of nurses' health in relation to their acceptance for training but again focused on tuberculosis and the 1930s. Deborah Dunsford, "'Too Hard a Life for a Girl': Becoming a Nurse at Auckland Hospital, 1913–1947," *Women's Studies Journal* 12, no. 1 (Autumn 1996): 27–42.

A study of Dunedin Hospital's response in another main city to the 1918 influenza epidemic did address nurses' health, noting that seventy-two nurses were admitted to the hospital in one month alone; in all, eighty-six nurses contracted the disease and four died. Judith A. Roddick, "Delirium and Fever in the Antipodes: Nursing and the 1918 Influenza Epidemic in Dunedin Hospital, New Zealand," *Journal of Research in Nursing* 11, no. 4 (2006): 363–64. Larger-scale studies of nursing beyond New Zealand have paid little attention to nurses' health. See, for example, its passing mention in Susan Reverby, *Ordered to Care: The Dilemma of American Nursing, 1850–1945* (Cambridge: Cambridge University Press, 1987), 64. A history of smallpox in Britain did note, however, that nurses' health was put at risk by doctors' occasional misdiagnosis of the disease. Margaret Currie, "Smallpox Nursing in Britain Part I: Disease, Patients, their Nurses and Places of Care," *International History of Nursing Journal* 6, no. 1 (2001): 48–54; "Part II: Nursing Care and Nurse Training," *International History of Nursing Journal* 6, no. 2 (2001): 59–65.

3. Francis S. Maclean, *Challenge for Health: A History of Public Health in New Zealand* (Wellington, NZ: Government Printer, 1964), 232.

4. William Irving, "Small-Pox and Vaccination," *Kai Tiaki* (October 1909): 139 (hereafter cited as *KT*). As volumes and issues for this journal were sometimes numbered incorrectly, the month and year are used in this article to designate issue and volume.

5. Figures adapted from Maclean, *Challenge for Health,* 223, 232, 281, 336.

6. See, for example, "Isolation Hospitals and Scarlet Fever" [letter to the editor], *Lancet* (1901): 316; "Scarlet Fever Mortality and Hospital Isolation," *Lancet* (1906): 1528–29; "Scarlet Fever Mortality and Hospital Isolation" [letter to the editor], *Lancet* (1907): 117; "Isolation Hospitals and Scarlet Fever" [letter to the editor], *Lancet* (1908): 967; "The Control of Scarlet Fever and Hospitals for Infectious Diseases" [letter to the editor], *Lancet* (1910): 953.

7. Margaret Currie, *Fever Hospitals and Fever Nurses. A British Social History of Fever Nursing: A National Service* (London: Routledge, 2005).

8. See for example "Infectious Diseases Hospital," *Otago Witness,* 14 August 1907, 17; "Charitable Aid Board," *Otago Witness,* 18 December 1907, 14.

9. "Hospital Board," *Otago Witness,* 4 March 1908, 18; John Angus, *A History of the Otago Hospital Board and its Predecessors* (Dunedin, NZ: Otago Hospital Board, 1984), 109.

10. Currie, *Fever Hospitals and Fever Nurses.*

11. "Register of Nurses," *New Zealand Gazette* (Wellington, NZ: Government Printer, 1910), 1: 403–28.

12. "Register of Nurses," *New Zealand Gazette* (Wellington, NZ: Government Printer, 1923), 1: 397–506. Although approximately 3,400 nurses were on the register at this time, some were no longer in active practice and some were living overseas.

13. "Training in Various Institutions," *KT* (July 1910): 94.

14. See, for example, "The Cubicle System in Infectious Hospitals," *British Journal of Nursing* 34, no. 893 (1905): 379 (hereafter cited as *BJN*); "Study of Scarlet Fever: Epidemiology and Prophylaxis," *Lancet* (1926): 617–18.

15. F. Graham Crookshank, "An Address on the Control of Scarlet Fever," *Lancet* (1910): 479, 480. See also "Professional Review. Practical Nursing," *BJN* 53, no. 1374 (1914): 105–6.

16. "The Barrier," *BJN* 52, no. 1360 (1914): 361.

17. James K. Watson, *A Handbook for Nurses* (London: Scientific Press, 1912), 293–94.

18. "Fever Nurses' Association. Examination for Certificate of Fever Training, October, 1919," *BJN* 63, no. 1652 (1919): 336; "Our Prize Competition," *BJN* 63, no. 1652 (1919): 337.

19. "Our Prize Competition," *BJN* 63, no. 1655 (1919): 376–77. For a similar topic for a later essay competition, see "Our Prize Competition," *BJN* 77, no. 1926 (1929): 5.

20. "College of Nursing, Ltd. Birmingham Three Counties Centre," *BJN* 67, no. 1740 (1921): 88–89.

21. Anne L. McDonald and Cicely Tulloch, *Wellington Hospital: Educating Nurses for More Than a Century 1883–1991* (Wellington, NZ: Wellington Hospital Nurses' Reunion Committee, c.1992), 10.

22. "State Examination of Nurses," *KT* (April 1910): 62–63. Dr. Alec Knyvett Gordon in Manchester preferred nurses to use a douche can with a separately boiled nozzle for each patient. See Alec Knyvett Gordon, "Some Aspects of the Nursing of Infectious Disease," *BJN* 31, no. 796 (1903): 5–6; Alec Knyvett Gordon, "Asepsis and Fever Nursing," *BJN* 52, no. 1362 (1914): 407–8.

23. "State Examination of Nurses," *KT* (October 1921): 172–73.

24. Alison Bashford, *Purity and Pollution: Gender, Embodiment and Victoria Medicine* (Houndsmills, UK: Macmillan, 2000), 137.

25. C. Burnie, "Infectious Diseases," *Australasian Nurses' Journal* 20, no. 9 (1922): 344 (hereafter cited as *ANJ*).

26. "Scarlet Fever," *KT* (April 1922): 62.

27. "State Examination of Nurses," *KT* (October 1913): 169.

28. "Nursing Precautions in Typhoid," *KT* (July 1916): 161.

29. "Department of Public Health, Hospitals and Charitable Aid Annual Report," *Appendices to the Journals of the House of Representatives* (Wellington, NZ: Government Printer, 1913): H-31, 13; Hester Maclean, *Nursing in New Zealand: History and Reminiscences* (Wellington, NZ: Tolan, 1932), 116–17.

30. "Smallpox Outbreak," *KT* (July 1913): 123; "The Smallpox Epidemic," *KT* (October 1913): 150. Between May 1913 and April 1914, an estimated 1,978 Maori and 116 settlers contracted smallpox, with probably 55 Maori dying. Maclean, *Challenge for Health*, 232.

31. "The Smallpox Campaign," *KT* (April 1914): 82–86.

32. See, for example, "Prevention Is Better than Cure," *KT* (April 1920): 70–72.

33. "Typhoid Nursing Among the Natives," *KT* (July 1911): 125.

34. "Some Camp Hospital Experiences," *KT* (October 1913): 146.

35. "Notes from District Nurses in the Back Blocks," *KT* (January 1918): 31–32.

36. "Obituary," *KT* (January 1911): 37–38.

37. "Obituary," *KT* (January 1917): 65; "Late Obituary Notice," *KT* (October 1919): 198.

38. "More Camp Hospital Experiences," *KT* (October 1913): 153.

39. "Obituary," *KT* (April 1908): 52.
40. "Deaths," *KT* (April 1909): 67.
41. Angus, *A History of the Otago Hospital Board,* 109.
42. Otago Hospital and Charitable Aid Board Miscellaneous Patients Register, DAHI D284 454, Dunedin Branch, Archives New Zealand.
43. See, for example, "The Nursing of Infectious Diseases" [book review], *KT* (October 1923): 175.
44. See, for example, Grace H. G. Dundas, *Text-Book for Fever Nurses* (Edinburgh: William Bryce, 1923).
45. See, for example, Francis J. Woollacott, *Lectures upon the Nursing of Infectious Diseases,* 3rd ed., ed. Dorothy C. Hare (London: Scientific Press, 1923), 24–26; Evelyn C. Pearce, *Fevers and Fever Nursing* (London: Faber & Faber, 1932), 51.
46. Woollacott, *Nursing of Infectious Diseases,* 24.
47. Edith Sandford, "Infectious Diseases," *Cassell's Science and Art of Nursing: A Guide to the Various Branches of Nursing, Theoretical and Practical,* vol. 3 (London: Waverley, n.d.), 91–118.
48. William T. Gordon Pugh, *Practical Nursing, Including Hygiene and Dietetics* (Edinburgh: William Blackwood, 1937).
49. Anna C. Maxwell and Amy E. Pope, *Practical Nursing: A Text-Book for Nurses* (New York and London: Putnam's, 1914), 669.
50. Pearce, *Fevers and Fever Nursing,* 42.
51. Eva C. E. Lückes, *Lectures on General Nursing,* 3rd ed. (London: Kegan Paul, Trench, 1888), 209–11.
52. "Enteric Fever Amongst Nurses," *ANJ* 10, no. 1 (1912): 6.
53. Alec Knyvett Gordon, "The Methods of Infection in Enteric Fever," *BJN* 40, no. 1031 (January 1908): 3–5. Cited excerpt reprinted in *KT* (April 1908): 53. Maclean notes that the entire *BJN* article was reprinted in *ANJ*.
54. "Untitled," *KT* (April 1908): 52–53.
55. "Scarlet Fever," *KT* (April 1917): 102. The writer is unidentified but the content and style indicate it was written by a physician. Descriptions of nursing fever patients on verandas in the sunshine are consistent with a New Zealand setting. Moreover, Maclean did not acknowledge this as an article reprinted from an overseas journal, which was her consistent practice.
56. See, for example, "The Eight Hour System," *KT* (January 1912): 31–33.
57. "Hospital Troubles" [editorial], *KT* (January 1911): 1–2.
58. "The Comfort of Our Nurses" [editorial], *KT* (October 1918): 169–70.
59. "The Nursing Profession," *KT* (April 1912): 18.
60. "Specialisation" [editorial], *KT* (July 1917): 128. Australian nurses in their first year at Sydney Hospital were also prohibited from attending patients with typhoid fever. "Enteric Fever Amongst Nurses," 6–7.
61. "Another Phase of the Badly-Used Probationer," *KT* (April 1921): 95.
62. "Minutes of Proceedings of Conference of Delegates of Hospital and Charitable Aid Boards, Held at Parliament Buildings, Wellington," *Appendices to the Journals of the House of Representatives* (Wellington, NZ: Government Printer, 1911): H-31, 197.
63. "The Eight Hour System," *KT* (October 1911): 155.
64. "Payment of Nurses and Probationers During Sick Leave," *KT* (October 1918): 204.

65. "New Zealand Trained Nurses Association—Wellington," *KT* (January 1911): 4. A "bawbee" was a Scottish term for a low-value coin.

66. "Nurses' Protection Against Accident and Sickness Fund" [advertisement], *KT* (January 1914): v.

67. "The Nurses' Protection and Savings Bank Fund," *KT* (January 1916): 51.

68. "Autotyphoid Inoculation Amongst Nurses," *KT* (July 1913): 126. See also "Sanitation and Typhoid Vaccine," *KT* (January 1914): 49.

69. "Vaccination Therapy in Typhoid Fever," *KT* (April 1911): 60.

70. "Anti-Typhoid Vaccination in the Winnipeg General Hospital," *ANJ* 11, no. 6 (June 1912): 194–95. This article was reprinted from the *Canadian Nurse.*

71. "Anti-Typhoid Vaccination for Hospital Nurses" [editorial], *ANJ* 11, no. 6 (June 1913): 181–82.

72. "Autotyphoid Inoculation Amongst Nurses," *KT* (July 1913): 126.

73. "Anti-Typhoid Inoculation," *KT* (October 1914): 181.

74. "Native District Nursing," *KT* (October 1915): 199.

75. "Nursing Precautions in Typhoid Fever," *KT* (July 1916): 161.

76. A. Raleigh, "Letter to the editor," *KT* (July 1911): 117.

77. Bashford, *Purity and Pollution,* 44–54; Reverby, *Ordered to Care,* 51–52, 57–58.

78. Douglas H. Scott and Mildred Hainsworth, "Infectious Diseases—A General Survey," *Modern Practical Nursing,* vol. 4 (London: Caxton, 1936), 18, 19.

79. "Discipline" [editorial], *KT* (January 1926): 1.

80. Mary I. Lambie, *My Story: Memoirs of a New Zealand Nurse* (Christchurch, NZ: N. M. Peryer, 1956), 10.

81. "Late Obituary Notices," *KT* (October 1919): 198.

82. Lückes, *Lectures on General Nursing,* 212.

Nurses Without Borders: The History of Nursing as U.S. International History

Julia F. Irwin
University of South Florida

Abstract. During World War I and its aftermath, thousands of U.S. nurses put their domestic careers on hold to work overseas. Many volunteered in the wake of war and disaster. Others worked as instructors in nursing schools and as the staff of fledgling public health agencies. This article charts the international travels of four especially mobile nurses, whose globetrotting careers took them to Europe, Asia, and the Caribbean. These women aspired to tackle world health issues, motivated by the conviction that the spread of U.S. professional nursing ideas stood to modernize the world. This article tells these nurses' stories and analyzes their ideologies of development and progress. In so doing, it demonstrates that professional women, working outside state channels, played a principal role in expanding U.S. influence in the world. Moreover, it makes the case for the centrality of nursing history to the history of U.S. foreign relations.

The past several years have been an exhilarating time for historians interested in the role of the United States in the twentieth-century world. In innumerable articles, panels, conferences, and monographs, historians of U.S. foreign relations have documented the spread of political, economic, and cultural influence to all parts of the globe.[1] The histories of nursing, medicine, and health have had much to contribute to this field of inquiry. Working in these areas, scholars have shown how the U.S. government embraced medical interventions and sanitation campaigns to complement political and diplomatic strategies.[2] They have analyzed the role of private institutions, such as the Rockefeller and Ford Foundations, in the spread and consolidation of American biomedical influence and ideas.[3] They have called attention to the role of biological, hygienic, and eugenic theories and practices in informing American understandings of other people and cultures and in shaping U.S. international relationships.[4] And a rising generation of scholars, incorporating transnational methodologies and pursuing research in multiple national archives, have begun to examine how populations on the receiving end of these medical interventions alternately received, resisted, and reinterpreted U.S. biomedical ideas.[5]

These newest histories of U.S. medical internationalism have tended to focus on the interactions between the United States and one nation or one region. Admittedly, a more limited geographical concentration is probably necessary. Otherwise, it would be difficult to attain a sufficiently thorough and intimate level of knowledge about a place, a prerequisite to understanding the complex and multifaceted interactions between U.S. reformers, state and local governments, private agencies, and the individuals whose bodies and mentalities these interveners hoped to influence. Scholars in history of medicine and health will benefit greatly from additional studies of medical internationalism from this vertical perspective, for these approaches show how American overseas medical and health interventions played out on the ground. Multi-archival, multilanguage local studies identify discrepancies between assumption and practice and consider how the targets of American reform experienced and reacted to efforts to change their social environments and individual behavior. These approaches bring voices to those outside the dominant power structure, adding nuance to our understanding of U.S. internationalism.

This article acknowledges the importance and intellectual excitement of this new turn in the field. But rather than considering the reformer/reformed, colonizer/colonized, United States/Them relationship, it takes a consciously lateral perspective: this is a study of U.S. nurses who worked across continents. Warwick Anderson has argued that alongside studies of on-the-ground relationships between Americans and others, we must also consider "the global circulation . . . of metaphor, assumption, and practice."[6] Even as we undertake detailed local studies, we must also chart the movement of ideas, personnel, and institutions across countries and continents. In short, we must look at medical internationalism on a horizontal as well as a vertical plane.[7]

Studying international history from a horizontal perspective makes the complex motivations and ideologies of U.S. international reformers far easier to recognize and analyze. Such an approach calls attention to material and intellectual similarities and patterns across time and space. Comparisons of contemporaneous U.S. health and medical interventions in Europe, the Caribbean, and Asia demonstrate that activities in diverse locales among diverse populations were not isolated or unconnected events, but formed part of a common process. Medical ideas and practices in U.S. territories such as Puerto Rico and the Philippines influenced medical interventions in Europe, Central Asia, South America, and other parts of the globe, and vice versa.[8] Ideas learned and practiced in the United States flowed out in multiple directions, and local actors transformed them according to their own agendas. These modified values and institutions then returned to the United States to influence domestic medical and health practices.

Recognizing these intellectual and material border crossings can provide evidence of a globalizing United States, paint a broader picture of "the Americanization of the world" in action, and help clarify the manner in which the United States consolidated its influence as it became a twentieth-century world power. While it is easy to point out the value of studying global connections, actually putting this approach into practice has proved a daunting task for historians in U.S. international history and foreign relations. As Isabel Hofmeyr noted in a 2006 *American Historical Review* roundtable, tracing "the movement of objects, people, ideas, and texts" provides a "key methodological challenge in any practice of transnational history."[9]

The history of nursing is in many ways ideally suited to confront this logistical problem. The archives, sources, and figures that are central to the field provide a ready means to trace the spread of U.S. global influence in the early twentieth century. The discipline should not be relegated to the peripheries of U.S. international history, therefore, but must be made central in any historical consideration of the United States in the world.

The History of Nursing as U.S. International History

To demonstrate how the history of nursing can inform the study of both U.S. international history and the broader history of medicine, this essay traces the careers of four nurses during World War I and the following decade. Pansy V. Besom, Helen L. Bridge, Kathleen D'Olier, and Alice L. Fitzgerald were among nearly 20,000 nurses from the United States who volunteered for overseas service with the American Red Cross (ARC) in World War I and the 1920s. These women graduated from U.S. hospital training schools during the first decade of the twentieth century and went to work as nurses in U.S. urban centers. As products of relatively new fixtures in U.S. nursing education, they were socialized as part of a generation of nurses committed to increasing professional and educational standards.[10] In their training and careers in Progressive Era United States, they developed a shared commitment to a distinctly U.S. vision of nursing and its complementary relationship to modern public health, a field characterized by its roots in the German bacteriological tradition but marked by emphasis on professional nursing, public health education, and preventive medicine. They believed that the expansion of professional nursing could improve hospital care and community health services, and, by extension, better the health of all individuals.[11]

This was no mere domestic goal. These nurses were committed to creating new professional and educational opportunities for women throughout the world. They believed that trained female nurses, physicians, teachers, and social workers, in cooperation with an educated, empowered female citizenry, held the power to lead their countries toward greater development and prosperity. Educated and independent women would fight to improve the health and welfare of their fellow citizens, uplifting their nations—and themselves—in the process. During and after the Great War, U.S. nurses worked to achieve this goal. Through the auspices of the ARC and other private and state agencies, they brought their ideas and institutions to Europe, the Caribbean, and Asia through nursing schools and public health campaigns.[12] As these women traversed national, continental, and cultural borders, they helped make U.S. nursing a global enterprise. At the same time—whether they knew it or not—they forged networks and relationships that undergirded the formation and consolidation of U.S. world power.[13]

Nurses' ability to cross geopolitical and professional borders depended on the simultaneous destabilization of another boundary: gender. In the United States, suffrage, changing social mores, and new career paths allowed many women to ignore and even erase barriers that had traditionally limited their opportunities. Working abroad, often without local male oversight, this generation of nurses and other female professionals found occasion to develop their careers and lead social reform initiatives. They blurred traditional boundaries to negotiate a new role for the United States in the world.[14]

These ARC nurses carried their experiences and assumptions about health, race, and civilization with them. Their ideas about sanitation and hygiene, learned in U.S. hospitals and university classrooms and practiced in U.S. urban centers, transferred readily (though not wholly intact) to the slums of Paris and Naples, villages and hamlets in Russia and Eastern Europe, and Asian capitals from Bangkok to Manila. The establishment of nursing schools and public health campaigns in these locales created material continuities in American medical interventions that transcended time and place.[15] If their methods were similar, so was the missionary ideology that underpinned them. Besom, Bridge, D'Olier, and Fitzgerald shared a modernizing impulse that ordered the world's people according to a hierarchy of levels of development and progress. Their worldview defined certain populations as easy and willing to reform and others as more difficult. Nevertheless, they believed that all populations could be improved if the United States took the lead in educational and environmental interventions.[16]

The faith that U.S. nursing, biomedicine, and culture stood to improve the world led nurses to try to implant their own values and norms among the populations with whom they worked. It would be a gross oversimplification, however, to cast these women as mere imperialists in progressive clothing. By improving public health and sanitation and creating opportunities for non-American women to pursue nursing education, they aspired to uplift and modernize the world. They acted under the conviction that improving social health and welfare was both a prerequisite to orderly, democratic society and a social justice issue. They believed, moreover, that the United States had a responsibility to exercise its growing political and economic clout in a manner that improved global health and well-being. If the spread of their ideas about public health, hygienic behavior, professional nursing, and preventive medicine was mission work for the modern age, these Progressive Era nurses saw themselves as nothing less than the couriers of the new gospels.[17]

The international careers of these women call attention to the informal global networks that gave form to U.S. internationalism in the 1920s.[18] In the wake of the war, the lines that had once organized diplomatic and economic power were in a state of flux. At the Paris Peace Conference, U.S. and Allied policymakers remapped Europe to create new borders and nation-states and debated the political future of European and U.S. colonial holdings. The boundaries that delineated power in the Old World began to dissolve, replaced by U.S. claims to world leadership.[19] In this chaos, the intercontinental spread of American nursing and medical ideas provided overarching unity to overseas engagements and justified the global expansion of U.S. power and influence as a benevolent, modernizing process.[20] U.S. nurses put forward a new vision for the role for the United States in the world, one that defined humanitarian engagement and assistance as the proper way to exercise influence beyond its borders. Ironically, their voluntary humanitarian interventions helped create a foundation for harder forms of American political and economic power in the decades to come.[21]

From Progressive Era United States to Wartime Western Europe and Russia

The date 6 April 1917 marked a radical break in U.S. diplomatic history. On that day, the United States entered the First World War as an associated power, negating Woodrow Wilson's promise to preserve neutrality and ending the country's longstanding refusal to intervene in European military affairs.

In the ensuing months, the nation struggled to mobilize a corps of citizen-soldiers.[22] Already in place was a mechanism to mobilize the army of nurses that would be required to care for wounded soldiers and allied civilians. The ARC had charged Clara D. Noyes, a graduate of the prestigious Johns Hopkins University nursing school and superintendent of the equally esteemed Bellevue Training School for Nurses, with recruiting and assigning the nearly 20,000 nurses and thousands of nurses' aides who served overseas on behalf of European civilians and the U.S. military.[23]

Overseas service allowed women from the United States the opportunity to advance their careers and act on their professional ambitions. At the same time, their interventions served the Wilson administration's propaganda needs by projecting an image of the United States as a benevolent and powerful nation that was prepared to revitalize the world by virtue of its generosity and the supremacy of its medical knowledge. One nurse whose work demonstrated these dual objectives was Alice L. Fitzgerald, who in December 1917 joined the ARC nursing service in France. A 1906 graduate of the Johns Hopkins University school, Fitzgerald had worked as a nurse at that institution, Bellevue, and Ellis Island. She enjoyed a successful career in the United States before the outbreak of war. Her work with wounded U.S. soldiers and French refugees fulfilled civic obligations then expected of professional women.[24]

Fitzgerald and the thousands of ARC nurses who served alongside her complemented U.S. military intervention by demonstrating U.S. alliance, improving sanitary conditions, and uplifting morale. Many nurses cared for U.S. forces, but their relief efforts for civilians were a particularly important part of the equation. U.S. nurses in France, Italy, and other Allied countries catered to the health needs of refugees and families of allied soldiers. They served as visiting health workers, built and ran tuberculosis dispensaries, established fresh air camps for children, and ran courses for local women on sanitation, hygiene, and nursing. Going beyond military assistance, ARC nurses carried multiple U.S. ideas about health, hygiene, and social reform out of the urban centers and rural hinterlands of Progressive Era United States and into the European war zone, packaged as U.S. humanitarian assistance.[25]

With peace came expanded possibilities. While most of her colleagues returned to the United States after the 11 November 1918 Armistice, Fitzgerald remained in Europe to pursue professional opportunities. In May 1919, the ARC appointed her chief nurse of its Commission to Europe. That November, she became director of the Nursing Service for the League of Red Cross Societies in Geneva, a coalition established to coordinate peacetime humanitarian and health interventions. During her tenure, Fitzgerald crossed the continent to organize schools of nursing and public health in Poland, Czechoslovakia, and Italy, and nurses' aide courses for women in Albania, Greece, Bulgaria, Romania, and Serbia. Staffed largely by U.S. nurses and physicians, these activities introduced U.S. ideas about health and hygiene and sought to create a generation of European women committed to those precepts.[26]

As Fitzgerald's wide field of work demonstrates, the twin processes of political and hygienic expansion extended far beyond the French and Italian war zones to Central and Eastern Europe. Russia was also a site for U.S. medical and military interventions. The 1917 Bolshevik Revolution came as a shock to many observers and prompted Allied governments to intervene on the side of Russia's anti-Bolshevik coalition forces. In August 1918, Wilson sent 10,000 troops to the port city of Vladivostok, in far eastern Siberia, to assist British, French, and Czech forces there. Preceding their arrival by several weeks was a contingent of physicians, nurses, and other volunteers representing the ARC Commission to Siberia. During the next year and a half, more than 200 U.S. nurses traveled to Vladivostok and cities along the 4,100-mile Trans-Siberian Railroad. As they had during the war, these women set up hospitals and dispensaries and waged campaigns against tuberculosis, typhus, and other infectious diseases. Their work offered a means to shore up civilian support for U.S. interests and modernize the medical landscape of Russia.

One of these nurses was Helen Bridge. A 1908 graduate of the Miami Valley Hospital School of Nursing in Dayton, Ohio, Bridge had worked as a nurse and an instructor of nursing in Ohio and Indiana and joined the ARC reserve corps in 1911. In May 1919, Clara Noyes, now chair of the ARC Nursing Service, assigned her to Vladivostok to work in a local ARC hospital. Bridge was soon organizing courses for Russian nurses' aides, and teaching basic professional skills and courses in home hygiene and care of the sick. By spring 1920, she had organized fourteen courses and enrolled more than 200 Russian women. As in Western Europe, ARC nurses took advantage of wartime upheaval to spread ideas about professional nursing and develop allegiance to U.S. models and principles of public health and sanitation.[27]

The successful, albeit limited, incorporation of U.S.-style nursing in Siberia stood to improve patient care and increase the number of skilled workers in the country, but more important, it promised to accelerate Russian moral and mental progress. U.S. guidance was key to this process. Russians had "lived in a state of war for such a long time they are stunned and have no initiative," explained one of Bridge's colleagues, "but can work and will do so readily if someone organizes and plans for them."[28] U.S. nurses saw an obligation to uplift their Russian sisters, both to increase their opportunities and to impart moral order in Russian society. "Our work has been infinitely worthwhile," Bridge reported, "not only because the standard of nursing care given the patients in our hospitals has been raised but because it has given us a hold on some of the Russian girls."²⁹ Bridge identified her students as "girls." By embracing professional, modern nursing, Russian girls could become Russian women, self-sufficient, disciplined, and ready to embrace modern conceptions of health and fitness.

A sense of racial and cultural hierarchy pervaded this maternal concern, codifying nursing education in the language of a missionary endeavor. Bridge saw Russian women as children who were eager to learn yet lagging in social and intellectual development. Winning their support for U.S. medical and cultural values required educators to act with compassion, not simply to force their values. "In order to work with them it is quite necessary for them to feel that you hold a deep personal interest in them," Bridge explained. "The girls are affectionate, sympathetic and sensitive and require a great deal of tact and soft handling." In spite of her optimism, teaching Russian women often tested Bridge's patience. After teaching there, Bridge concluded that she was prepared "to teach a group of Hottentots . . . without so much as the quiver of an eyelash."³⁰ In consigning Siberian peasants and indigenous South Africans to the same imperial imaginary, Bridge likened Russian nursing education to mission work in contemporary colonial sites. According to this logic, Russian peasants could advance and develop, but only with professional, sympathetic oversight. Women from the United States declared it their duty to guide Russians on this path to progress.

From Relieving Wartime Allies to Rebuilding Postwar Central and Eastern Europe

World War I and the Russian Civil War had provided an opportune moment for nurses to intervene in European society and extend their professional ambitions across the Atlantic. After military forces had withdrawn, however, nurses continued to influence European structures of medicine and health. More than four years of war had left European society in disarray. U.S. citizens stepped in to tackle immediate material needs and rebuild crumbled structures of civil society, motivated jointly by a sense of compassion and a fear that continued social upheaval would breed political unrest and Bolshevism. Most notably, Congress appropriated $1 million to Herbert Hoover's American Relief Administration for food shipments to Central and Eastern European nations after the war. The ARC complemented Hoover's efforts with child health centers, dispensaries, and nursing schools. The institutions and approaches employed to improve the public's health in Progressive Era U.S. towns and cities had structured wartime civilian assistance. In the war's wake, U.S. nurses again transplanted this public health infrastructure in an effort to rebuild and reorder postwar society.[31]

In the 1920s, the ARC turned to the project of creating graduate nursing schools in Eastern Europe. Echoing recent U.S. debates between working nurses and advocates of higher professional standards, the elevation of graduate nursing in Europe extended the U.S. fight to raise standards overseas.[32] This project sounded valuable to Helen Bridge. After teaching for sixth months in Vladivostok, Bridge had joined the ARC "Great White Train," a mobile typhus disinfection unit that carried nurses and physicians to towns and cities along the Trans-Siberian Railroad. Her labors were cut short in May 1920, however, when Bolshevik military advances compelled the ARC to evacuate. Not ready to return home, Bridge accepted an assignment to Warsaw to cooperate with local officials in organizing "a modern school of nursing." In May 1921, the Warsaw School of Nursing opened with Bridge as its director.[33]

The Warsaw School mirrored contemporary U.S. professional nurse training programs to foster "a more rational system of caring" in Poland. Potential candidates had to be at least eighteen years old and have completed two years of high school. The school itself included four classrooms equipped "for complete and scientific instruction." Graduate nurses from accredited U.S. training schools, local physicians, and University of Warsaw faculty gave lectures and mentored students. The complete course took two years and required 559 hours of theoretical instruction and practical work in a Warsaw hospital.[34] These efforts to rationalize Polish nursing brought the fight for professionalization to Eastern Europe. Bridge said of her students, "I feel sure that the standards of the profession in Poland will be safe with them, if we can educate them wisely."[35] Sister schools in Krakow, Prague, and Bajina Bašta, Serbia, aspired to similar ends.

Like the schools in the United States on which they were modeled, the schools imposed strict moral and physical standards, considering them essential if Eastern European civilians were to accept professional nursing as a legitimate endeavor for women. Students had to "be of average height and weight and free from organic defects." They had to be Christian and present three certificates of good character, including from their school principal and church pastor.[36] Bridge believed it was "necessary to chaperone our students very carefully." Since "practically every hospital nurse is the mistress of some physician, one feels that they have need of the eyes of an eagle and the wisdom of a serpent."[37] Increasing the respectability of professional nursing demanded maternal oversight and strict control of professional and personal standards, which U.S. nurses assumed as a central part of their efforts.[38]

The class and ethnic assumptions that pervaded Bridge's assessments of her students suggested her reluctance to consider them her equals. Nevertheless, she remained optimistic that Polish and U.S. nurses would one day become peers if they had access to education and proper guidance. "In spite of the fact that nurses have always been held to be women of low moral standards," Bridge argued, they would "be able to do much to change these conditions . . . if we can educate them wisely." With U.S. guidance, Eastern European women would ultimately attain the cultural power and autonomy required to lead their nations to progressive modernity. "What they make of themselves and of their countries," Noyes agreed, "will depend far more than the world can realize upon the help we shall give them to help themselves." With U.S. assistance and the transformative power of education, women could be the driving force in leading Europe to a new and better place.[39]

U.S. nurses remembered their recent efforts to win legitimacy for professional nursing as a period of selfless struggle. They not only expected Polish women to emulate their curricular and moral standards, but also demanded that they be ready to give themselves fully to the cause of professional nursing. "All the sacrifice and devotion should not be on one side," Noyes contended. "As many American women in our pioneer stage gave freely of their time and strength toward the development of nurse education, so the women of Poland may also be obliged to give."[40] But excessive guidance had its limits. U.S. "pioneers" had blazed a path for Polish women to follow, but only through autonomous leadership and local struggle would professional nursing prevail.

While Bridge and her colleagues worked to develop the nursing profession in Central and Eastern Europe, other nurses from the United States focused on child and maternal health. These were major public health issues in early twentieth-century United States. Influenced by principles of positive eugenics and a commitment to preventive medicine, health professionals urged active intervention in the health of young populations to increase the fitness of future U.S. citizens. Better breeding and decreased disease and mortality promised stronger, more industrious populations prepared for the rigors and responsibilities of democratic citizenship.[41]

The ARC extended this logic to Poland, Czechoslovakia, and the Balkan States in the years following the Armistice. Working through the ARC and with European state and private agencies, U.S. medical, nursing, and welfare professionals enacted a widespread child health campaign and built nearly 500 child health stations in the region. These centers provided free clinical care to children from birth to age fourteen. They also offered prenatal and postnatal exams for mothers and courses for local women in nutrition, childhood diseases, and proper feeding and care of children—the tenets of "scientific motherhood."[42] By aiding children, teaching their mothers, and creating a more permanent health infrastructure, U.S. nurses hoped to make a lasting impression on health on the continent.[43]

Kathleen D'Olier and Pansy Besom were two of the dozens of nurses who engaged in this child health work. From 1919 to the end of 1920, D'Olier, a public health nurse and graduate of Rochester General Hospital, volunteered for the ARC in Athens, Greece, to develop the child welfare program for that city. Pansy Besom, a 1905 graduate of the Delaware Hospital School of Nursing, had built her career as a public health nurse in Stamford, Connecticut, and as a child welfare nurse in Boston. Besom worked in both Poland and Czechoslovakia as an operating room nurse, dispensary nurse, and instructor in nursing courses at an ARC school. She quickly rose through the ranks to become director of the ARC Nursing Service in Czechoslovakia. In this capacity she oversaw the construction and administration of child health centers in the region, an endeavor she found difficult but professionally and personally satisfying: "It seems no time since we started this work and while I have at times been very home sick and tired of it all, it has been very interesting and I believe worth while."[44]

Although this work aimed to improve the wellbeing of individual children, it was part of a much larger mission to know the state of health in Eastern Europe. Armed with extensive data and statistics on population health, the ARC claimed the authority to control and reorganize the structures of civil society. Ultimately, the goal was that "every child will be under the eye of the health authorities; every child, be it sick or well or in good social surroundings or bad will be examined by a physician."[45] In Czechoslovakia, for example, Besom and her staff gathered four-page medical and social histories of 47,500 children in an attempt to create a complete medical and social record for each child in the country.[46] Throughout Eastern Europe, nurses and social workers surveyed the state of regional charities, hospitals, and related social institutions and set in motion efforts to bring them up to their own professional standards.

The health centers and other aspects of the child health program thus served multiple functions. Basic health care, physical examinations, and health classes produced knowledge about the needs and physical conditions of local populations while diffusing U.S. ideals and methods of hygiene and social work. Reconstructing Europe was not just an effort to rebuild ruined buildings and feed rumbling stomachs. It was a chance to reinvent the bodies and minds of Europe's newest democratic citizens in accordance with contemporary U.S. principles of public health.[47] In many ways, postwar nursing schools and child health centers, like their wartime predecessors, were scientific missionary endeavors, sites to reconstruct and modernize European bodies and mentalities. U.S. nurses worried about the toll of war on physical and political health and believed they could remedy both concerns by winning European allegiance to biomedical and hygienic practices.

Although it is easy to discuss this growing global influence of U.S. ideas in the decades following World War I in the abstract, it is important to recognize the role individual U.S. citizens played in this transition. Besom, Bridge, D'Olier, and Fitzgerald provided clear material and ideological continuities in wartime and postwar relief efforts and linked progressive international interventions across time and space.

From Postwar Eastern Europe to the 1920s American Empire

Nurses certainly hoped to leave a legacy for their work, yet most did not intend to remain overseas permanently. As conditions in Europe stabilized and local personnel took up the work, justification for extensive intervention waned. In June 1922, with the health centers up and running, U.S. personnel ceded direction of them to local agencies and ministries of health. Helen Bridge remained director of the Warsaw Training School until 1928, but this length of stay was rare; most ARC volunteers returned to their careers in the United States at this juncture. At first glance, the move out of Europe confirms the traditional characterization of the 1920s as a decade in which the United States retreated from both the international community and Progressive Era social commitments. Some, however, considered new ways to direct their professional and reforming ambitions abroad.

Nurses had implemented educational and health reforms throughout Europe and Siberia. In the 1920s, the global circulation of medical ideas and practices bridged sites of formal and informal U.S. empire. As their colleagues headed back to the United States, some nurses looked farther afield, eager to apply the methods they had learned and practiced in Europe to the Philippines, Puerto Rico, Thailand, China, and other sites of strategic economic and political interest to the United States.[48] Nurses found further opportunities to develop their careers abroad; in the process, they transplanted their knowledge and experiences to new sites. The scientific missionary impulse, already evident with Russians and Eastern Europeans, grew more strident as nurses interacted with populations they deemed even less developed.

Perhaps because of their own transnational experiences, nurses believed that the effort to improve public health was not to be limited by national borders; it demanded a global approach. In 1921, after a two-year term as director of the League of Red Cross Societies Nursing Service, Alice Fitzgerald resigned to work for the Rockefeller Foundation International Health Board in the Philippines. Fitzgerald's work among immigrants to the United States and among Europeans taught her that people and pathogens crossed borders readily. Efforts to improve the health of Filipinos and other potential U.S. immigrants, therefore, "should begin on the other side."[49] Although Fitzgerald left the ARC to pursue new international health work, some of her colleagues did so from within the organization. In 1921, Kathleen D'Olier transferred to Puerto Rico to implement a child health program under the auspices of the local ARC chapter. And in late 1923 Pansy Besom traveled to Manila to become director of nursing for the ARC Philippines chapter. In far-flung territories and provinces, these nurses worked to extend their professional and social commitments to the world.[50]

Besom, D'Olier, and Fitzgerald transported the methods and philosophies of child welfare nursing they had learned in Progressive Era United States and put into practice in Great War–era Europe to their posts in the outlying regions of the American empire. As a surveyor of sanitary conditions and an advisor to the U.S. governor-general in the Philippines, Fitzgerald lobbied for sanitary reforms and improved standards for nursing education in the archipelago. Besom, D'Olier, and their staffs organized prenatal and child health clinics, treating thousands of patients per month. They offered physical examinations and health care for babies and young children and gave demonstrations and classes for mothers on care and feeding. They appointed visiting nurses to distribute publicity, establish health clinics and community gardens, and inspect homes and schools. And they staffed mobile clinics to bring dental and health services throughout the islands. "A carefully thought-out program is under way for the improvement of community life," Besom explained, "a program of sanitation and public health in the backward provinces."[51]

The concern with uplifting "backward" populations had provided conceptual unity to health reform efforts, whether in the United States, Western Europe, Eastern Europe, or Siberia. It took on even greater importance in the postwar American empire. In the 1920s, heated debates raged in the United States and its territories regarding the political status of indigenous residents of U.S. colonial holdings. Some members of the U.S. civic body argued that those populations lacked the capacity for self-governance and required continued political oversight and tutelage. Others maintained that these civilians had a right to either autonomous governance or treatment as full and equal members of the U.S. civic body. Many progressives—Besom, D'Olier, Fitzgerald, and Noyes among them—tended toward the second position, favoring legislation that would transfer political control from U.S. to local authority and end formal political oversight. At the same time, they assumed a moral responsibility to ensure that indigenous populations possessed the requisite physical and civic fitness to assume that independent status, a conception based on a decidedly U.S. vision of modernity. "The ideals we are striving to inculcate are American ideals," explained one of Besom's colleagues. "We are giving them to a people but a short time removed from tribal conditions."[52] Nurses defined their reforms as a gift to U.S. citizen-subjects and a necessary prerequisite to their eventual independence.[53]

Even though nurses perceived Filipinos and Puerto Ricans as lagging behind their U.S. and European peers, they believed that efforts to foster local autonomy were paramount. As in Europe, they aspired to develop the nursing profession and nurture local leadership. Stressing "the necessity of having all work undertaken by Porto Ricans," D'Olier arranged nursing and social work courses at the University of Porto Rico and established an autonomous nursing school in San Juan.[54] Besom sponsored nursing conferences and scholarships and looked to new graduates of Philippines nursing schools to replace their U.S. counterparts. She instructed her staff that their participation in Filipino public health projects "should be in the nature of a demonstration, and that every effort should be made to urge the assumption of responsibility for the conduct of these services by properly supervised agencies as soon as wise and practical."[55] In their efforts, these nurses envisioned a world in which every major city boasted a Johns Hopkins, a Bellevue, and a department of health to rival its U.S. counterparts. Yet securing the acceptance of U.S. biomedical and nursing ideas throughout the world, they realized, required more than faithful replication of U.S. institutions and ideas. Only by nurturing local leadership and developing authentic support for their ideas and practices could they achieve their long-term goals.

While this scientific missionary impulse was greatest in the Philippines and Puerto Rico because of their colonial relationship and perceived dependence on U.S. guidance, it readily transferred to other "backward" regions in which the United States and its citizens held interests. In 1925, after several years in the Philippines, Alice Fitzgerald returned to work for the League of Red Cross Societies in Geneva. She continued to take interest in the ARC plans to expand wartime nursing efforts to fields beyond Europe and the U.S. colonies. "South America is a stupendous field for future nursing developments," she advised Clara Noyes. "With its record of splendid achievement in Europe cannot the America Red Cross see its way to continue its good work by spreading out to South America? If you do not take a hand in the future of nursing down there, then I can see only chaos ahead for those poor people."[56] Continued ARC expansion was vital to the global advancement of professional nursing. Also at stake, however, was the potential for U.S. nurses to instill order in purportedly less developed areas of the world.

Fitzgerald carried this mentality with her when she moved to Bangkok in 1926 to serve as director of nursing at a Rockefeller Foundation hospital. As a consultant, Fitzgerald had championed the establishment of professional nursing in non-European nations. Her attitude shifted once she engaged personally in the task. She described her work as "full of difficulties and quite the hardest nut I have ever been asked to crack." Fitzgerald faulted cultural immaturity and different religious traditions as the key impediments to her work. "A poligamous country is not ready for advanced education for women," she contended, "as the men do not want them to become emancipated and refuse poligamy which they would of course do."[57] On hearing of these struggles, Noyes too questioned the feasibility of the international nursing mission. "In a country where the women are still regarded as having no souls, not to mention rights, I am wondering whether it is actually possible to introduce a modern system of nurse education. A modern system . . . calls for students of education, intelligence and social background. . . . I am wondering, therefore, what you have to build upon."[58]

Everywhere they were introduced, U.S. nursing and medical interventions were defined as a means to uplift women and, by extension, to stimulate progress and nurture civilization. As nurses traveled farther from their zones of comfort, however, their cultural and ethnic assumptions about the capacities of local populations limited their sense of possibility. Nurses negotiated vast geopolitical, gendered, and professional borders in their work, but cultural and racial presumptions sometimes limited their quest to spread U.S. values across the world, to nurture true autonomy, and to embrace the full potential of the international equality they espoused.

Crossing Borders in U.S. History and Historiography

In the twentieth century, the United States became a world power through ideological expansion more than through landed conquest, a process based on physical transferal and ultimate acquiescence to U.S. political, economic, and cultural values and institutions—nursing, medicine, and health among them. It relied on the development of an empire by consensus, built by private individuals who exercised soft forms of power. This was not an abstract phenomenon, but one carried out by actual individuals—often non-state actors—engaged in on-the-ground interactions across multiple sites.[59] The international spread of nurses and their ideas, as this essay makes clear, is no mere sideshow to this story—it is fundamental to it. As nurses transported training schools, child health programs, and hygienic ideas from U.S. cities to the European war zone to myriad sites of U.S. strategic interest, they created tangible links that facilitated U.S. expansion in other realms as well. Recovering the history of their international careers, therefore, demonstrates important material and intellectual processes at work in forging global U.S. influence and consolidating U.S. American nursing's global power.

Whereas nursing and public health methods and institutions created material continuities in U.S. global expansion, cultural assumptions about race, civilization, and U.S. responsibility provided conceptual unity. Descriptions of civilians in Vladivostok, Manila, and Warsaw echoed one another because nurses from the United States conceived these populations as lacking elements of knowledge and culture characteristic of an advanced, modern people. Wherever they were introduced, U.S. ideas and practices regarding health, hygiene, and professional nursing held a common promise for the populations who consented to them. Nurses believed that acquiescence to the hegemony of U.S. medical and professional ideals would assure individual and collective improvements; resistance indicated a stubborn, illogical reaction that nurses interpreted as evidence of a population's backwardness. To progress, local populations required hygienic reforms, improved nutrition and sanitation, the liberation and education of women, and, above all, the guidance of committed U.S. professionals to achieve these ends.

The growth of U.S. power in the world depended fundamentally on this scientific missionary enterprise. The centrality of nurses to this endeavor calls attention to the significant role female professionals played in forging U.S. world power and the global spread of U.S. nursing. It points, moreover, to the power of constructed feminine gender roles in this process. The expansion of U.S. political, cultural, and economic influence, in rhetoric though not always in practice, was defined as a benevolent process. U.S. policymakers and private citizens hoped to project an image of the United States as a new type of world power, defined by its generosity and modernity. The avowedly humanitarian nature of U.S. nurses' assistance projects served as valuable cultural diplomacy. Their provision of voluntary expert assistance to remedy local health issues, coupled with efforts to nurture local professionals, helped legitimize the spread of U.S. cultural and political influence by masking the more violent and aggressive aspects of American empire and defining U.S. influence in the world as a force for good.

As they bolstered U.S global expansion, nurses benefited individually through the new career and leadership opportunities they enjoyed. Moreover, they elevated the status of professional nursing throughout the world. U.S. women enhanced the power and prestige of the United States and in so doing advanced their own interests.

Yet it would be a grave disservice to cast these nurses as mere agents of empire or shallow careerists. Besom, Bridge, D'Olier, and Fitzgerald believed that by staging biomedical interventions and uplifting the status of women, they would eventually improve the health of all citizens. They were firmly committed to the idea that health and education were universal rights and international social justice issues. In some important respects, their health and nursing interventions represented a distinctly liberal path, especially when compared to contemporary alternatives. These nurses lived in a nation whose military occupied several Caribbean nations and whose territorial governments forced sanitary, hygienic, and educational reforms in Puerto Rico and the Philippines.[60] Because they worked through private agencies outside the government, nurses lacked the state authority to impose change by force of law or arms. Instead, they had to win allegiance to Western nursing and biomedicine by force of example. They undoubtedly benefited from their status as professionals and as U.S. citizens, which bestowed a level of cultural authority and coercive power. Nonetheless, the voluntary nature of their interventions required at least some level of cultural negotiation and compromise, setting them apart from counterparts working within the colonial infrastructure.

They also placed substantial faith in the capacities and interests of local populations, virtues many of their contemporaries were unwilling to concede. In a period marked by conservative attempts to dismantle local self-government initiatives and tainted by a fierce biological racism that declared some populations incapable of progressing to a more "civilized" state, they tried to foster local leadership and to replace U.S. citizens in positions of direct political and social oversight with indigenous counterparts. Although they agreed with many of their contemporaries that populations on the margins of U.S. citizenship were not yet prepared for self-government, they tended to be optimistic in predicting how long it would be before their reforms took root, imagining in some cases that they could succeed in little more than a generation.

Simultaneously, then, these nurses rationalized U.S. international guidance and expansion even as they offered viable, less violent alternatives for its execution. By considering these nuances, and taking into account both the motivations and intent of nurses and the broader consequences of their efforts, a picture of the workings of U.S. global power emerges that is more complicated—yet arguably more satisfying—than one constructed using a less nuanced analytical frame. Too often, historical assessments of humanitarian interventions center on their inherent prejudices and power dynamics, thereby smearing assistance as indistinguishable from imperialism. At the other end of the spectrum, analyses that focus solely on their virtues tread perilously into apologia or glorification. Neither approach does justice to the practitioners of 1920s voluntary welfare assistance, their intentions, or the political and cultural outcomes of their activities. The history of international nursing, viewed from a lateral perspective, nicely underscores the tensions and the complexities of the history of U.S. global expansion.

The postscript to this story suggests, finally, that the circulation of U.S. ideas was never a one-way diffusion from the United States to the world outside its borders. The nurses in this story, like most of their counterparts, did not remain abroad permanently. They returned to the United States and often continued their nursing careers. There is fertile ground for further research into the post-international lives of these and other nurses, for their biographies might reveal how assumptions formed outside the United States trickled back to inform U.S. discourses about nursing, medicine, race, civilization, and the U.S. humanitarian mission.[61]

Pansy Besom left the Philippines in 1932 but continued to work in nursing and social welfare. During the Great Depression, she served as county supervisor for the New York State Federal Emergency Relief Administration and other New Deal relief projects. She served as assistant director for the Scranton, Pennsylvania, Visiting Nurse Society in 1937–1942, and assistant director of the ARC North Atlantic Area Nursing Service until 1948. Alice Fitzgerald likewise built a successful nursing career in the United States after her time overseas. After employing her for several years in Bangkok, the Rockefeller Foundation sent her to survey the state of nursing at Peking Union Medical College Hospital in China and the general state of nursing in Singapore. In 1929 she returned to the United States. She was appointed to survey the state of nursing in Maryland and later became directress of nurses at Polyclinic Hospital in New York.[62] Helen Bridge returned from Warsaw in 1928 to marry. Although she retired from nursing to devote herself to housekeeping, she volunteered her services to an ARC sanitary unit after the German invasion of Poland in 1939. The place of the nursing profession in the international community continued to be of interest to these women long after they returned to their lives within U.S. borders.[63]

Taking the histories of U.S. nurses into account and highlighting their centrality to the study of U.S. international history invites a reconsideration of the history of U.S. foreign relations in new and vital ways. These nurses—Besom, Bridge, D'Olier, Fitzgerald, and many others—*are* our U.S. international history, for they were the actual, physical embodiments of the United States in the world. Their letters, writings, and biographies are an invaluable archive for scholars interested in examining the on-the-ground workings of U.S. influence and soft power.[64] Like Besom, Bridge, D'Olier, and Fitzgerald, U.S. historians must take steps to transcend borders—in this case, the all-too-rigid disciplinary boundaries that sometimes blind us to other fields and alternate modes of inquiry—if we are to fully understand the rise and role of the United States as a world power.

Julia F. Irwin
Assistant Professor
Department of History SOC 107
University of South Florida
4202 E. Fowler Ave
Tampa, FL 33620

Notes

1. A sampling of overviews and edited anthologies demonstrates the vibrancy and breadth of this field. See Thomas W. Zeiler, "The Diplomatic History Bandwagon: A State of the Field," *Journal of American History* 95 (March 2009): 1053–73; Thomas Bender, ed., *Rethinking American History in a Global Age* (Berkeley: University of California Press, 2002); Robert E. Hannigan, *The New World Power: American Foreign Policy, 1898–1917* (Philadelphia: University of Pennsylvania Press, 2002); Ann Laura Stoler, ed., *Haunted by Empire: Geographies of Intimacy in North American History* (Durham, N.C.: Duke University Press, 2006). For Europe, see, e.g., Daniel T. Rodgers, *Atlantic Crossings: Social Politics in a Progressive Age* (Cambridge, Mass.: Harvard University Press, 1998), chap. 9; Robert W. Rydell and Rob Kroes, *Buffalo Bill in Bologna: The Americanization of the World, 1869–1922* (Chicago: University of Chicago Press, 2005); Victoria de Grazia, *Irresistible Empire: America's Advance Through Twentieth-Century Europe* (Cambridge, Mass.: Belknap Press of Harvard University Press, 2005). For the Caribbean and Pacific, see, e.g., Julian Go, *American Empire and the Politics of Meaning: Elite Political Cultures in the Philippines and Puerto Rico During U.S. Colonialism* (Durham, N.C.: Duke University Press, 2008); Emily Rosenberg, *Financial Missionaries to the World: The Politics and Culture of Dollar Diplomacy* (Cambridge, Mass.: Harvard University Press, 2004).

2. Several good examples are Warwick Anderson, *Colonial Pathologies: American Tropical Medicine, Race, and Hygiene in the Philippines* (Durham, N.C.: Duke University Press, 2006); Laura Briggs, *Reproducing Empire: Race, Sex, Science, and U.S. Imperialism in Puerto Rico* (Berkeley: University of California Press, 2002); Amy Fairchild, *Science at the Borders: Immigrant Medical Inspection and the Shaping of the Modern Industrial Labor Force* (Baltimore: Johns Hopkins University Press, 2003).

3. Marcos Cueto, ed., *Missionaries of Science: The Rockefeller Foundation in Latin America* (Bloomington: Indiana University Press, 1994); John Farley, *To Cast Out Disease: A History of the International Health Division of the Rockefeller Foundation, 1913–1951* (Oxford: Oxford University Press, 2004); Matthew Connolly, *Fatal Misconception: The Struggle to Control World Population* (Cambridge, Mass.: Harvard University Press, 2008).

4. Nayan Shah, *Contagious Divides: Epidemics and Race in San Francisco's Chinatown* (Berkeley: University of California Press, 2001); Alexandra Minna Stern, *Eugenic Nation: Faults and Frontiers of Better Breeding in Modern America* (Berkeley: University of California Press, 1995); Johanna Schoen, *Choice and Coercion: Birth Control, Sterilization, and Abortion in Public Health and Welfare* (Chapel Hill: University of North Carolina Press, 2005), chap. 4.

5. Anne-Emanuelle Birn, *Marriage of Convenience: Rockefeller International History and Revolutionary Mexico* (Rochester, N.Y.: University of Rochester Press, 2006); Ceniza Choy, *Empire of Care: Nursing and Migration in Filipino-American History* (Durham, N.C.: Duke University Press, 2003); Steven Palmer, *From Popular Medicine to Medical Populism: Doctors, Health, and Public Power in Costa Rica, 1800–1940* (Durham, N.C.: Duke University Press, 2003), chap. 7; Marcos Cueto, *Cold War, Deadly Fevers: Malaria Eradication in Mexico, 1955–1975* (Baltimore: Johns Hopkins University Press, 2007).

6. Warwick Anderson, "Where Is the Post-Colonial History of Medicine?" *Bulletin of the History of Medicine* 72, no. 3 (1998): 522–30.

7. For ideas about this global approach, see Emily Rosenberg, "Walking the Borders," in *Explaining the History of American Foreign Relations*, ed. Thomas Paterson and Michael Hogan (Cambridge: Cambridge University Press, 1991), 24–35; David Thelen, "The Nation and Beyond: Transnational Perspectives on United States History," *Journal of American History* 86, no. 3 (December 1999): 965–75; and Ian Tyrrell, *Transnational Nation: United States History in Global History Since 1789* (New York: Palgrave Macmillan, 2007). For examples of these approaches outside medical history, see Akira Iriye, *Global Community: The Role of International Organizations in the Making of the Contemporary World* (Berkeley: University of California Press, 2004); Leila J. Rupp, *Worlds of Women: The Making of an International Women's Movement* (Princeton, N.J.: Princeton University Press, 1997); Erez Manela, *The Wilsonian Moment: Self-Determination and the International Origins of Anticolonial Nationalism* (New York: Oxford University Press, 2009).

8. One model is Farley's *To Cast Out Disease*. His thorough institutional history ably demonstrates the movement of American medical personnel and ideas across borders.

9. Isabel Hofmeyr, "*AHR* Conversation on Transnational History," *American Historical Review* 111 (December 2006): 1440–64.

10. For the professionalization of nursing, see Susan Reverby, *Ordered to Care: The Dilemma of American Nursing, 1850–1945* (Cambridge: Cambridge University Press, 1987); Karen Buhler-Wilson, *No Place like Home: A History of Nursing and Home Care in the United States* (Baltimore: Johns Hopkins University Press, 2003).

11. For what is distinctive about American medicine in this period, see, e.g., Ronald L. Numbers and John Harley Warner, "The Maturation of American Medical Science," in *Sickness and Health in America: Readings in the History of Medicine and Public Health*, ed. Judith Walzer Leavitt and Numbers (Madison: University of Wisconsin Press, 1997), 130–42; Nancy Tomes, *The Gospel of Germs: Men, Women, and the Microbe in American Life* (Cambridge, Mass.: Harvard University Press, 1999), pts. II and III, 91–236.

12. Americans could participate in overseas nursing through a wide array of organizations such as the Rockefeller Foundation International Health Board, U.S. territorial agencies, and charities and agencies in host countries. In the early twentieth century, especially during World War I and its aftermath, the ARC became recognized as one of the dominant U.S. players in international relief and assistance. Privately funded and administered but benefiting from a special relationship with the U.S. government, the ARC was the "official volunteer" agency of the United States. Before World War II, it served as an institutional home for many Americans who wanted to work in global health and welfare initiatives, including the four nurses in this story. Politicians recognized privately administered aid as a valuable form of cultural diplomacy and a way to foster global stability and development without committing state resources. The White House and Department of State thus lent enthusiastic support to the ARC international assistance projects. For more on this relationship, see Julia F. Irwin, "Humanitarian Occupations: International Relief and Assistance in the Formation of American International Identities, 1898–1928" (PhD diss., Yale University, 2009).

13. For an overview of the diplomatic and political side of this process, see Hannigan, *The New World Power*.

14. For changes in women's political and social lives, see Nancy F. Cott, *The Grounding of Modern Feminism* (New Haven, Conn.: Yale University Press, 1989). For professionalization of nursing, see Reverby, *Ordered to Care;* Buhler-Wilson, *No Place like Home*. For the rise of women in other social professions, see, e.g., Ellen Fitzpatrick, *Endless Crusade: Women Social Scientists and Progressive Reform* (New York: Oxford University Press, 1990); Elizabeth N. Agnew, *From Charity to Social Work: Mary E. Richmond and the Creation of an American Profession* (Urbana: University of Illinois Press, 2003); John Louis Recchiuti, *Civic Engagement: Social Science and Progressive Reform in New York City* (Philadelphia: University of Pennsylvania Press, 2007).

15. For contemporary American ideas about sanitation and hygiene, see Tomes, *The Gospel of Germs;* Dorothy Porter, *Health, Civilization, and the State: A History of Health from Ancient to Modern Times* (London: Routledge, 1999), chap. 9.

16. For American ideological conceptions about the links between health, hygiene, race, civilization, and democratic citizenship, see Natalia Molina, *Fit to Be Citizens? Public Health and Race in Los Angeles, 1879–1939* (Berkeley: University of California Press, 2006); Fairchild, *Science at the Borders;* Hannigan, *The New World Power,* chap. 1; Michael H. Hunt, *Ideology and U.S. Foreign Policy* (New Haven, Conn.: Yale University Press, 1987); Matthew Jacobson, *Barbarian Virtues: The United States Encounters Foreign People at Home and Abroad, 1876–1917* (New York: Hill and Wang, 2001), chaps. 3, 4; Gail Bederman, *Manliness and Civilization: A Cultural History of Gender and Race in the United States, 1880–1917* (Chicago: University of Chicago Press, 1996). On the growing faith in the influence of environment over biology, see Elazar Barkan, *The Retreat of Scientific Racism: Changing Concepts of Race in Britain and the United States Between the World Wars* (Cambridge: Cambridge University Press, 1993).

17. For Progressive tensions between their own expertise and the goal to build democratic, autonomous leadership, see Leon Fink, *Progressive Intellectuals and the Dilemmas of Democratic Commitment* (Cambridge, Mass.: Harvard University Press, 1997), esp. chaps. 1, 8. On the secular missionary impulse and connections between improved health and modernity, see, e.g., Cueto, ed., *Missionaries of Science;* Ruth Rogaski, *Hygienic Modernity: Meanings of Health and Disease in Treaty Port China* (Berkeley: University of California Press, 2004); Anderson, *Colonial Pathologies.*

18. For other efforts at American cultural internationalism in the 1920s, see Emily S. Rosenberg and Eric Foner, *Spreading the American Dream: American Economic and Cultural Expansion, 1890–1945* (New York: Hill and Wang, 1982), chaps. 5–8; Akira Iriye, *Cultural Internationalism and World Order* (Baltimore: Johns Hopkins University Press, 2000), chap. 2.

19. See Neil Smith, *American Empire: Roosevelt's Geographer and the Prelude to Globalization,* California Studies in Critical Human Geography 9 (Berkeley: University of California Press, 2004), chaps. 5, 6.

20. For the construction of American expansion as a benevolent process, see Laura Wexler, *Domestic Visions in an Age of U.S. Imperialism* (Chapel Hill: University of North Carolina Press, 2000); Ian Tyrrell, *Woman's World/Woman's Empire: The Woman's Christian Temperance Union in International Perspective, 1880–1930* (Chapel Hill: University of North Carolina Press, 1991); Eileen J. Suárez Findlay, *Imposing Decency: The Politics of Sexuality and Race in Puerto Rico, 1870–1920* (Durham, N.C.: Duke University Press, 2000).

21. Joseph S. Nye pioneered the phrase and concept "soft power." See his *Bound to Lead: The Changing Nature of American Power* (New York: Basic Books, 1991); *Soft Power: The Means to Success in World Politics* (Cambridge, Mass.: Public Affairs, 2004); "Soft Power," *Foreign Policy* 80 (Fall 1990): 153–71.

22. David Kennedy, *Over Here: The First World War and American Society* (Oxford: Oxford University Press, 1980); Jennifer D. Keene, *Doughboys, the Great War, and the Remaking of America* (Baltimore: Johns Hopkins University Press, 2001).

23. "Life of Miss Jane A. Delano," 1919, Box 1, Jane Delano Collection, Accession 91–0030, Hazel Braugh Archives, Lorton, Virginia (hereafter HB); "Brief Outline of the Professional Life of Jane A. Delano," Jane Delano Folder, Box 20, RG200, Ser. 1, National Archives, College Park, Maryland (hereafter NACP); "Biographical Sketch of Clara D. Noyes," 1936, Clara D. Noyes Folder, Box 68, Historical and WWI Nursing Files, RG200, Ser. 1, NACP; Lavinia L. Dock, *History of American Red Cross Nursing* (Washington, D.C.: American Red Cross Nursing Service, 1922), 232–25.

24. For American civic voluntarism, particularly the construction of women's wartime obligations, see Chris Capozzola, *Uncle Sam Wants You: World War I and the Making of the Modern American Citizen* (Oxford: Oxford University Press, 2008), 6–9, chap. 3.

25. For ARC work among civilians, see Henry P. Davison, *The Work of the American Red Cross During the War* (Washington, D.C.: American National Red Cross, 1919); Henry P. Davison, *The American Red Cross in the Great War* (New York: Macmillan, 1919); Fisher Ames, Jr., *American Red Cross Work Among the French People* (New York: Macmillan, 1921); June Richardson Lucas, *The Children of France and the Red Cross* (New York: Frederick Stokes, 1918).

26. "Alice L. Fitzgerald Receives the Florence Nightingale Medal," press release, 12 September 1927, Alice Fitzgerald Folder, Box 31, RG200, Ser. 1, NACP; Dock, *History*

of American Red Cross Nursing, 583–84, 872, 1082, 1129, 1137–46. For the League of Red Cross Societies, see John F. Hutchinson, *Champions of Charity: War and the Rise of the Red Cross* (Boulder, Colo.: Westview, 1996), chap. 6.

27. Biographical sketch of Helen Bridge, typescript, Helen Bridge (Pohlman) Folder, Box 73, RG200, Ser. 1, NACP; Dock, *History of American Red Cross Nursing,* 936.

28. Annie L. Williams, "Entering Russia Through the Back Door," memoirs, Box 4, Annie L. Williams Collection, Foreign War Relief Collection: Siberian Commission, Accession 1991–2004, HB.

29. Helen Bridge to Clara Noyes, 14 November 1919, Box 73, RG200, Ser. 1, NACP.

30. Ibid.

31. "Joint Statement by Mr. Hoover and Col. R. E. Olds, Chief Commissioner of the Red Cross, 15 April 1919"; Robert E. Olds, "Memorandum to Form Basis for Instructions to American Red Cross Representatives on the Subject of Co-Operation with American Relief Administration Representatives," 1919; Herbert Hoover to Henry P. Davison, 22 February 1919; Robert Olds to Hoover, 15 February 1919, all in Folder 430–1, Box 430, American Relief Administration European Operation Records, Accession 23001–9.07, Hoover Institution Archives, Palo Alto, California. For the ARA, see Bertrand M. Patenaude, *The Big Show in Bololand: The American Relief Expedition to Soviet Russia in the Famine of 1921* (Palo Alto, Calif.: Stanford University Press, 1992).

32. For contemporary American standards, see Reverby, *Ordered to Care,* 121–42; Buhler-Wilson, *No Place like Home;* Barbara Melosh, *The Physician's Hand: Work Culture and Conflict in American Nursing* (Philadelphia: Temple University Press, 1982), 33–34. For simultaneous efforts to establish professional nursing schools overseas, see Susan McGann, "Collaboration and Conflict in International Nursing, 1920–1939," *Nursing History Review* 16 (2008): 29–57; Anne Marie Rafferty, "Internationalising Nursing Education During the Interwar Period," in *International Health Organisations and Movements, 1918–1939,* ed. Paul Weindling (Cambridge: Cambridge University Press, 1995); Farley, *To Cast Out Disease;* Sarah Elise Abrams, "Dreams and Awakenings: The Rockefeller Foundation and Public Health Nursing Education, 1913–1930" (PhD diss., University of California, San Francisco, 1992); Choy, *Empire of Care,* chap. 2.

33. Helen L. Bridge, "The Warsaw School of Nursing," typescript [1923?], Box 863, RG200, Ser. 2, NACP; Clara Noyes to Helen Bridge, 28 February 1921, Box 73, RG200, Ser. 1, NACP.

34. Bridge, "The Warsaw School of Nursing."

35. Helen Bridge to Clara Noyes, 2 August 1921, Box 863, RG200, Ser. 2, NACP.

36. "Rules for School of Nursing" (Warsaw), 8 February 1921, Box 863, RG200, Ser. 2, NACP.

37. Bridge to Noyes, 2 August 1921.

38. Marion Parsons to Miss Shelton, 27 July 1921, Box 890; RG200, NACP; "Rules for School of Nursing" (Warsaw).

39. Bridge to Noyes, 2 August 1921; Clara D. Noyes, "Endowed Training Schools to Meet the World's Need for Nurses," draft article for *Johns Hopkins Nurses Alumnae Magazine,* 11 April 1921; Noyes, "Red Cross Nurses from America: Lifting Nursing to a Higher Plain in Europe," draft article for *The Delineator,* 1921; Box 3, RG200, Ser. 2, NACP.

40. Clara Noyes to Helen Bridge, 16 February 1924, Box 863, RG200, Ser. 2, NACP.

41. Alisa Klaus, *Every Child a Lion: The Origins of Maternal and Infant Health Policy in the United States and France, 1890–1920* (Ithaca, N.Y.: Cornell University Press, 1993); Laura Lovett, *Conceiving the Future: Pronatalism, Reproduction, and the Family in the United States, 1890–1938* (Chapel Hill: University of North Carolina Press, 2007), chap. 6; Richard A. Meckel, *Save the Babies: American Public Health Reform and the Prevention of Infant Mortality, 1850–1929* (Ann Arbor: University of Michigan Press, 1998); Daniel J. Kevles, *In the Name of Eugenics: Genetics and the Uses of Human Heredity* (Cambridge, Mass.: Harvard University Press, 1998); Stern, *Eugenic Nation*.

42. For "scientific motherhood," see Rima Apple, *Mothers and Medicine: A Social History of Infant Feeding, 1890–1950* (Madison: University of Wisconsin Press, 1987); Rima Apple, *Perfect Motherhood: Science and Childrearing in America* (New Brunswick, N.J.: Rutgers University Press, 20066); Julia Grant, *Raising Baby by the Book: The Education of American Mothers* (New Haven, Conn.: Yale University Press, 1998); Molly Ladd-Taylor, *Mother-Work: Women, Child Welfare, and the State, 1890–1930* (Urbana: University of Illinois Press, 1994).

43. Ernest P. Bicknell, *With the Red Cross in Europe, 1917–1922* (Washington, D.C.: American National Red Cross, 1938), chap. 20.

44. For D'Olier, see Dock, *The History of American Red Cross Nursing*, 1181–82. For Besom, see Elizabeth H. Vaughan, "Biographical Information on Pansy V. Besom," 1922, Pansy Besom Folder, Box 6, RG200, Ser. 1, NACP; Pansy Besom to Clara Noyes, 14 March 1922, Box 890, Records of the American National Red Cross, RG200, Ser. 2, NACP.

45. Henry O. Eversole, "Twenty-One Child Health Centers Organized and Established by the American Red Cross," 1922, Box 889, RG200, Ser. 2, NACP.

46. Henry O. Eversole, "Our Children: Child Health Work in the Czecho-Slovak Republic," 1922; Elsie M. Bond to Eversole, 1922, Box 892, RG200, Ser. 2, NACP.

47. "American Red Cross Resume of Child Health Work (July 1, 1921 to December 21, 1921)," manuscript, 1921, Box 837, RG200, Ser. 2, NACP.

48. Historians of U.S. internationalism have discredited the 1920s as a period of isolationism. They demonstrate that international involvement remained steady and even increased through economic and cultural exchanges. See, e.g., Frank Costigliola, *Awkward Dominion: American Political, Economic, and Cultural Relations with Europe, 1919–1933* (Ithaca, N.Y.: Cornell University Press, 1984); Alan Dawley, *Changing the World: American Progressives in War and Revolution* (Princeton, N.J.: Princeton University Press, 2003); de Grazia, *Irresistible Empire*, chap. 1.

49. Clara Noyes to Rockefeller Foundation International Health Board, Recommendation for Alice Fitzgerald, 11 January 1922, Box 31, RG200, Ser. 1, NACP.

50. Vaughan, "Biographical information on Pansy V. Besom"; Kathleen D'Olier, "Report on Nursing Service in Porto Rico, 1 July 1922–23"; Olympia Torres, "Report on Home Hygiene Classes in Porto Rico, for Year 1925–26," 1926; Box 667, RG200, Ser. 2, NACP; Dock, *The History of American Red Cross Nursing*, 1201–2.

51. Pansy V. Besom, "Radio Talk," 15 May 1929, Box 666, RG200, Ser. 2, NACP.

52. Mary Concannon to Arthur Dunn, 8 August 1925, Box 666, RG200, Ser. 2, NACP.

53. For the concept of "capacity," see Paul A. Kramer, *The Blood of Government: Race, Empire, the United States, and the Philippines* (Chapel Hill: University of North Carolina Press, 2006), 310–18. For ideas about "probationary citizen-subjects," see Anderson, *Colonial Pathologies*.

54. "Projects of the Service Organization, Insular and Foreign Division," 24 September 1920, Box 215, RG200, Ser. 2, NACP.

55. Pansy Besom to Elizabeth Fox, 10 July 1929, Box 666; "Report on Health Activities of Red Cross in the Philippines," 1929, Box 666; RG200, Ser. 2, NACP.

56. Alice Fitzgerald to Clara Noyes, 29 September 1925, Box 31, RG200, Ser. 1, NACP.

57. Alice Fitzgerald to Clara Noyes, 17 February 1927, Box 31, RG200, Ser. 1, NACP.

58. Clara Noyes to Alice Fitzgerald, 5 April 1927, Box 31, RG200, Ser. 1, NACP.

59. Nye, *Soft Power.*

60. See Mary Renda, *Taking Haiti: Military Occupation and the Culture of U.S. Imperialism, 1915–1940* (Chapel Hill: University of North Carolina Press, 2001); Kramer, *Blood of Government.*

61. As Amy Kaplan, Mary Renda, and Kristin L. Hoganson have argued, interactions with the world outside U.S. borders have a return influence on domestic culture. These transactions reshape the way U.S. residents think about national identity and the U.S. place in larger global networks. Amy Kaplan, *The Anarchy of Empire and the Making of U.S. Culture* (Cambridge, Mass.: Harvard University Press, 2002); Mary Renda, *Taking Haiti;* Kristin L. Hoganson, *Consumer's Imperium: The Global Production of American Domesticity, 1865–1920* (Chapel Hill: University of North Carolina Press, 2007).

62. Biographical notes on Alice Fitzgerald, typescript, Alice Fitzgerald Folder, Box 31, RG200, Seri. 1, NACP.

63. Bridge, then 54, was not called to serve. Helen Bridge to Clara Noyes, 15 April 1928, RG200, Ser. 1; Bridge Pohlman to Mary Beard, 8 September 1939, Box 862, RG200, Ser. 2, NACP. As yet, I have been unable to trace Kathleen D'Olier's activities. She remained in Puerto Rico for most of the 1920s, but it is unclear what happened to her afterward.

64. For these archives, see American National Red Cross Historical and WWI Nursing Files (RG200, Ser. 1) and the general records of the American National Red Cross (RG200, Ser. 2–5), NARC. Also see individual manuscript collections at Hoover Institution Archives, Palo Alto, California, and Hazel Braugh Archives, Lorton, Virginia.

Gender, Politics, and Regionalism: Factors in the Evolution of Registered Psychiatric Nursing in Manitoba, 1920–1960

Beverly Hicks
Brandon University

Abstract. In Canada, psychiatric nursing care is provided by two kinds of nurses. East of Manitoba, it is provided by registered nurses who may or may not have specialized psychiatric nursing education. In the four western provinces, a distinct professional group, registered psychiatric nurses, also provide care. Saskatchewan was the first province to achieve distinct legislation, in 1948, followed by British Columbia in 1951, Alberta in 1955, and Manitoba in 1960.

Several factors coalesced to sway Manitoba to adopt the distinct profession model. First, there was little interest by the general nursing body in mental hospital nursing. Second, the other three western provinces had formed a Canadian Council of Psychiatric Nursing that encouraged mental hospital attendants and nurses in Manitoba. Third, a group of male attendants took on leadership roles supported by the mental hospital superintendents. Finally, Manitoba was culturally and geographically more aligned with western than eastern Canada.

In Canada, for more than sixty years, psychiatric nursing care has been provided by two different kinds of nurses. In the east, registered nurses (RNs), who may or may not have specialized education in psychiatric nursing, provide psychiatric nursing care. In the four western provinces of Manitoba, Saskatchewan, Alberta, and British Columbia, a distinct professional group, registered psychiatric nurses (RPNs), also provide care. Canada thus is in the unique position of having two kinds of psychiatric nurses who form uneasy alliances and, at times, conflict.

Veryl Tipliski has examined the history of this dual system. She explored in detail the evolution of psychiatric nursing in three provinces from 1909 to 1955. Ontario, east of Manitoba, developed psychiatric nursing as a specialty of general nursing. Saskatchewan, to the west, followed the distinct profession model. Tipliski ends her history in 1955, a time when, she concludes, the province of Manitoba could have tilted to the east or to the west.[1]

Previously sealed documents, public government documents, records of general and psychiatric nursing organizations in Manitoba, and oral interviews reveal a picture of a complex coalescence of events that tilted Manitoba to the west. I argue that four sets of factors came together to sway Manitoba to the western Canadian distinct profession model. First, few RNs worked in mental hospitals, and the general nursing licensing body, the Manitoba Association of Registered Nurses (MARN), showed little interest in such nursing. On the other hand, when the provincial government introduced licensed practical nursing (LPN) into Manitoba in 1945, a good relationship developed between the mental hospital schools of nursing and the LPN advisory council. Second, western Canada had an alternative model of psychiatric nursing and an increasingly active national group, the Canadian Council of Psychiatric Nursing (CCPN), which supported and encouraged Manitoba mental hospital attendants and nurses to seek legal recognition. Third, a group of willing male attendants took on leadership roles, and provincial psychiatrists and politicians supported the creation of an alternative workforce. Finally, regionalism and geography played a part.

Psychiatric Nursing in Canada

Psychiatric nursing arose in asylums, usually at the behest of the medical superintendents, as insanity became medicalized in the late nineteenth and early twentieth centuries.[2] The construction of insanity as a medical condition created a new medical specialty, and the physicians who took an interest in the mentally ill and their care and treatment modeled their practice after that of their colleagues in general hospitals. This included turning asylums into hospitals, inmates into patients, and attendants into nurses.[3]

As treatment shifted to a medical model, the medical superintendents required skilled nurses to assist with popular treatments such as hydrotherapy and insulin coma. In some situations, the medical superintendents created their own specialized workforce; in others, general nurses were encouraged to take up the new specialty of psychiatric nursing. The recruitment, education, and control of the new workforce became a contested space that resulted in the evolution of two kinds of psychiatric nurses in a Canadian context marked by distinct regional differences.

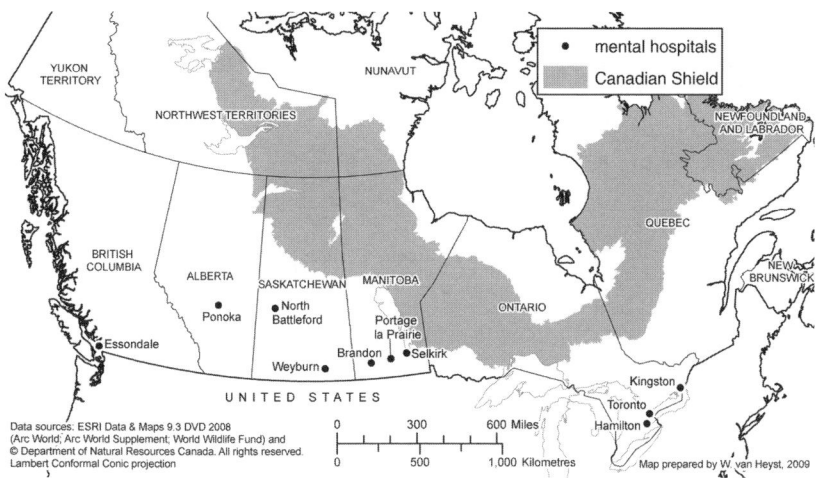

Figure 1. Canadian shield.

East of Manitoba: The Model of Psychiatric Nursing in Ontario

In Ontario the Kingston, Toronto, and Hamilton mental hospitals established schools of nursing between 1905 and 1909. This action coincided with the formation of the Graduate Nurses Association of Ontario (GNAO). The schools of nursing in the mental hospitals were under the control of the superintendents, who saw the value of having the students also affiliate at a general hospital in order to be eligible for registration with the GNAO. Affiliations were not always easily attained, but the GNAO was committed to this idea and cooperated with the superintendents. When the GNAO gained their registration legislation in 1922, which gave them control over the registration of nurses, the graduates of the specialty schools of nursing were included under the act.[4]

West of Manitoba: The Model of Psychiatric Nursing in Saskatchewan

The western province of Saskatchewan developed the distinct profession model partly because of a different relationship with the nursing regulatory body, the Saskatchewan Registered Nurses Association (SRNA). Saskatchewan led the way in many social movements in the late 1940s, with the reforms implemented by the Co-operative Commonwealth Federation government of Thomas (Tommy) Douglas.[5] This socialist-leaning government had come to power in 1944 following a decade of drought, depression, and war. It promised sweeping social and economic changes for the people of Saskatchewan, and reform of the psychiatric system was high on the agenda. The mental hospitals at North Battleford and Weyburn, not unlike other mental hospitals, were plagued by overcrowding, lack of standards, and lack of staff.[6] The staff had little training, although the attendants at North Battleford and Weyburn had been receiving rudimentary training since 1930 and 1931, respectively. A three-year training course was instituted beginning in 1937, and the government presented graduates with a diploma signed by the minister of health and the hospital superintendent.[7] But, like many other such training programs, the curriculum and teaching were inconsistent, controlled by medical superintendents, and not recognized beyond the institution.

Training of attendants and improvement in care for the mentally ill was interrupted by World War II, but in 1946 commissioner of mental health services for Saskatchewan Donald McKerracher, a psychiatrist from Ontario, was appointed to head up the much-needed reforms. This marked the beginning of changes not only in the mental health system, but also in the evolution of psychiatric nursing. McKerracher identified the overcrowding and lack of treatment as direct results of the shortage of psychiatrists to treat and discharge patients. Improving treatment and discharge rates also required skilled nursing care. Recruiting general nurses to work in the mental hospitals was difficult, but McKerracher saw the value of training for both male and female staff. He approached the SRNA seeking affiliation for the mental hospital nurses. But the complexity of arranging for the students to be away at a general hospital for any length of time, coupled with SRNA caution regarding their background knowledge, created barriers too difficult to overcome.[8] McKerracher instead recommended the establishment of an alternative workforce. The timing was fortuitous.

In 1944 the United Civil Servants of Canada (UCSC) unionized the Weyburn hospital staff, including the psychiatric attendants. At North Battleford, attendant William Vowles saw the poor conditions under which attendants and nurses worked, and believed a union was the only way to improve working conditions. He did not wish to join a general trade union such as the UCSC and instead formed a Trade Union of Hospital Employees. Despite the desire to remain separate from the larger union, the group was eventually forced to affiliate with the USCS.[9] Working conditions improved, but the economic goals of the union did not fit with the burgeoning professional aspirations of the psychiatric attendants.

Attendants from North Battleford and Weyburn who were active in the union occasionally met on union business. They also discussed the need for more recognition and status for attendants, and the idea of a professional association gradually evolved. In 1947, when McKerracher turned to Vowles to assist in his ambition of having a trained workforce in the two mental hospitals, these professionalization goals fit with his. The Psychiatric Services Branch, the government department that managed the provincial mental hospitals, developed a 500-hour curriculum for attendants. The next step was recognition through legislation.[10]

Premier Douglas supported the legislation, and Alex Connon, Member of Legislative Assembly for the Battlefords, presented the bill.[11] This direct government involvement assured its smooth passage. Inevitably, when the SRNA learned of the proposed legislation, it was concerned about the use of the term "nurse." Vowles, however, argued that the term "psychiatric" preceding "nurse" clearly distinguished between the two groups, and pointed out that he had deliberately refrained from using the term "registered."[12] Despite writing Douglas directly, the SRNA was unable to stop or even delay the bill, and "psychiatric nurse" became the title.[13] Tipliski describes the swift passage of the legislation on 25 March 1948 as a "stunning victory."[14] The training program established by this legislation and conducted by mental hospital staff was considered a solution to the staffing difficulties. It also became the foundation of an emerging professionalism, which was growing not only in Saskatchewan but also in the provinces to the west, Alberta and British Columbia.

West of Manitoba: Psychiatric Nursing in British Columbia

Although Saskatchewan achieved the first legislation for psychiatric nurses in Canada in 1948, British Columbia had, a year earlier, established an association of psychiatric nurses registered under the British Columbia's Societies Act.[15] Essondale, the largest mental hospital in the province, had first introduced training for attendants in the 1930s, and in 1937 a three-year course was established that led to a diploma in psychiatric nursing.[16] But without standards the training was contingent on the availability of staff to take the training, and it was disrupted during the war years. After World War II the training became more organized and professional aspirations grew. Two male psychiatric nursing education instructors from Essondale, Wilfred Pritchard and Richard Strong, arranged meetings to discuss the formation of a professional association. The minutes of the meetings in the spring and summer of 1947 describe a need to set standards, gain professional standing and recognition, and be properly registered. The attendants saw themselves as specialists of a kind, but they had no organization and faced powerful opposition from the RNs, who they believed did not look favorably on them. The minutes record their awareness that they needed to demonstrate they "could give as good, if not better service to the mentally ill, than the comparatively inexperienced registered nurses."[17]

At the official organizational meeting the group, led by Pritchard and Strong, established aims and objects. Their first goal, "to promote, improve and maintain an enlightened and progressive standard of psychiatric nursing," was the same wording used thirteen years later when Manitoba established its objectives. The deliberations culminated in the formation of an association with the blessing of Arthur Crease, director of mental health services in British Columbia.[18] The British Columbia Psychiatric Nurses Association was registered under the Societies Act on 4 September 1947. In 1950, the association embarked on a program to gain legal recognition, and with government support and assistance, achieved the 1951 legislation that became known as the Psychiatric Nurses Act of British Columbia. The term "attendant" was replaced with "nurse," and the legislation required that all psychiatric nurses be licensed.[19]

West of Manitoba: Psychiatric Nursing in Alberta

The next province to achieve legislation for psychiatric nurses was Alberta. Psychiatric nursing in Alberta developed along similar lines and encountered some of the same challenges as the groups in Saskatchewan and British Columbia. In the 1930s, Charles Baragar, previously superintendent at Brandon Mental Hospital in Manitoba, came to Alberta as commissioner of mental health and superintendent of Ponoka Mental Hospital. Baragar hoped to establish in Alberta what he had not been able to accomplish in Manitoba—a combined training program for psychiatric nurses. In 1931, he developed a training plan, but without consulting the Alberta Association of Registered Nurses (AARN). When he sought its approval, it responded with dismay. In its review and subsequent report the AARN determined that there were not sufficient bed patients to sustain a training school; the curriculum was unsatisfactory; as the students had to work twelve-hour days, there was not sufficient time for instruction; and there were no trained nurses to supervise students on the wards. The report concluded that the course should be discontinued, and proposed instead that a postgraduate course for general nurses, affiliation for third-year general nursing students, and employment of Alberta's unemployed general nurses would be sufficient to provide nursing staff for the mental hospitals.[20]

Baragar, highly incensed, immediately appealed to minister of health George Hoadley, and vehemently refuted each point in the report.[21] The Senate of the University of Alberta quickly made the necessary adjustments and approved the school. (In Alberta at that time, the university senate was responsible for monitoring and approving the education of professionals such as nurses even if they were not educated at the university.) Baragar then arranged for the general hospital affiliations and developed a four-year course, two years at the mental hospital followed by two years in a general hospital. Five female nurses graduated from the first course in 1936, and this combined program continued into the 1960s.[22]

The male attendants were not permitted to take this course. Instead, a three-year course led to a diploma in psychiatric nursing.[23] Ten years later, one of these attendants, Edward (Ted) James, supported by Randall McLean, director of mental health services, organized a meeting to discuss the formation of a professional association. The Saskatchewan and British Columbia psychiatric nurses sent letters of encouragement.[24] The Alberta Psychiatric Nurses Association was registered under the Alberta Societies Act in May 1950. The Psychiatric Nurses Training Act of Alberta became law in 1955.

A strong camaraderie developed among the male leaders of these three provincial associations. They bonded around the issue of seeking recognition for themselves, although they may not have fully distinguished between union and professional activities at the time. Many of the men had been active in their provincial unions, and when the national group started in 1951, letters were often signed *fraternally yours*, a term more frequently associated with unions than with professional associations.[25] Nevertheless, these were the men who worked to establish professional bodies in their own provinces and who subsequently formed an association in western Canada.

Psychiatric Nursing in Manitoba

The Province of Manitoba assumed responsibility for the care and control of its citizens when it was incorporated in May 1870. This included those identified as mentally ill, feebleminded, criminal, or who otherwise who did not fit easily into society. It built three large institutions over a four-year period: an Insane Asylum at Selkirk in 1886, a Home for Incurables at Portage la Prairie in 1890, and also in 1890 a Home for Delinquent Boys in Brandon.[26] In 1891, the government turned the Brandon reformatory into a second asylum.[27]

For the next thirty years, the institutions at Brandon and Selkirk were run by physicians assisted by a variety of attendants. There seem to have been no particular qualifications or educational requirements for the keepers or attendants, and about equal numbers of men and women were employed. The institutions were relatively self-supporting through farms and gardens, with labor usually provided by patients.[28] The farms also served as a form of therapy for the patients. The institutions provided local employment, and they became part of the social and economic landscape of the communities.[29]

Very little changed in the management of the provincial institutions until 1915, when a new liberal reform government under Tobias Norris came into power.[30] This professional, idealistic administration quickly instituted reforms that included giving women the right to vote and establishing a public health nursing system.[31] The government also created a Public Welfare Commission to oversee public institutions. In 1918, the commission invited Charles (C. K.) Clarke, and Clarence Hincks of the Canadian National Committee for Mental Hygiene to conduct a survey of the Manitoba mental hospitals. The National Committee had been established after World War I in Toronto to address the needs of ailing returned soldiers and monitor the conditions of the nation's mental hospitals.[32] Clarke and Hincks were critical of mental health care in Canada generally; the Manitoba asylums were singled out for their particularly poor conditions, and sweeping reforms were recommended. The report made particular note of the lack of trained nurses.[33]

The Norris government, probably already aware of the conditions of the mental hospitals, took the opportunity to institute much-needed reforms. In 1920, it appointed a provincial psychiatrist, Alvin Mathers, who in turn appointed new superintendents for the Selkirk and Brandon asylums, now renamed hospitals. Edgar Barnes, a psychiatrist from Ontario, became superintendent of Selkirk Hospital for Mental Diseases, and Charles Baragar assumed the responsibility at Brandon Hospital for Mental Diseases.[34] These new superintendents had vision and ambition. Like their colleagues in other parts of Canada, their psychiatric skills had been honed during World War I. They saw the care of the insane as a medical specialty and the role of the superintendent as that of clinician rather than custodial manager.[35] Having trained nurses was vital to the vision.

Psychiatric Nursing Schools in Manitoba

The superintendents of the two mental hospitals in Manitoba established training schools for psychiatric nurses, Selkirk's in 1920 and Brandon's in 1921.[36] The programs of the two institutions operated independently, without consistent standards beyond what each superintendent felt was necessary for the operation of his own institution As often as not, educational needs of the students were subverted to service needs, and the graduates received no legal recognition.

While similarities existed between the training programs at Brandon and Selkirk, there were also important differences. Baragar, from the outset, hoped that nurses trained at Brandon would be eligible for registration with the licensing body, the Manitoba Association of Graduate Nurses (MAGN), later the Manitoba Association of Registered Nurses (MARN). A small victory was achieved in 1927 when three nurses from Brandon affiliated at St. Boniface Hospital in Winnipeg, to take a general nursing course that made them eligible to write registration exams with MAGN. But no further affiliations took place at that time.[37]

In Canada, some mental hospitals provided training only for female staff in the desire to make asylums seem more like hospitals.[38] However, Brandon and Selkirk provided training to both male and female staff.[39] Brandon, for example, began training men in 1921; between 1924 and 1946, 103 male attendants graduated, only a small portion of the male attendants.[40] In 1947 the course was made compulsory.[41] Many of the men with this training became ward supervisors on the male side of the hospital, and it is from this group that the leaders emerged who wished for more recognition and status for the psychiatric nurses. As much as possible, female RNs supervised the infirmary and admission wards.

Little information exists on the instruction provided to male attendants at Brandon, but in the 1950s it increased to 358 hours. In 1956 anatomy and physiology received 50 hours of instruction, nursing arts 72 hours, psychiatric nursing only 42 hours. Psychiatry, first aid, drugs, medical-surgical nursing, occupational therapy, and ethics made up the remainder of the classroom time.[42] The rest of the three-year course was spent on various wards of the hospital, and service always preceded learning. Any clinical teaching was provided by the male ward supervisors, who had been trained at the institution. Many of these supervisors became adept at managing medical treatments such as insulin coma, and they passed on these skills. Two male nurses spoke positively of the instruction and skill development received from these ward supervisors.[43]

The education of the female students in the mental nursing diploma course of the 1940s and 1950s is not much better documented. The number of hours of instruction is recorded, but the content is unclear. Again, there was heavy emphasis on nursing skills. For example, in 1943 the subject called psychiatric nursing received 20 hours of instruction and 150 hours in nursing arts. Even the subject called medical surgical nursing received more hours than psychiatric nursing.[44]

The heavy emphasis on nursing skills may have resulted from a number of factors. First, Brandon had always been able to hire a small number of RNs as teaching staff, some but not all of whom had additional psychiatric nursing training. No doubt, they were familiar and comfortable with basic nursing skills and emphasized these skills. Second, the psychiatric nursing knowledge of the time seemed limited to descriptions of behavior and its management. One graduate of the early 1960s recalled the instruction she received as a student nurse: to provide reassurance to the patients but to avoid any discussion of problems and always refer patients' concerns to their psychiatrist.[45] In reality, the patient may only have seen the psychiatrist once a week for a short visit. Third, the medical superintendents taught the student nurses psychiatry, which no doubt reflected their own view of what they thought psychiatric nurses needed to know.[46] Finally, the major theories of the causes of mental illness in the 1940s and 1950s were physiological, and this model directed the complex and labor-intensive physiological treatments such as lobotomies and insulin coma. These treatments required skilled nursing care, although they were restricted to a limited number of newly admitted and diagnosed patients. Physically ill patients had to be cared for in the infirmary, and patients with tuberculosis, in special wards.[47] However, the majority of patients either languished on back wards or were employed in hospital-based activities such as farming, housework, gardening, or crafts.

Brandon finally achieved a long hoped for affiliation with a general hospital in 1942, when it entered into an arrangement with the Winnipeg General Hospital (WGH) to have eligible female students take two years additional training. This combined program provided the opportunity for these student nurses to gain the experience, knowledge, and skills to write the licensing exams to become RNs. The graduates of this program had dual qualifications: a psychiatric nursing diploma from Brandon and an RN from MARN. The nurses who returned to Brandon were given supervisory or teaching positions.[48]

The Brandon affiliation with WGH continued until 1947 and was replaced with a more integrated affiliation with Brandon General Hospital (BGH). This new combined program demonstrated good cooperation and collegiality between the instructors of the two Brandon hospitals. The director of nursing education at BGH had at one time been an instructor at Brandon Mental Hospital and was sympathetic toward the nurses there. Having most of the teaching in the home town of Brandon was probably an advantage as well. This arrangement also provided a reciprocal agreement for general nursing students from the affiliating hospitals to come to Brandon for psychiatric nursing education and experience. Affiliation in psychiatric nursing was not mandatory in Manitoba at the time, so the program was particularly progressive.[49]

Unfortunately, the superintendents who controlled psychiatric nursing education decided to discontinue the BGH combined program just two years after the first class graduated in 1952.[50] The RN portion of the program was to be replaced with the same LPN program that the female students were already receiving at the Portage Home and Selkirk. This training would now be available to all female students, not just the few selected for the RN combined program. The decision was pragmatic. Staffing the mental hospitals was the priority of the superintendents.[51] That MARN did not protest the termination of this combined program perhaps indicates how little interest was taken in nursing care of the mentally ill in the provincial mental hospitals. When Julia Hannah, matron of Brandon, notified the MARN board that the program was to be replaced by a combined psychiatric nurse/LPN program, it is recorded that "the president thanked Mrs. Hannah for the information." There is no record of any further discussion.[52]

The Portage Home for Incurables

The third psychiatric nurse training program, established in 1936 at the Portage Home for Incurables, is another facet of psychiatric nursing in Manitoba. Portage has been described by one historian as "an unhappy conglomeration of idiots, imbeciles, epileptics, senile, and mentally normal people suffering from incurable diseases."[53] It also became the last resort for some patients when Selkirk and Brandon became overcrowded.[54] For its first forty years the institution had nonmedical superintendents, one of whom was noted for planting trees, and another for building a fine herd of Holstein dairy cows.[55] Physicians from the town of Portage La Prairie provided required medical care during this time.

This situation changed with the appointment in 1930 of the first medical director, Henry Atkinson, an energetic young physician from Selkirk. In his glowing first annual report he laid out his vision of an idyllic life for mentally handicapped children. He arranged for the removal of the elderly and frail to other facilities and set about his reforms. Although he often stated that his patients were not sick, he did see the need for skilled nursing care for them, especially those who suffered from epilepsy and other physical disabilities. One of his reform goals was the establishment of a nurse training school.[56]

When his plan came to the attention of MARN, its president wrote to the minister of health and welfare that MARN was responsible for nursing education in the province, and that it did not support the establishment of training at the Portage Home.[57] In an unpleasant exchange, MARN made suggestions as to how the program should be run. When the minister inquired as to whether MARN would register these graduates, the reply was no. The minister then asked, rather testily, what concern it was of theirs. He informed them that it had been impossible to secure the services of general nurses who would stay for any length of time, and therefore the superintendent had to develop his own staffing solutions.[58] Portage continued for another ten years with in-house training as best it could until another political decision again changed the psychiatric nursing landscape in Manitoba.

Licensed Practical Nursing and Psychiatric Nursing

The Manitoba government established the licensed practical nursing program to solve the post–World War II nursing shortage. The students needed ten years of schooling to enter the program, which provided ten months instruction in basic nursing skills. An advisory council of nursing instructors and Department of Health and Welfare officials managed the program.[59] At one of the early meetings of the advisory council, the minister of health and welfare, medical superintendents, and instructors from the three mental hospital schools of nursing discussed the possibility of including the female students from these institutions in this training. Brandon could not participate at the time as it was still involved in combined psychiatric nurse/RN training, but it seemed a good opportunity to provide additional training in general nursing skills for the female staff at the Portage Home and Selkirk. The training would also provide the female students with a legally recognized qualification. The instructors already teaching at Selkirk were RNs and therefore met the requirement that RNs teach in the LPN program, at least at Selkirk. The necessary arrangements for affiliation at general hospitals were made. The program commenced at Selkirk in 1946 and made a brief beginning at Portage.[60]

At Portage, two students expressed dissatisfaction with the general hospital experience, and persuaded their classmates to request they not affiliate. Superintendent Atkinson supported this minor rebellion by telling them they certainly did not need the general affiliation for mental nurse training. When the students were advised by the registrar of the LPN advisory council that without the LPN diploma their careers would begin and end in the mental hospital, they relented, but Atkinson did not. He told the advisory council his students would not be able to comply with the LPN training requirements, and no further Portage students participated at that time.[61] Four years later, in 1950, Atkinson allowed the female students to participate and inquired if the male students could also do so.

The Portage and Selkirk institutions benefited from the association with the LPN program in a number of ways. The advisory council had developed a Manual for Administrators of Schools of Practical Nursing, which set out an orderly and detailed curriculum of the ten general nursing courses under the headings topic, content, objectives, expected outcomes, learning activities, and student application.[62] The psychiatric nursing portion of this program was not articulated so clearly. But, because of the interest taken by the advisory council in the mental hospital students and the good working relationships between the council and the mental hospital instructors, greater attention was eventually paid to the psychiatric nursing curriculum. By 1953 a Manual for Psychiatric Schools of Nursing, similar to the Manual for Administrators of Schools of Practical Nursing, established a minimum curriculum for the four psychiatric nursing subjects: psychiatry, psychiatric nursing, psychology, and occupational therapy.[63] The plight of the male students also concerned the LPN advisory council, and this benefited the male attendants in the mental hospitals. In August 1959, the male students at Brandon began receiving the same number of hours of instruction as the female students in the LPN program except for maternal, infant and child care, and nutrition.[64]

These initiatives improved the quality of the training and provided a curriculum framework that imposed order on psychiatric nursing instruction and resulted in province-wide standards. The nursing instructors also benefited from this relationship. It provided them with a forum for discussing curricula with colleagues outside the control of the medical superintendents. This may well be why John Kellie noted, "this was the first time standards were applied to the training of psychiatric nurses in Manitoba."[65]

By 1957, therefore, psychiatric nursing education in Manitoba had achieved some consistency. But Manitoba psychiatric nursing was legally and professionally isolated in the center of Canada. It did not fit either the eastern model of general nurses providing mental health care, or the western model of a distinct profession. The support and encouragement of the recently formed Canadian Council of Psychiatric Nursing (CCPN) in western Canada, the male camaraderie among the leaders of this group, and the political will to establish the new profession finally tilted Manitoba to the west.

The Canadian Council of Psychiatric Nursing

When Saskatchewan and British Columbia were the only two provinces in Canada with any sort of association of psychiatric nurses, it was inevitable that they would form an alliance. Wilfred Pritchard, president of the British Columbia Psychiatric Nurses Association, wrote to William Vowles, president of the Saskatchewan Psychiatric Nurses Association, "Dear Bill lets start an association."[66] These two men, eager to see psychiatric nursing gain professional status and recognition, believed that a national association would benefit their aspirations.

In June 1950, the first joint meeting of the two provincial organizations took place at North Battleford, Saskatchewan. They explored the aims and purposes of the association and how they could cooperate for their mutual benefit. They made plans to form a Canadian council of psychiatric nurses, set standards and policies, and combat common problems as they affected psychiatric nurses and psychiatric nurses associations that might later join them. They established committees to draw up regulations and by-laws and a common pledge.[67] A year later Alberta joined them and a national body was formed, the CCPN. The group held its first annual meeting in 1951, and two Manitoba representatives attended as observers.[68] The CCPN continued to hold annual meetings. Two major themes dominated the proceedings from 1954 to 1957: the need to get an association organized in Manitoba, and the relationship with the Canadian Nurses Association (CNA), who proposed the development of a combined psychiatric nurse/RN training program.[69]

The Canadian Nurses Association and a New Combined Program Proposal

A proposal to establish a combined psychiatric nurse/RN training program arose out of the growing CNA recognition and concern that psychiatric nursing in Canada was evolving into two models.[70] The CNA, in an effort to deal with the issue, recommended the development of combined psychiatric nurse/RN training and selected Essondale Mental Hospital in British Columbia for a pilot project. A committee chosen to develop the recommended program included nursing instructors from Essondale and a number of general hospitals and representatives from the University of British Columbia, the Registered Nurses Association of British Columbia, and the British Columbia Psychiatric Nurses Association. The large committee was divided into two subcommittees to develop the psychiatric and general nursing sections of the combined course. They established the central objective that the program would train an individual who could function in both general and psychiatric nursing. The subcommittees worked throughout 1956, but one of the difficulties they seemed to have from the outset was the practice of meeting independently to discuss the two portions of the proposed curriculum. Despite obvious goodwill in trying to arrive at a combined program, the process lacked integration. The muddled thinking revealed in the minutes suggests that separation rather than integration marked the deliberations. No minutes of meetings after December 1956 have been located. Nevertheless, this project represents one of the first recorded efforts of the national bodies of psychiatric nurses and RNs to work together to solve the psychiatric nursing issue at a national level.[71]

The CCPN executive body had been invited to Ottawa in both 1954 and 1955 to meet with the CNA to discuss the project. CCPN president Richard Strong reported to the annual CCPN meeting at North Battleford, Saskatchewan, in June 1955. He agreed that the plan for a combined program gave the psychiatric nurses a "good deal."[72] A year later, at the June 1956 meeting in Oliver, Alberta, he gave a comprehensive and favorable report of the work of the committee, although he cautioned, "We still must be constantly on guard and wary of proposals which might be detrimental to psychiatric nurses."[73] The project was briefly alluded to at the 1957 CCPN meeting in Essondale, British Columbia, but it never appears again in the minutes of the meetings of this body. Strong later reflected that it had been a long, arduous chore that got bogged down because several key people left, and a very ideal project fell flat.[74] What started out as a promising venture simply faded away.

Politics of Psychiatric Nursing in Manitoba, 1957–1960

No doubt the executive of the CCPN, taken up with the events in Ottawa and the proposed combined program in British Columbia, had little time for local matters. At the 1955 annual meeting Strong apologized for the lack of progress on the establishment of the distinct profession in Manitoba. Efforts had been made by mail to interest the mental hospital staff in Manitoba, but with little response.[75] At the 1956 annual meeting it was noted that further efforts needed to be made to interest Manitoba graduates in forming an association and that Saskatchewan, the nearest province, should send a delegation to help organize them.[76]

Initially, Manitoba seemed reluctant, and there are no records of early efforts to develop an association. This reluctance is curious, but one speculation is that as the nursing educators and directors of nursing in the mental hospitals all had MARN licensure, perhaps they discouraged the process or saw no need of further licensing. The majority of the female ward staff at the three provincial institutions now received an LPN diploma and may not have seen the need for any other credentials. The male staff, however, remained without legal recognition.

Some of the senior attendants were active in the Manitoba Government Employees Association (MGEA). This union represented all government employees, including attendants and nurses, and addressed any concerns regarding working conditions.[77] However, like their counterparts in the other western provinces, the mental hospital attendants felt the union did not exactly meet their professional aspirations. At Selkirk, Alfred Barnett, a long-term attendant and strong union man, suggested that an association rather than a union would be better for the psychiatric nurses.[78] But it was at Brandon, not Selkirk, that the first recorded organizational meeting of psychiatric nurses took place.

Other events were pulling Manitoba in a westerly direction. In May 1957, Gladys Fitzpatrick, RN, was appointed superintendent of nursing at Brandon. She had been the matron at North Battleford and had also worked at Weyburn.[79] Familiar with the separate profession and organization of psychiatric nursing in Saskatchewan, she spoke to the chief attendant, Arthur Russell, and another senior attendant, David Gibson, about forming an association.

The promised visit to Manitoba by the executives of the CCPN also took place in summer 1957. Max Schreder and Duke Leflar, president and secretary-treasurer, who both resided in Weyburn, met with the MGEA as well as with psychiatric nurses in Brandon, Selkirk, and Winnipeg. The visit was reported in the *Bison*, the MGEA newsletter, along with an article that praised the Saskatchewan psychiatric nurses for establishing standards for the profession and suggested Manitoba might consider doing the same. The writer noted that not only would the individual psychiatric nurses benefit but the standard of care would be raised.[80]

Following the information meetings of summer 1957, Russell and Schreder established a correspondence. In September Schreder wrote to Russell further encouraging him to get Manitoba organized because prestige, opportunities, and even pay would be increased. Schreder ended on an optimistic note that it would also be another step toward the formation of a dominion Association of Psychiatric Nurses.[81]

But it was not only the CCPN and the senior attendants who were interested in organizing psychiatric nursing in Manitoba. In further correspondence Schreder reported that the superintendents had made their own inquiries.[82] This must have bolstered the emerging group, and in February 1958 an organizational meeting was held in the auditorium at Brandon Mental Hospital. Russell informed the group that "Miss Fitzpatrick said Sask standards much higher than Manitoba [sic]."[83] It is not known who was in attendance, but no such meeting would have taken place on hospital property without the written or tacit approval of the medical superintendent.

Russell notified provincial psychiatrist Thomas Pincock of the plans to form an association of psychiatric nurses. Pincock replied that he very much wanted to see such an organization and wished to cooperate intelligently and effectively.[84] He did not add that in fact he and the superintendents had already made plans for an association of psychiatric nurses. He had not only made inquiries about different forms of legislation from the other three western provinces, but he had already decided the form the legislation should take. In November 1958 Pincock informed the superintendents that he had looked into the legislation from the other three provinces and determined that the Alberta legislation would suit Manitoba's purposes better than the others.[85] Pincock wanted the psychiatric nurses to have responsibility for their association, but the curriculum and rules and standards for training would remain with the superintendents.

The control exerted by the superintendents is further illustrated by the fact that Pincock asked the government lawyer to draw up a bill to form a psychiatric nurses' association. The psychiatric nurses were without legal representation at that point, and in their naivety seemed content to allow the government lawyer to make legal decisions for them. It was this government lawyer who informed them they needed to hire their own lawyer.[86] In May 1959 they retained the services of James Wilson, who reviewed the draft prepared by the government lawyer. Wilson sent a copy of a proposed bill to Pincock, who was not pleased with the new draft, which suggested that one act combine management of association affairs and control of education.[87] In the end the politicians and superintendents prevailed and two bills passed through the legislature and received royal assent on 26 March 1960.[88]

The first bill gave the governance of the Psychiatric Nurses Association of Manitoba to its members. The second placed the education of psychiatric nurses in the hands of a committee comprised of the provincial psychiatrist, the mental hospital superintendents, and the superintendents of nursing, but not the directors of education or the chief male attendants, the equivalent of the superintendents of nursing. (The superintendents of nursing were RNs whereas the chief male attendants were not.) The men who had provided so much leadership and service in the formation of the association were, at this point, shut out of the psychiatric nursing educational process.[89]

Conclusion

The history of the evolution and professionalization of registered psychiatric nursing in Manitoba, as indeed in western Canada, illustrates the contextual, contingent, political, and gendered nature of its origins. The achievement of legislation in each province was dependent on political good will and the support of the mental hospital superintendents. Had they not supported, indeed, encouraged the establishment of the separate profession, it is unlikely it would have happened. It has been argued that the superintendents were controlling and powerful. Indeed that may be true, but they also needed trained staff for the mental hospitals.

The desire of many of the male attendants for professional status fueled the drive for recognition and legislation in Manitoba and western Canada. The sense of camaraderie that developed among the male leaders of the four western provinces also contributed to the success of the movement to professionalize mental hospital work.[90] Manitoba, the last of the provinces to organize an association, benefited from the experience of the three other provinces.

The relationship with the nursing regulatory bodies in the western provinces was uneasy. The nursing bodies wanted to maintain control of the title nurse, and nursing education, as was their mandate, but with the inability to attract RNs to the mental hospitals the immediate problem of the superintendents was adequate staffing, not the maintenance of the RN professional goals. Even the popular combined program in Manitoba failed to produce sufficient numbers of nurses who stayed on at the mental hospitals. While staffing the mental hospitals may have been the initial goal of the superintendents in the development of a specialized workforce, the psychiatric nurses soon developed their own agenda, becoming members of a respected, distinct, and self-governing profession.

In Manitoba geography may also have played a role. The 1957 visit of the CCPN executive from Weyburn, Saskatchewan, was accomplished in a comfortable three-hour drive to Brandon and a further two to Winnipeg. Toronto is a formidable two-day drive through the Canadian Shield. There was no pull from the east for the psychiatric nurses of Manitoba to adopt the eastern Canadian model. Had psychiatric nursing in Manitoba not aligned with the three western provinces, it would have been isolated in the middle of Canada.

But beyond political will, the wishes of the superintendents, and the aspirations for professional recognition and regional compatibility, a nursing space existed in the mental hospitals in which few others were interested. It was this unclaimed space that the male and female attendants appropriated, and that turned the work into a profession.[91]

BEVERLY HICKS
Retired Assistant Professor
Psychiatric Nursing Program
Brandon University
137 Victoria Avenue
Brandon, MB R7A 0Z2
Canada

Acknowledgments

This paper is based on a presentation made at the International History of Nursing Conference sponsored by the Canadian Association of the History of Nursing, Toronto, Ontario, 5–8 June 2008.

Notes

1. Veryl Margaret Tipliski, "Parting at the Crossroads: The Development of Education for Psychiatric Nursing in Three Canadian Provinces, 1905–1955," (PhD diss., University of Manitoba, 2002), 484.

2. The construction of insanity as a medical condition is not without controversy. See Michel Foucault, *Madness and Civilization: A History of Insanity in the Age of Reason*, trans. Richard Howard (New York: Random House, 1965); R. D. Laing, *The Divided Self: A Study of Sanity and Madness* (Harmondsworth, UK: Penguin, 1965); Thomas Szasz, *The Myth of Mental Illness* (New York: Harper and Row, 1961).

3. Asylum literature and early psychiatric nursing literature are closely related. See James E. Moran, "Keepers of the Insane: The Role of Attendants at the Toronto Provincial Asylum, 1875–1905," *Social History* 28, no. 55 (1995): 51–75; Patrick J. Connor, "Neither Courage Nor Perseverance Enough: Attendants at the Asylum for the Insane, Kingston, 1877–1905," *Ontario History* 88, no. 4 (1996): 251–72; Cheryl Krasnick Warsh, *Moments of Unreason: The Practice of Psychiatry and the Homewood Retreat, 1883–1923* (Montreal: McGill-Queen's University Press, 1989); Patricia O'Brien D'Antonio, *Founding Friends: Families, Staff and Patients at the Friends Asylum in Early Nineteenth-Century Philadelphia* (Bethlehem, Pa.: Lehigh University Press, 2006); Geertje Boschma, *The Rise of Mental Health Nursing: A History of Psychiatric Care in Dutch Asylums, 1890–1920* (Amsterdam: Amsterdam University Press, 2003); Tipliski, "Parting at the Crossroads"; Catherine Mary (Kate) Prebble, "Ordinary Men and Uncommon Women: A History of Psychiatric Nursing in New Zealand Public Mental Hospitals, 1939–1972" (PhD diss., University of Auckland, 2007); Peter Nolan, "Psychiatric Nursing, Past and Present: The Nurses' Viewpoint" (PhD diss., University of Bath, 1989); Mick Carpenter, "Asylum Nursing Before 1914: A Chapter in the History of Labour," in *Rewriting Nursing History*, ed. Celia Davies (London: Croom Helm, 1980); Alexander Walk, "The History of Mental Nursing," *Journal of Mental Science* 107 (January 1961): 1–17; Beverly Hicks, "From Barnyards to Bedsides to Books and Beyond: The Evolution and Professionalization of Registered Psychiatric Nursing in Manitoba, 1955–1980" (PhD diss., University of Manitoba, 2008); Susan T. Wood, "Changing Times: A Historical Review of Psychiatric Nursing in the Province of Saskatchewan" (master's thesis, University of Regina, 1998); Angela Martin, "Determinants of Destiny: The Professional Development of Psychiatric Nurses in Saskatchewan" (master's thesis, University of Regina, 2003); Christopher Patrick Dooley, "When Love and Skill Get Together: Work, Skill and the Occupational Culture of Mental Nurses at the Brandon Hospital for Mental Diseases 1919–1946" (master's thesis, University of Manitoba, 1998).

4. Tipliski, "Parting at the Crossroads," chap. 4.

5. Harley D. Dickinson, *The Two Psychiatries: The Transformation of Psychiatric Work in Saskatchewan, 1905–1984* (Regina: Canadian Plains Research Centre, University of Regina, 1989); Duane John Mombourquette, "A Government and Health Care: The Co-operative Commonwealth Federation in Saskatchewan, 1944–1964" (master's thesis, University of Regina, 1990).

6. Dickinson, *The Two Psychiatries*, 77; Tipliski, "Parting at the Crossroads," 281.

7. F. H. Kahan, *A Different Drummer: The History of the Saskatchewan Psychiatric Nurses' Association, 1948–1973* (Regina: Saskatchewan Psychiatric Nurses Association, 1973), 2.

8. Tipliski, "Parting at the Crossroads," 281–82.

9. Kahan, *A Different Drummer*, 7; Dickinson, *The Two Psychiatries*, 106.

10. Kahan, *A Different Drummer*, 11; Dickinson, *The Two Psychiatries*, 109.

11. Kahan, *A Different Drummer*, 13; Tipliski, "Parting at the Crossroads," 293. Battlefords, which Connon represented in the provincial legislature, was the district in which the North Battleford mental hospital was located.

12. Kahan, *A Different Drummer*, 13–14.

13. Ibid.

14. Ibid., 300.

15. The Societies Act governed the business of benevolent, social, recreational, and artistic organizations and was the only option for incorporation and recognition of the Psychiatric Nurses Association at the time. Professional legislation came later.

16. History compiled by Mrs. M. L. McKay, RN, n.d., College of Registered Psychiatric Nurses of British Columbia (CRPNBC), Port Moody. Documents located by the author in May 2007 in the CRPNBC offices in a box of memorabilia donated by the family of a well-known psychiatric nurse, Catherine Murray (hereafter CRNBC, Murray memorabilia).

17. Handwritten minutes of meetings at New Westminster, British Columbia, 22, 27 May, 2 June 1947, CRPNBC, Murray memorabilia.

18. Richard Strong, History of the Psychiatric Nurses Association of British Columbia, manuscript, n.d., CRPNBC, Murray memorabilia.

19. History compiled by Mrs. M. L. McKay RN, CRPNBC, Murray memorabilia.

20. Final Report on the Establishment of a School of Nursing at the Ponoka Mental Hospital, College of Registered Psychiatric Nurses of Alberta (CRPNA), Edmonton, Historical File, n.d. A handwritten notation states, "Sent to Dr. Baragar by Miss Kate S. Brightly, RN Registrar A.A.R.N (Alberta Association of Registered Nurses)."

21. Baragar to Hoadley, CRPNA, Historical File. The document is not dated but is obviously in response to the AARN report.

22. Ian H. Clarke, "Public Provisions for the Mentally Ill in Alberta, 1906–1936" (master's thesis, University of Calgary, 1973), 153; author unknown, "History Provincial Mental Hospital School of Nursing," n.d., CRPNA, Historical File. Baragar did not live to see this first graduation.

23. Geertje Boschma, Olive Yonge, and Lorraine Mychajlunow, "Gender and Professional Identity in Psychiatric Nursing in Alberta, Canada, 1930–1975," *Nursing Inquiry* 12, no. 4 (2005): 243–55.

24. Letter from Frank Jones (Saskatchewan Registered Psychiatric Nurses Association) to Campbell Evans (Ponoka, Alberta), 16 September 1949, suggesting they may be interested in forming an association similar to the one in Saskatchewan; letter from W. L. Pritchard (British Columbia Psychiatric Nurses Association) to C. W. Evans (Ponoka, Alberta), 30 March 1950, congratulating Alberta on its progress toward legislation and offering help, CRPNA, Historical File.

25. The Canadian Council of Psychiatric Nurses (CCPN) Archives are maintained at the offices of the Registered Psychiatric Nurses Association of Saskatchewan, Regina, Saskatchewan. The minutes of the 1955 annual meeting record that Fraternal Greetings were brought by Mr. Kenwood, delegate from BC, and by Mr. James, delegate from Alberta.

26. Kurtland I. Refvik, *History of the Brandon Mental Health Centre, 1891–1991* (Brandon, Manitoba: Brandon Mental Health Centre [BMHC] Historical Museum, 1991), xi.

27. Ibid., 2.

28. The Department of Public Works Annual Reports, 1892–1920, Manitoba Legislative Library, Winnipeg, provide detailed information on size of dairy herds, amount of vegetables harvested, and general condition of barns and stables. Labor provided by patients is dutifully recorded.

29. Christopher Dooley, "Mental Hospitals: 'Asylum Towns' in Prairie Canada, 1925–1975" (paper presented at Annual Meeting of the Canadian Historical Association, Congress of the Social Sciences and Humanities, York University, Toronto, June 2006).

30. W. L. Morton, *Manitoba: A History* (Toronto: University of Toronto Press, 1957); James Jackson, *The Centennial History of Manitoba* (Toronto: Manitoba Historical Society and McClelland and Stewart, 1970).

31. John Kendle, *John Bracken: A Political Biography* (Toronto: University of Toronto Press, 1979), 27.

32. David MacLennan, "Beyond the Asylum: Professionalization and the Mental Hygiene Movement in Canada, 1914–1938," *Canadian Bulletin of Medical History* 4 (1987): 7–23.

33. Refvik, *History of the Brandon Mental Health Centre*, 45; MacLennan, "Beyond the Asylum," 14; Cornelia Johnson, "A History of Mental Health Care in Manitoba: A Local Manifestation of an International Social Movement" (master's thesis, University of Manitoba, 1980).

34. Thomas A. Pincock, "A Half Century of Psychiatry in Manitoba," *Canada's Mental Health* 14 (May 1970): 4–10.

35. J. Matas, "The Story of Psychiatry in Manitoba," *Manitoba Medical Review* (June–July 1961): 360–64.

36. Department of Health and Public Welfare Annual Reports, Selkirk Mental Hospital (SMH) and Brandon Mental Hospital (BMH), 1921, Manitoba Legislative Library.

37. Handwritten register of all students who graduated from any of the training programs at Brandon between 1920 and 1995 (hereafter Register), BMHC Museum. Note that in 1927 three nurses had gone to St. Boniface Hospital for training and graduated with an RN. Refvik, *History of the Brandon Mental Health Centre*, 51.

38. Connor, "Neither Courage Nor Perseverance Enough." Connor explores this issue at the Kingston Mental Hospital in Ontario.

39. Department of Health and Public Welfare Annual Reports, SMH and BMH, 1920s and 1930s, Manitoba Legislative Library.

40. Notation in Register that a course had commenced for male attendants, 200.

41. Notation in Register that the course was now compulsory, 197.

42. McKee Archives, Brandon University, Brandon, Manitoba, BMHC Collection. A meticulously compiled document by an unknown author identifies the number of hours of instruction and number of weeks of clinical experience for each of the six educational programs conducted at BMH between 1920 and 1970 (hereafter referred to as the Curriculum Document).

43. Remi Beaudette, interview with author, 27 November 2006; Walter Tetzlaff, interview with author, 1 February 2007. Transcripts in McKee Archives; tapes in possession of author.

44. Curriculum Document, diploma course for female students, 1943.

45. Marlene Brichon, interview with author, 22 October 2006.

46. Stuart M. Schultz, M. D., *Notes on Psychiatry*, 1 December 1956, Provincial Archives of Manitoba (PAM), GR 6224, Q12344.

47. Revik, *History of the Brandon Mental Health Centre*, 86–87.

48. Register. Seven classes graduated with a total of 32 graduates; only a few remained at BMH.

49. Tipliski, "Parting at the Crossroads," 470.

50. These men were provincial psychiatrist Thomas Pincock, Selkirk superintendent Edward Johnson, Brandon superintendent Stuart Schultz, and Portage superintendent Henry Atkinson.

51. Schultz to Elliott, 10 October 1952, PAM, GR 157, H-14–21–1B.

52. Minutes of MARN Board Meeting, 31 May 1954, College of Registered Nurses of Manitoba Archives, Winnipeg, Canada.

53. Barry Edginton, "Moral Treatment to Monolith: The Institutional Treatment of the Insane in Manitoba, 1987–1919," *Canadian Bulletin of Medical History* 5 (1988): 176.

54. Ibid.

55. Vera Stokes, "Articles of Interest: The Evolution of the Manitoba School for Mental Defectives, Portage la Prairie 1890–1943," n.d, Manitoba Developmental Centre Museum, Portage la Prairie, Manitoba (formerly School for Mental Defectives or Portage Home for Incurables).

56. Department of Health and Public Welfare Annual Report, Provincial Mental Hospitals, 1930, Manitoba Legislative Library.

57. Minutes of MARN Board Meeting, 1 October 1937, Winnipeg, CRNM Archives.

58. Minutes of Special Meeting, 1 November 1937, CRNM Archives. The MARN Board seemed to be concerned that the proposed program had been designated as nurse training.

59. History of Licensed Practical Nursing in Manitoba, PAM, P4565, File 19.

60. Minutes of LPN Advisory Council, 11 February 1946, PAM, P4562.

61. Minutes of LPN Advisory Council, 9 September 1946, PAM P4562.

62. Advisory Council, Licensed Practical Nurses, Department of Health and Public Welfare, Manual for Administrators of Schools of Practical Nursing, November 1952, PAM, GR 157, S-14–21–1B.

63. Manual for Schools of Psychiatric Nursing, 1953, McKee Archives, BMHC Collection, SB 47.

64. Minutes of LPN Advisory Council, 6 December 1956, PAM, P4562; notation in Register, 194.

65. John Kellie, "A History of the School of Nursing: The Manitoba Developmental Centre," manuscript, 1988, College of Registered Psychiatric Nurses (CRPNM) Archives, Winnipeg, Manitoba.

66. *Dear Bill, Let's Start an Association . . . A Tribute to the Psychiatric Nurses Association of Canada on the Occasion of Its 25th Anniversary* (Port Moody: British Columbia Registered Psychiatric Nurses Association, 1976), CRPNM Archives.

67. "The History and Future of Psychiatric Nursing," *Canadian Journal of Psychiatric Nursing* 24, no. 4 (October–December 1983): 6–10.

68. "Psychiatric Nurses Association of Canada," *Prism* (July 1980): 7–16; Minutes of Meeting, 15–16 June 1951, Essondale, British Columbia, CCPN Archives.

69. Minutes of Annual Meetings, 17–18 June 1954, Essondale, British Columbia; 16–17 June 1955, North Battleford, Saskatchewan; 14–15 June 1956, Oliver, Alberta; 13–14 June 1957, Essondale, British Columbia, CCPN Archives.

70. Tipliski, "Parting at the Crossroads," 447–52.

71. Minutes of Committee Meetings, 11 January, 21 March, 11 April, 14 November, 17 December 1956; List of Committee Membership, Objectives of the Psychiatric Nursing Portion of the Program, n.d.; Philosophy Combined Course in Psychiatric and General Nursing, February 1957. CRNBC, Murray memorabilia.

72. President's report, Minutes of Meeting, 16–17 June 1955, North Battleford, Saskatchewan, CCPN Archives.

73. President's report, Minutes of Meeting, 14–15 June 1956, Oliver, Alberta, CCPN Archives.

74. Richard Strong, History of Psychiatric Nurses Association of British Columbia, ca. 1965, CRNBC, Murray memorabilia.

75. Minutes of Meeting, 16–17 June 1955, North Battleford, Saskatchewan, CCPN Archives.

76. Minutes of Meeting, 14–15 June 1956, Oliver, Alberta, CCPN Archives.

77. Doug Smith, Jock Bates, and Esyllt Wynne Jones, *Lives in the Public Service: A History of the Manitoba Government Employees' Union* (Winnipeg: Manitoba Labour Education Centre; Manitoba Government Employees' Union, 1993), 110. Both Alf Barnett from Selkirk and Art Russell from Brandon were active in union affairs in the 1950s.

78. Alf Barnett, handwritten notes, n.d., CRPNM Archives, File, Old Correspondence.

79. Annual Report (Hospital Copy), 1957, PAM, GR 6224. Miss Gladys Fitzpatrick was hired as Matron of BMH, 1 May 1957, *The Bison* 10, no. 2 (July 1957): 14.

80. *The Bison* 10, no. 2 (July 1957): 6.

81. Schreder to Russell, 23 September 1957, CRPNM Archives, File, Old Correspondence.

82. Schreder to Russell, 16 December 1957, CRPNM Archives, File, Old Correspondence. Schreder informed Russell that provincial psychiatrist Dr. Pincock "had made inquiries re establishing psychiatric nurses association."

83. Art Russell, handwritten notes of first meeting of psychiatric nurses, Brandon, Manitoba, 20 February 1958, CRPNM Archives, File, Old Correspondence.

84. Pincock to Russell, 2 May 1958, CRPNM Archives, File, Old Correspondence.

85. Pincock to superintendents, 24 November 1958, attached to letter from Schultz to BMH senior staff, CRPNM Archives, File, Old Correspondence.

86. Barnett to Sprowl at Portage la Prairie, 14 May 1959. Barnett informed Sprowl that a meeting was arranged with the government lawyer and that they needed their own lawyer, CRPNM Archives, File, Old Correspondence.

87. Wilson to Barnett, 10 June 1959, CRPNM Archives, File, Old Correspondence; Wilson to Minister of Health and Welfare, 23 June 1959, PAM, GR 459, File Psychiatric Nurses Act 1959–1968.

88. Legislative Assembly of Manitoba, *Debates and Proceedings* 4, 56 (26 March 1960): 2009, Manitoba Legislative Library.

89. Hicks, "From Barnyards to Bedsides to Books and Beyond." Over the next twenty years, men assumed numerous leadership roles. The first five presidents of the Psychiatric Nurses Association of Manitoba were men. Subsequently men achieved positions as directors of nursing and directors of nursing education at all three provincial institutions.

90. It would be unfair to say that no general nurses were supportive of psychiatric nursing. In each of the four western provinces there was at least one stalwart general nurse who supported and encouraged psychiatric nursing, and their stories have yet to be told. It was the organized professional nursing bodies that seemed disinterested.

91. http://www.rpnc.ca. The profession in western Canada has continued to survive and thrive. Currently more than 5,000 RPNs are employed in a variety of positions.

Political Dreams, Practical Boundaries: The Case of the Nursing Minimum Data Set, 1983–1990

Jennifer Hobbs
VA San Diego Healthcare System

Abstract. The initial development of the Nursing Minimum Data Set (NMDS) was analyzed based on archival material from Harriet Werley and Norma Lang, two nurses involved with the project, and American Nurses Association materials. The process of identifying information to be included in the NMDS was contentious. Individual nurses argued on behalf of particular data because of a strong belief in how nursing practice (through information collection) should be structured. Little attention was paid to existing practice conditions that would ultimately determine whether the NMDS would be used.

In 1985, a small group of highly educated and motivated nurse administrators and faculty from across the United States met to identify and develop a nursing-specific data set.[1] The group intended the data set to provide administrators and researchers a means for evaluating the delivery of nursing care. This was a tall order, made more difficult by the group's choice of application and use of the Nursing Minimum Data Set (NMDS) in no fewer than five settings where nurses practiced: hospitals, ambulatory care, home care, community, and long-term care. This data set was to be a collection of information about nursing practice arranged into specific categories. Each category, for instance patient demographics, was given a narrow definition that provided a means of consistency (in theory) regardless of who collected the data or where.

However, a data set is never isolated from the beliefs and biases of the individuals who create it. Any data set provides an interesting window into what members of a given group think about their work; the NMDS provides a unique opportunity to analyze a particular perspective on nursing work. The NMDS was an attempt to create an altogether different record of patient care, one that promoted and represented the work of nursing rather than medicine. If the nurses involved succeeded in getting the NMDS adopted and disseminated, this alternative record would fully recognize that another provider besides physicians delivered essential care to patients as it offered information about the work of nurses.

This article examines the pre-conference planning, actual conference, and post-conference debates surrounding the creation of the NMDS. The study is based on primary sources from the two nurses responsible for convening the NMDS conference, Drs. Harriet Werley and Norma Lang.[2] The documents reviewed shaped the particular story surrounding the creation of the NMDS and was largely told from the perspective of these two individuals through memos, papers, letters, meeting minutes, and conference proceedings.

Lively discussions erupted over what information to include in the data set, how to organize it, and, perhaps most important, why certain types of information were necessary. Many of the nurses involved with the NMDS staked their careers on how the data set developed and how it might be used. They also prioritized, organized, and promoted certain aspects of practice though their information choices. These choices were illustrative of their beliefs about practice, and a reflection of the context in which the choices were made. Examining the things people created in order to better control their social environment, particularly those aimed at organizing clinical information, illuminates perceptions about clinical authority and social power. These factors in turn elucidates the means by which nurses attempted to shape patient care.

Nurses involved with the NMDS ardently believed that if they had more clinical information, they could better understand—and, more important, have power over—clinical practice. Using this power, these nurses believed they would have the capacity to thwart attempts to dictate the work of nurses by groups like medicine.[3] They believed that by using information contained in the NMDS they could facilitate policy changes, gain bureaucratic representation within health care organizations, and ultimately help organize the work of nurses. These were logical assumptions about how this information could be applied, but the nurses failed to deal directly with the political nature of their proposal.

Background of the NMDS

After the passing of the 1965 Social Security Act Amendments that launched the Medicare and Medicaid programs, and subsequent additions to that law in 1972, the U.S. government experienced dramatic increases in health care costs.[4] Implementing these social services, which facilitated access for the elderly and individuals with particular ailments such as end-stage renal disease, contributed greatly to rising health care expenditures. The initial setup of these programs had virtually no caps on spending. If a hospital wanted to increase profits, all it had to do was increase patient volume and the diversity of services offered.

Patients were beginning to feel empowered to make decisions about their care and to anticipate high-quality care.[5] This expectation manifested an anticipation of cure, access to all the latest technology, and skillful expertise not only from physicians but also from nurses. Thus, while cost evaluation on the part of hospitals and government-sponsored programs was important, so was the need for hospitals to evaluate the quality of services delivered.

This need to evaluate both costs and quality of service prompted development of two levels of information practices aimed at evaluating practice or service provision at the local and national aggregate level. Locally derived practices focused on streamlining data collection to evaluate and then improve practice. During the late 1970s and early 1980s, a plethora of charting tools were introduced. Some of the more popular tools, several of which are still in use, were the SOAPE (subjective, objective, assessment, plan, and evaluation) charting format, the POMR (problem-oriented medical record), and the nursing process known as ADPIE (assessment, diagnosis, plan, intervention, and evaluation).[6] These tools served to identify some of the care nurses and physicians delivered to patients, and also provided a means to deal with increasing complexity of practice.[7]

Nationally, information practices focused on making the work surrounding patient care visible. This was a necessary step for physicians and nurses alike if, under the new federally funded programs, physicians desired continued reimbursement for services and nurses desired the opportunity to cost out their services and determine staffing.[8] Information associated with treatment decisions that involved specific levels of care, technology, or other types of billable services provided the means to evaluate practice on an aggregate level. The information then served as a proxy for practice in terms of what was done for patients. Although the stated purposes of these information practices were quality assurance and cost evaluation (with control of costs to follow), many, if not most, initially had to identify practice. To a certain extent, there was a void of information about the general types of services offered to patients.

Professional organizations such as the American Psychological Association (APA), government agencies, and groups such as the American Hospital Association (AHA) were all working to develop information practices to evaluate services in terms of cost.[9] It was during this time that the Department of Health and Human Services (DHHS) developed the hospital discharge data set, first put together in 1974 and revised in 1979 and 1984.[10]

Nurses were looking into designing a data set as well. However, in contrast the AHA or APA, it was not a nursing professional organization like the American Nurses Association (ANA) that took on the task of designing the NMDS. Throughout the development period, the ANA was struggling with budgetary and membership issues. It was losing members to emerging specialty organizations poised to meet the needs of nurses working in areas that required specialized skills and knowledge such as critical care, nephrology, and oncology. As the areas of specialization grew, the ANA's struggle to maintain responsibility over the scope, standards, and certification of nursing practice intensified. These persistent problems kept the organization preoccupied with staying financially viable and limited its participation in the design of information practices.

Given this lack of centralized leadership in nursing, many nurses working independently of the ANA sought ways to capitalize on public and government interest in health-related information. One of the numerous information practices proposed during the period was a Minimum Data Set (MDS). An MDS held particular appeal because, as the name signifies, it was the least amount of information needed to evaluate a given service.[11] Most MDSs designed in the 1970s and 1980s identified the services provided to patients and evaluated costs. Additionally, each data set needed to be useful for most if not all potential users, contain no duplicate data (data contained in another MDS), be reasonably easy to collect, and, as was the case with health-related data sets, protect the identity of patients.

The Pre-Conference Planning Phase: 1983–1985

In 1983, Harriet Werley, a professor of nursing at the University of Wisconsin–Milwaukee, sought out likeminded nurses to plan a conference to identify an NMDS. Werley was a well-known nurse educator and researcher who before entering academia had a long and distinguished military career. At the Walter Reed Army Institute of Research, she participated in conferences initiated by IBM to identify data processing needs in health care.[12] These experiences shaped her understanding of nursing's need for data to study and improve clinical practice. Werley asked for the collaboration of her dean, Norma Lang, who agreed to co-chair this yet-to-materialize conference. Lang's background, including service on Wisconsin's Professional Standards Review Organization

(PSRO) Hospital Review System and a much longer academic career path, was very different from Werley's.[13] In the late 1970s Lang worked to identify and develop cost and quality measures for the state. Lang and Werley held similar interests with regard to information tools and practice issues, and they were committed to developing an NMDS that represented nursing practice.

Pre-conference planning began in 1983 in anticipation of a formal conference in 1985.[14] The local planning group was comprised of colleagues of Werley and Lang, the majority of whom resided in the immediate geographical area of Milwaukee. Within the planning group, there were two main groups interested in the NMDS: hospital nursing administrators interested in accounting for nursing care delivery and faculty interested in researching the clinical activities of nurses. The local planning group made numerous requests for funding from the National Center for Health Statistics, Weston National Center for Health Services Research, and the DHHS Division of Nursing, but all rejected the requests, stating that the NMDS was not a funding priority.[15]

Despite financial difficulties, Werley and Lang continued planning for the conference, holding meetings throughout the summer, fall, and winter of 1983. At the 11 July 1983 meeting the group quickly came to a consensus that the intent of the NMDS was "professional control of practice." Participants argued that the NMDS would enable management of practice through establishment of norms, standards, and cost of nursing services. The group believed that dictating the information collected was the way to determine priorities of nursing work, going so far as to equate "control of practice [with] control of information."[16]

Because this type of financial and professional control was so incredibly valuable, many discussions erupted at the local planning meetings about the future content of the NMDS. The nurses saw this as an opportunity to represent nurses' work through information, and each tried to advocate for his or her particular view of the profession via inclusion of specific data points. While Werley believed in the importance of information, she continually reminded the group that they were "not talking about establishing a professional identity."[17]

But the nurses working on planning for the NMDS believed they *were* trying to establish a professional identity. The planning group was determining what information was representative of nursing practice when deciding on different points of data that best captured nursing's work. Members purposely selected information that "delineate[d] [the] discipline's scientific knowledge," leaning heavily toward academic aspects of practice.[18] At one of the meetings just prior to the NMDS conference, a member commented that the data points identified to date "might not provide adequately for the inclusion of . . . worker related variables" and of "data of interest to nurse administrators . . . thus the NMDS might not reflect the context of nursing care."[19]

This comment goes beyond addressing the simple notion of disconnect between nursing service and education, and emphasizes the type of information choices being made by the group. Including data points that highlighted nurses' decision-making capacity and scope, in contrast to those that captured nursing resources (staffing, skill mix), essentially promoted a particular perspective of nursing practice. The NMDS was intended to create a record of care that recognized the critical services nurses delivered to patients. Separating the nurse from the costs of the hospital room was a common refrain and emblematic of the group's motivation. Formal identification of nursing services was nonexistent in bureaucratic terms, so the potential power associated with the idea of the NMDS was substantial.[20]

One of the more heated discussions surrounded the review of commissioned papers. It was decided early in the planning phase that select attendees would be asked to present papers on topics related to the NMDS. Prior to the conference, the planning committee collected and vetted forty-three papers from colleagues and members of the planning group who held likeminded positions about the construction of a NMDS.[21] Two papers in particular addressing the use of nursing resources drew animated conversation at the January 1984 meeting.

One of these controversial papers identified variables for measuring the cost-effectiveness of nursing care delivered.[22] It proposed a number of measures that examined nursing services in terms of cost, and therefore framed potential solutions in terms of cost cutting. Such measures would be handy for nurse administrators who were responsible for hospital-wide budgets, but the measures carried risks. Framing nursing care in terms of costs rather than profit placed these services at risk each time budgetary crises emerged. This, along with the fact that the measures were not singularly nurse dependent, prompted doubts over the usefulness of these data points.

The second and more political of the two papers examined measures to assign a monetary value to nursing services in terms of revenue generated.[23] At the time the only other providers viewed in this manner were physicians and surgeons. For nurse administrators, this was a double-edged sword. If their areas of responsibility demonstrated profit, their power might increase within their organizations. In addition, if hospitals or government payers collected data on the cost of nursing services across the country, nurses could use the information to change the dynamics of state and national negotiations about health care spending. However, the prospect of selling this data collection strategy to hospitals or government payers was limited for the same reasons. Assigning a monetary value to nursing services challenged the bargaining power of other providers, namely physicians, who largely laid claim to revenue generation. If the data collection strategy was successful, it would force hospitals to negotiate with nursing. Despite the political nature of the proposed paper, it was accepted as one of thirty to be presented at the conference.[24]

At times it was unclear whether there would be a conference at all. The planning committee continued to search for funding throughout the spring and summer of 1983 without success. They solicited financial support from the Robert Wood Johnson Foundation and the Health Care Financing Administration; both declined.[25] Early in the fall Roy Simpson, a member of the planning committee and director of hospital systems support for the Hospital Corporation of America, suggested that the group seek funding from his organization's foundation.[26] Werley quickly pulled together a grant application and sent it off.

With funding issues still unresolved, the planning group focused on further selection of potential information to include in the NMDS. The nurses reviewed existing MDSs for ideas about what information to include in theirs. During this review they first wrestled with what would become a formidable issue: the fact that the data set proposed by Werley and colleagues was overtly provider specific.[27] The DHHS had fueled the creation of MDS by favoring development of patient-specific, and in some cases site-specific, MDSs. This made sense because the agency was attempting to evaluate costs of services rather than costs of specific providers such as nurses or physicians.

Still, each of the data sets sanctioned and collected by facilities for the DHHS did contain provider information (either physician or surgeon). So, although the expectation that labeling the data set nursing specific made the information no more provider specific than the ambulatory or discharge data sets promoted by the DHHS, it did not conform to the commonly understood standard. The idea of removing the *nurse* identification embedded in the data set was not well received, especially by Werley, who halted any discussion on the matter.[28]

In January 1984, the planning committee revisited the Hospital Corporation funding application.[29] Werley had contacted Simpson numerous times about the status of the application, and he had not replied. Werley's frustration showed in her communications to the planning group as she lamented the lack of response.

Revamping Health Care Reimbursement

Werley's frustration was understandable since the momentum that had fueled the identification of information practices like the NMDS had stalled with the rollout of the Diagnosis Related Group (DRG) program. With the passing of the 1982 Tax Equity and Fiscal Responsibility Act and its implementation in 1983, the primary assumption embedded in the government's cost containment effort was that all patients with the same or related diagnoses required the same care.[30] Essentially, the care provided had to comply with an established set of standards linked to a particular diagnosis or cluster of diagnoses known as a DRG. The government set standards and payment based on what was considered appropriate treatment, length of stay, and service intensity for a given diagnosis. Hospitals and providers were busy dealing with the details of the new DRG billing procedure, and organizations that might have supported the NMDS conference were instead attending to this new information demand.

Later the following year, the DHHS revision of its Hospital Discharge Data Set occupied the planning group discussions.[31] Conference planners were interested in two major revisions of physician identifiers: one that split the attending physician and surgeon into separate categories and one that indicated the type and date of procedures.[32] The latter revision included a notation about the risks associated with surgical intervention. These risks were identified by the categories *procedural*, *anesthetic*, or *specialized training*. These physician identifiers generated discussion about how nurse identifiers would be used in the NMDS.[33]

The opportunity to differentiate the type of nurse delivering care to patients was important. The creators of the NMDS wanted to distinguish between registered and unlicensed nurses, and to identify nurses who were prepared at the diploma, associate, baccalaureate, and master's level.[34] The administrators on the planning committee resisted this, preferring instead to measure hours of (generic) nursing care given to patients. They feared that identifying the type of nurse might limit their discretion to use less costly staff if links were made between improved patient outcomes and more highly educated nurses. This was a very politically charged notion and a difficult one to mandate in terms of data collection. Unlike a physician or surgeon who took care of patients across a hospitalization, a patient might receive care from numerous nurses or their delegates such as nurses' aides.

Furthermore, identifying patient risk in terms of nursing care delivered was a challenge. Risk was important, because greater patient risk meant higher levels of services consumed and higher costs associated with the nursing care provided. The planning group debated several proposals that argued for one or another mechanism for risk evaluation, but all framed risk in terms of patient acuity.[35] Patient acuity was defined somewhat differently depending on when the evaluation was completed and who designed the particular tool, but generally speaking the tools measured the amount of nursing care needed by a patient. The planning group reviewed several popular acuity tools, but did not choose one. All involved with the group did, however, agreed that a risk evaluation measure would be included, and the decision was tabled until the conference.

In December 1984, conference planners finally received good news regarding funding. The Hospital Corporation of America Foundation agreed to partially fund the event with a conference grant; these funds were in addition to the University of Wisconsin School of Nursing support already being used.[36] The IBM Corporation, contacted through Werley's old military connections, was also brought on as a small sponsor and agreed to provide computers for use during the conference.[37]

The NMDS Conference: 1985

Conference planners extended invitations to a select group of sixty-five individuals including nurses, information systems experts, and health records specialists.[38] Sixty-four of the invitees attended the conference, held in Milwaukee, 15–17 May 1985. In the conference proceedings submitted for publishing later that year, Werley gave the impression that the attendees were a diverse group that included clinicians, administrators, researchers, and faculty, and that this group represented the concerns of the staff who would be called upon to collect a large portion of the information required by the data set. However, the only three clinicians in attendance were advanced practice nurses, and probably not the type of nurse responsible for collecting information. Essentially, the makeup of the group was not so different from other groups formed during the time period who worked on designing information tools: elite and highly educated nurses, none of whom could reasonably be considered representative of the average nurse practicing in a hospital.

Werley's opening plenary remarks reviewed the planning committee's work and highlighted the main challenge associated with the creation of the NMDS—meeting the needs of multiple data users in multiple clinical sites.[39] Further complicating the design challenges was the diversity in skill and educational training of nurses at the five sites. To put the scope of this data set into perspective required considering newly adopted responsibilities of nurses. Nurse practitioners were diagnosing and treating patients, and staff nurses in specialty areas were increasingly intervening on patients' behalf, often relying on standing orders and their independent decision-making skills rather than physician interaction. The important point, as it relates to the NMDS, is that nurses adopted the various skills and knowledge needed to execute these activities, and these skills were variable not only within a given clinical area such as acute care but most certainly across different areas. If the NMDS was to be useful or even simply reflective of the care being given, it had to be relevant not only across this variability but also to different types of nurses.

Perhaps Lang was more sensitive than Werley to the challenges that faced the NMDS. Lang's opening comments reflected what she considered the biggest challenge facing participants: that of achieving consensus in an era of specialization and differentiation.[40] Her statements reflected both her experiences in writing the ANA Social Policy Statement and the realities of practice. The ANA Social Policy Statement had been released in 1981 as an attempt on the part of Lang, other members of the committee responsible for its creation, and the ANA to describe nursing's contribution to patients.[41] The statement's release was met with an intense push back from practicing nurses, whose immediate clinical experiences were not reflected in it. Their practice realities were such that patients were requiring increasingly specialized care. For all intents and purposes, the NMDS was moving in the opposite direction from nursing and health care, which were moving toward specialization. Lang, while certainly supporting the work of the NMDS, made it very clear that the time ahead would be challenging.[42]

The conference itself focused on thirty papers commissioned by the planning group. Participants who presented papers addressed different elements of the NMDS, including a wide range of topics such as data set integration, regulatory requirements, and general upkeep of the NMDS, once it was defined. Werley portrayed these papers as representative of the presenters' individual perspectives, but conference planners had heavily edited all the papers prior to acceptance, going so far as to request revisions to significant portions of the content.[43] The papers were used as jumping-off points for discussion about the NMDS content, and participants reached a consensus rather quickly with regard to the general types of data acceptable for inclusion. Task forces formed around each of the six topic areas: demographics, assessment, diagnosis, intervention, outcomes, and acuity/intensity.[44] It is within the task forces that participants addressed the most contentious issues and critical decisions of the conference.

The Demographic Task Force

One of the main points of contention concerned demographic data. Joyce Anderson, an administrator at Memorial Medical Center, Long Beach, California, chaired the task force that had selected patient identifier, medical diagnosis, sex, race, ethnicity, date of birth, and so forth as demographic items.[45] These data points were reasonable inclusions, except that they were duplicated in two DHHS data sets already in wide use: the Ambulatory Care Data Set and the Uniform Hospital Discharge Data Set. This violated a generally accepted standard for information of this type.

Many of the attendees argued for dropping the patient, facility, and medical demographic data, but Werley halted discussion on the matter.[46] With some support, she pushed for the inclusion of all demographic data regardless whether it was duplicated elsewhere. This was motivated in part by pragmatic issues arising from the intended use of the NMDS in five clinical areas. If the NMDS was to become a viable information practice, the demographic data were needed for eventual linkages comparison to other MDSs. But the decision was also strongly motivated by professional pride. The object of nursing care was and remains the patient, and the demographic task force selected patient data points that were "most discriminating regarding nursing (process) resource or services required (utilized)."[47] Members viewed selection of patient, facility, and staff demographics as self-defining for nursing. Naming aspects of the patient that were pertinent to nursing care, aspects of the facility that were critical to nursing, and aspects of the nurse that were critical to the profession were not areas where Werley entertained compromise.

This desire to make nursing a visible entity in bureaucratic terms was a strong motivator, but also a detriment. The DHHS basic standard for MDS information practice was very clear—MDSs were designed to complement, not replicate, each other. The insistence on inclusion of all demographic information in the NMDS created difficulties for anyone considering adopting it. For hospitals, it meant that the burden of information collection would not be lessened but possibly increased by the adoption of the NMDS. Despite these very straightforward issues, the participants, under Werley's insistence, moved forward with inclusion of the data. Also addressed in the demographic task force meetings was the problem of mechanism to identify the nurse providers involved with a patient's service use. Again the scope of the data set forced inherent problems to the surface and made the task challenging. Because the NMDS was to be used in five different service areas, identifying a single data point (or even a cluster of data points) to recognize the nurse provider was nearly impossible. The task force was keen to identify nurse practitioners (NP) because this type of nurse had expanded practice boundaries compared to other nurses. But the task force also had to consider providers in areas such as long-term care, where a registered nurse or unlicensed personnel (e.g., a nurse's aide) delivered the majority of care. The NMDS creators were faced with first identifying the types of nurses caring for the patient and then deciding how many of the nurse providers to identify.

Unlike physicians, whose episode of care extended across a patient's service use or was limited to discrete interventions, nurses' work was not easily anchored to a single patient or point in time. Patients relied on nurses for twenty-four-hour care, and therefore it took more than one nurse to care for a hospitalized patient. If the nurses designing the NMDS wanted to capture the care delivered, they needed to decide whether they were going to give each nurse a provider number, or group types of providers by skill level. Ultimately they chose neither of these, and instead decided to identify a primary nurse for an entire episode of care, such as an NP or a specialized registered nurse. This identification was ultimately geared toward identifying nurses with greater responsibility, like NPs or nurses with specialized training, to ease cost capture.

The Assessment Task Force

The assessment task force started its session by developing a consensus statement stressing the importance of the information collected during the course of a physical exam.[48] The group noted that patient information generated from physical assessment was the foundation of the nursing information system. This statement was well accepted among the nurses involved with the NMDS, but its broad scope was also at odds with the purpose of the NMDS—to identify the minimal amount of information needed to evaluate services provided to patients. Throughout the conference the members struggled to balance the scope of the data set with their desire to make nursing visible. The urgency to affect nurse identification through information collection meant that the NMDS constantly pushed its own purpose boundaries. The nurses wanted the data set to be a decision-support system used in real time, just as much as they wanted a post-service data collection tool. If there was any awareness about inherent incompatibility of these information demands, it was not reflected in the decisions made by the group.

Despite this, the assessment task force attempted to choose from among four standardized physical examination forms: a checklist, Gordon's Functional Health Patterns, the Classification of Nursing Diagnosis Taxonomy, and a five-page general health assessment form from the University of Iowa.[49] Using assessment categories from each of the samples, the task force tried to come up with a list of around fifteen items. The difficulty they experienced was evident in their report to the main group, which highlighted difficulties with selecting items to represent physical exam information relevant across the five settings where the NMDS was to be used. The task force struggled to select data points that made sense for a medical-surgical patient as well as a patient in critical, long-term, or ambulatory care.[50] Anderson continually returned to the idea that the NMDS should support nurse decision making in a variety of settings, although again this was not a function of an MDS. In the end, the creators decided to drop assessment from the data set altogether, opting instead to place this information in a clinical abstract.

The clinical abstract was fast becoming an additional information tool being developed by the group. At this point in the conference, the purpose of the clinical abstract might be best defined as an information catchall, as it was the category where any information that did not fit easily into the standardized NMDS was placed. It included some narrative information like a general statement about patient issues upon admission, and checklists like the assessment tools mentioned above. The abstract was also intended to give some context for the information in the data set, functioning like a clinical story that chronicles the patient's episode of service. For the time being, the task force left the general category of assessment information in the abstract, with no decision about what specific assessment information to include.[51]

The Assessment and Diagnosis Joint Task Force

The definition of nursing diagnosis selected and approved by the diagnosis task force, chaired by Christine Tanner of Oregon Health Sciences University, was the same as that in the ANA Social Policy Statement, which defined nursing practice as treatment of patient's responses to illness, not the illness itself.[52] That statement was highly controversial, especially for nurses in advanced practice roles. NPs and other nurses affected by the need for specialization saw the nursing diagnosis definition as a step backward, yet despite this opposition and the ANA removal of the statement from the Social Policy Statement four years prior to the NMDS conference, the NMDS nurses accepted it without much discussion.

The topic that generated the most discussion was which nursing diagnoses of the numerous sets available should be included in the NMDS. Because the creators of the NMDS agreed that nursing diagnosis was the end product of assessment, conference organizers asked the assessment and diagnosis task forces to work together to address this issue. However, the two task forces could not agree. The diagnosis group saw significant differences between assessment categories and nursing diagnosis, where the assessment group did not.[53] The assessment task force wanted fourteen to sixteen classification categories from which to select a diagnosis for a particular patient, rather than using a specific nursing diagnosis. For example, there were three general categories of assessment: functions, behaviors, and conditions, all of which broke into subcategories of data. The subcategories were items such as self-care management, emotion, and cognition. The diagnosis group, in contrast, wanted a specific nursing diagnosis identified, even though multiple nursing diagnoses were often used across a patient's service use. Moreover, the specificity of the nursing diagnosis (when compared to the generality of the assessment categories) was problematic because it left little room for the homegrown nursing diagnoses that facilities actually used.

The intense debate surrounding nursing diagnosis was largely owed to the composition of the diagnosis task force, which included many influential members of the North American Nursing Diagnosis Association (NANDA). NANDA saw itself as responsible for sanctioning nursing diagnosis and creating the Classification of Nursing Diagnosis,[54] though it was struggling to adopt an overarching framework for the classification while keeping control over the nursing diagnosis production process. The group was considering adopting a controversial nursing theory, and members of NANDA in attendance at the NMDS conference saw potential for conflict if any other framework was adopted. By promoting individual nursing diagnosis over a classification, NANDA was free to continue pursuing its preferred organizing framework for its taxonomy.

The assessment task force took a different approach, modeling the organization of nursing diagnosis around categories that cut across the different service settings the NMDS intended to represent. For example, the self-care category would apply in each setting, but the assessment data included there would be different if the patient was hospitalized versus using home health services. This approach gave the NMDS flexibility to include nursing diagnosis generated from other nursing groups, such as the Omaha system designed for use in community-oriented areas of practice like home health. Openness to consideration of other diagnosis classifications, however, was threatening to the NANDA group, which was trying to gain recognition from the ANA as *the* organization responsible for production and approval of nursing diagnosis. Conference organizers, who also attended some of the NANDA conferences, did not want to see the NMDS meeting derailed, so they tabled further discussion, intending to revisit the issue at the post-conference meetings.[55]

The Intervention Task Force

Karen Rieder, who worked in the Veterans Administration (VA) system and chaired the intervention task force, oversaw the development of sixteen categories of nursing interventions during the conference. While this topic and its associated subcategories did not generate much discussion, one interesting item removed early from the list of interventions was "monitoring equipment."[56] Use of monitoring equipment as part of patient care was growing at a rapid pace, and nurses were expected not only to be able to use a given piece of equipment but also to understand what actions to take based on the information generated by that tool. Even technology previously used by nurses, for example, blood pressure cuffs, were now used differently or more frequently as monitoring tools. In other words, nurses' time was increasingly occupied with not only operating equipment, but also recording and acting on the information generated.

Since monitoring equipment was used to gather information, and that information was often used to assess patient condition, the NMDS group subsumed this topic under surveillance, a category that encompassed physiological and psychological assessment. What is interesting about this category is that the creators of the NMDS seemed to fail to recognize that just this one topic represented a mountain of data work for the average nurse. This omission reflected not only the academic and administrative composition of the task force, but also a subtle resistance to the technology itself. Superficially, applications of technology were equated with a task orientation to the work of nursing, which held a negative connotation for the NMDS group. The group continued to identify additional data points without much consideration of how the sheer volume of data would influence the work of nurses.

The Outcomes Task Force

The outcomes task force defined the outcomes associated with nursing care as nursing treatment's influence on consumer health status. Barbara Given, task force chair and a faculty member at Michigan State University College of Nursing, presented the three general categories subsumed under health status: role resumption, health management, and activities of daily living (ADL).[57] Role resumption attempted to measure a patient's ability to resume his or her job, health management examined a patient's ability to manage his or her illness, and ADL considered how well a patient was able to execute personal hygiene, feeding, and so forth. The ADL and health management indexes were measured as independent, interdependent, or dependent, while role resumption was qualified as immediate, delayed, or adaptive.

For the most part the task force took a pragmatic approach to the three categories, with one major reservation: if these outcomes were associated with nursing care, how then could the influence of the institution and other professionals involved with patient care be separated? The group raised this question in part because, like the nurses involved with NANDA, the nurses who worked on the NMDS wanted to contribute to the differentiation of nursing care from medical care.[58] Of particular concern was how care rendered by physicians was framed by existing data sets as independent of outside influence and attributable to one person, whereas nursing care was subsumed under room costs and involved more than one nurse for any given patient. For the time being, the task force accepted the categories and moved on to the final section of the NMDS.

The Acuity/Intensity Task Force

Sue Ellen Pinkerton chaired the acuity/intensity task force, which met in two sessions over the course of the conference. Pinkerton was a nurse administrator who later went on to be chief nursing officer for the University of Florida Medical Center in Gainesville. In the first session the task force produced a general definition of acuity/intensity: the amount and level of nursing resources an individual patient required in a single episode of hospitalization, day of stay, or encounter.[59] The several qualifiers defining *episode* were necessary due to the scope of the NMDS, with its five service areas. But they was also a point of confusion because the NMDS group used acuity/intensity, a largely hospital-based measure of resource use, to represent service use in areas such as home health, community care, and long-term care.

Also discussed under the umbrella of acuity/intensity was the caregiver's skill level. Although how and where to include skill level had already been debated under the demographic category, it was revisited here because of the assumption that the sicker the patient or the more complex the management, the higher the skill level required of the nurse.[60] Again, while this conceptualization of service use worked well in the hospital, it did not necessarily apply in the other areas covered by the NMDS. Furthermore, it did not take into consideration nurses not directly involved with patient care activities, like nurse administrators or case managers, or nursing care delivered by more than one type of nurse. As with most of the discussions where the answer was not clear, Werley stepped in and made the decision. In this case, she determined that the reporting of staff mix/skill level would be determined by agency, tabling any further discussion to the post-conference meeting.

The Close of the Conference

In the interim between the close of the NMDS conference in May 1985 and the September 1985 post-conference meeting, participants who had presented papers were again asked to revise and resubmit their work to Werley for review.[61] She intended to solicit interest from various nurse-friendly academic book editors in the hopes of publishing a volume of conference proceedings. However, despite the apparent progress of the group, problems began to surface in the months leading up to the post-conference. It seemed that after the May meeting Werley had the sense that the data set was getting away from her and responded by tightening control over the remaining NMDS communications and meetings.[62]

This sense manifested itself first in Werley's editing style, which included a broad editorial purview and acute attention to the content, specific word usage, due dates, and general details of the manuscripts submitted to her.[63] While this strained her relations and collaboration with the authors (most submissions included profuse apologies each time an author turned something in for review), Werley's manner was perhaps most troubling for Lang, who bore the brunt of it because she was coeditor with Werley and responsible for reviewing all the papers. A continual stream of handwritten and typed letters from Werley flooded Lang's desk in the four months leading up to the post-conference. Werley tracked when a manuscript was delivered to Lang, when it was returned, and to what degree the editing was satisfactory. She also sent detailed notes to Lang critiquing her comments and questioning each decision she made. While Werley was known for her no-nonsense editorial style, the feedback she provided Lang was unsolicited.[64]

The Post-Conference

The post-conference was held in Chicago in September of 1985. The task force leaders revised and submitted reports summarizing their conference sessions, and the issues left unresolved created the agenda for the post-conference meeting.[65] The content and purpose of the clinical abstract, selection of a nursing diagnosis classification, and ownership of the data set were all on the agenda. Each task force leader and others in attendance at the conference sent comments ahead to Werley, hoping to influence the remaining decisions to be made surrounding the NMDS.

The post-conference meeting started with a discussion about the general purpose of the NMDS. Werley stressed repeatedly that the data set was not designed to support clinical decision making, but rather was to represent clinical practice after it was delivered.[66] This clarification was needed because much of what the NMDS nurses focused on was how clinicians might use the data set in practice as a decision-making tool. This focus was understandable; Werley and the other nurses used conference time for concurrent discussions of nursing information systems designed to support clinical decision making. Still, the data set the group was trying to develop remained a post-service use data collection tool, not an active charting tool. Werley, adding to the mixed messages, pushed for keeping many elements in the NMDS that were duplicated in other MDSs because in her view doing so moved nurses closer to a universal model for documentation.

After refocusing the group, Werley moved on to a discussion about the clinical abstract. To date, the clinical abstract had been the catchall for data points that either did not fit into one of the NMDS categories or did not lend themselves to discrete consistent categories, for instance, patient assessment data. The discussion of the clinical abstract brought to the surface concerns about the sheer size of the NMDS and the potential poor acceptance of the information practice because of its enormity.[67] It was suggested that the clinical abstract was actually a more appropriate and manageable representation of the nursing care delivered, and participants suggested that it should function as a face sheet to be completed at the end of a patient's service use. Again, as with previous challenges, Werley tabled the discussion and moved to review the decision to place assessment in the abstract.

There were many concerns about the removal of assessment data from the NMDS. Academic nurses believed that leaving out these data points made it difficult to convey the clinical effectiveness of the interventions delivered to the patient. Nurse administrators argued for excluding assessment because they worried about the size of the NMDS and the inconsistency with which nurses applied assessment skills. Standardizing a particular level of assessment meant that many nurses employed under the administrators automatically fell short because of lack of training. After much discussion a vote was called, resulting in a 6–5 vote in favor of excluding assessment from the data set entirely, followed by unanimous support for including the data in the clinical abstract.[68]

The group next addressed the issue of nursing diagnosis. At the close of the conference, the remaining issue was how nursing diagnoses would be arranged in the NMDS, and two arguments were made: either organize diagnoses by the sixteen assessment categories selected by the NMDS group or choose one of several diagnosis classifications in development. Those in favor of using the sixteen categories associated with assessment argued for leaving the nursing diagnosis category open, citing inconsistencies with application and general development of nursing diagnosis. Moreover, if the section were left open, each facility could decide for itself which classification best represented its practice area. Werley called a straw vote on the matter to limit discussion, with results largely split along NANDA membership lines, and no decision was reached.[69]

Discussion moved on, and the data category of nursing interventions was reviewed. The group decided, with little protest, to remove interventions from the NMDS and place them in the clinical abstract.[70] Some expressed concern over duplicate information in the demographic and acuity/intensity sections. After a brief discussion, the information describing service elements was removed from the demographic section. Although this move addressed the duplicate information in the data set, the issue of the same elements contained in multiple other data sets was not resolved. Werley, taking a stubborn stance, refused to change the demographic information or remove elements that were already collected in other sets like the Hospital Discharge Data Set.

The final issue taken up at the post-conference was that of ownership of the NMDS. During the meeting sessions group members voiced concerns regarding licensing.[71] Many felt that licensing would hinder the uptake of the NMDS by limiting interest to those who could afford to purchase it. Overwhelmingly the post-conference group felt that it was most appropriate to allow for free use or public ownership of the data set. The group agreed that the University of Wisconsin–Milwaukee School of Nursing would house the data set, with Werley and Lang supporting its dissemination though various means.

Communication about the data set by Werley and Lang to members of the nursing profession had already occurred prior to the post-conference meeting. Lang, because of her strong connection to the ANA, was often a point of contact for many of the elected leadership of the organization and had given several presentations on the NMDS. This began to upset Werley, who prior to the post-conference meeting communicated her concern over Lang's involvement in a series of notes attached to her general formal school business communication with Lang.[72] The tenor of the notes reflected a growing perception by Werley that she was losing some control over the data set. It is unclear whether the spontaneous decision by the NMDS post-conference participants to have Werley and Lang disseminate the NMDS, or some other unidentified issue, pushed Werley to accuse Lang of taking credit for the NMDS.[73]

Troubles with Dissemination of the NMDS, 1986–1990

After the events in Chicago, Werley focused on producing a manuscript of the conference proceedings. She found an editor interested in publishing the manuscript and continued to follow up with authors of the conference papers for their revisions.[74] In addition to the manuscript, there were three planned dissemination strategies for the NMDS: to raise awareness about the data set within the nursing community through various professional conferences, solicit government agencies to adopt the data set, and apply for funding to conduct research on the data set.[75]

The interaction between the general nursing community and the NMDS was minimal. Werley solicited feedback from colleagues. A few had misgivings about the selection of the NANDA classification; almost all voiced concern about repeating elements in the data set.[76] Barbara Gallant, a nurse administrator, attended one of Werley's presentations on the NMDS and pressed Werley to address the information burden the data set placed on staff nurses.[77] Gallant felt that staff nurses would bear the brunt of the data collection required by the NMDS. Werley disregarded Gallant's and others' comments, again leaving the duplicate elements intact.

That decision proved to be a major hurdle as Werley turned her sights to gaining government acceptance of the data set. Werley's work history was one of distinguished service to the armed forces. This service was well recognized, and her status in the nursing community was one of a certain level of reverence. She used her accomplishments and connections from her previous work to gain access to many government leaders and organizations. In particular, Werley worked closely with Faye Abdellah, deputy surgeon general and chief nurse officer of the U.S. Public Health Service, to gain access to the DHHS Health Information Council, charged with overseeing the development of a variety of information practices aimed at evaluating health care services.[78] Due to Abdellah's assistance, the Health Information Council invited Werley and Lang to submit a letter outlining the benefits of the NMDS, including how this data set addressed the federal government's information needs.

Per Abdellah's instructions, the letter succinctly outlined the purpose of the NMDS and its potential benefit to the DHHS. Although Werley and Lang were cosigners to this letter, Lang offered only cursory edits. Werley's first draft was disappointing, as it contained a litany of reasons why the NMDS was important for nursing, but little about its usefulness to the government. Abdellah reviewed the letter and sent it back to Werley for revisions, stressing again the need to make the case for the data set in terms of its value to the government, not just nursing. Werley made minimal changes to the letter and submitted it to the council for consideration.

The letter was submitted in August 1986 to DHHS assistant secretary Robert Windom and routed for review to Ronald Blankenbaker, chairman of the National Committee on Vital and Health Statistics.[79] At Windom's request, the DHHS granted Werley a review meeting in Washington, D.C., in October 1987 at which the NMDS was considered for adoption. Werley's long-time colleague Elizabeth Devine, rather than Lang, accompanied her to the meeting of the National Committee on Vital and Health Statistics in Washington, D.C.

The committee commented primarily on the inclusion of nursing diagnoses, the profession-centric nature of the data set, and the duplicate data contained in the NMDS. The committee stressed that "considerable attention needed to be given to inconsistencies with nursing diagnosis" if the data point was to be used to capture costs.[80] The committee was referring to the weak connection between nursing diagnosis and patient needs or resource use, a connection that was not measured by a single nursing diagnosis. If the relationship was explicated, the use of nursing diagnosis "might be particularly beneficial to current efforts to define severity of illness." Additionally, the committee noted with concern that the NMDS was specific to services rendered by a particular profession rather than practice setting. Last, the committee commented that the DHHS would have to remove the duplicate data if it accepted the data set for use.

Months passed after the committee hearing and Werley kept in frequent contact with Abdellah, hoping for word about the DHHS decision. In April 1987, Werley received a letter from Assistant Secretary Windom informing her that "no programmatic or administrative needs" were identified that would "warrant the promulgation within all programs for the department, the NMDS."[81] Werley was understandably frustrated, as the phrase "no programmatic or administrative needs" was becoming an increasingly familiar refrain.

While awaiting the DHHS decision, Werley had been communicating with Ron Norby, Associate Chief of Staff for Nursing at the VA San Diego Healthcare System throughout the spring of 1987, in the hopes that the facility might consider using the NMDS as part of its information system.[82] As Norby recalled, he was interested in the data set, but due to the highly cumbersome, labor-intensive data collection that would be required, he made the decision not to mandate its use at his facility.[83] Norby suggested that Werley contact Vernice Ferguson, chief nursing officer for the VA system, to see whether other facilities might be interested. Just as Norby had done, Ferguson entertained the idea of the NMDS, but in the end did not adopt it.[84]

Simultaneously, Werley continued to seek funding for the NMDS project. She obtained more support from the Hospital Corporation of America Foundation to support projects testing and refining the NMDS at two local Milwaukee acute care facilities, as well as for several yet-to-be-identified dissemination projects.[85] The funding was a welcome relief for Werley, who had little results obtaining other forms of support.[86]

The support the University of Wisconsin–Milwaukee contributed, totaling over $85,000, was pulled shortly after the post-conference.[87] In a letter to Ursula Springer, chief executive officer of Springer Publishing, and Ruth Chasek, the Springer editor, Werley blamed her school's administration (indirectly accusing Lang) for her lack of productivity. Werley reflected, "I had a terrible time since June . . . I lost my secretary on June 30th, then learned they will cut back the time to only a 50% slot, when the secretary could not keep up even at 100%. Then I discovered . . . that 'they' did not give a contract to a research assistant who is crucial to our ongoing research—testing and refinement of the NMDS."[88]

In addition to the waning financial support by the school, Werley was having increasing difficulty rallying support for the NMDS project from colleagues within the school. Lang completed the coediting of the conference proceedings, working through Werley's comments such as instructing Lang to "be precise and scholarly in your work so I do not need to check everything in such detail."[89] However, once the proceedings had been edited, Lang avoided further involvement, refusing to feel "brow beaten."[90] The collaboration that brought the NMDS project to fruition five years earlier was now absent and had been replaced by tolerant respect.

Conclusion

Despite disputes over ownership that erupted at the conclusion of the post-conference meeting, the NMDS was a shared information practice. The content of the data set was not original to any of the numerous individuals who lent their time and talent to its creation. Rather, the elements were *common* political representations of nursing practice that were largely representative of the participants' particular perspectives. Nursing diagnosis signified nurses' outward claimed process of clinical reasoning and subsequent expanded practice boundaries. The inclusion of the demographic section was important because it recognized nursing services previously unacknowledged and laid claim to the patient. The notion of costing out nursing care in terms of acuity-intensity ratings was another popular representation of nursing practice that aimed to identify nursing services in billable terms.

When attempting to combine all these and the other items of the NMDS together, organizers had important political choices to make. On the one hand, they could mandate the elements of the data set and leave the particular data points open to customization by the facility; alternatively, they could mandate across the board both the element category and specific data points. In most cases, choices were made that embedded inflexible data points or standards in the data set that disregarded the larger nursing community's investment in the information, and failed to consider the context in which the NMDS would be used. This made seeking funding, recognition, or other forms of uptake exceedingly difficult because it was rather easy to find an objectionable data point or category.

Throughout this process, little attention was paid to existing practice conditions that ultimately determined whether the NMDS would be used. The information choices made by NMDS nurses reflected emerging aspects of practice that were not widely accepted standards. Individual nurses who argued on behalf of a particular piece of data or form of data did so because of a strong belief in how nursing practice (through information collection) *should* be structured. The choices largely represented the academic and administrative backgrounds and preparations of the nurses who named the content of the NMDS.

Ironically, the rollout of the DRG program potentially positioned the prospect of adoption of the NMDS well. The financial upheaval left the health care industry looking for ways to meet the information demands of government payers, who in turn were looking for ways to standardize information collected for billing purposes. Despite this timing, the NMDS was generally not well received. An argument can be made that the changes in the financial context were simply too great and that the window of opportunity was missed. However, this addresses only part of the story surrounding the NMDS, especially given that dozens of data sets were created, tested, and adopted during the time period.

The opportunity to prioritize certain aspects of nursing practice was and remains a powerful notion. The group's struggle to maintain a focus on creating a post-service evaluation tool versus a real-time clinical tool was in part evidence of the inherent power attributed by the group to the information practice they designed. The idea that the NMDS could be all things to all nurses, or that the structure of the NMDS alone should structure the information demands of nurses, was simply incompatible with practice demands. In the end, repeated unilateral decisions by conference organizers about the content and form of the NMDS hindered its clinical utility and disabled uptake. The story of NMDS is illustrative of issues surrounding control in clinical information systems: how initiatives can fail when consensus is not desired or sought after and how difficult it can be to flip from an entrepreneurial ideal to practical application.

JENNIFER HOBBS
VA Post-Doctoral Nurse Fellow
VA San Diego Healthcare System
3350 La Jolla Village Drive
San Diego, CA 92161

Acknowledgments

The author wishes to thank Julie Fairman, Joan Lynaugh, Nathan Ensmenger, Patricia D'Antonio, and the anonymous reviewers for their thoughtful comments and suggestions on this manuscript.

Portions of this article were first presented at the American Association for the History of Nursing Annual Conference, September 25–28, 2008, Philadelphia, Pennsylvania.

This work was supported by the Department of Veterans Affairs, Veterans Health Administration, Office of Academic Affiliations, Post-doctoral and Pre-doctoral Nurse Fellowship Program; the American Association for the History of Nursing; and the Gamma Gamma and Xi Chapters of Sigma Theta Tau International.

Notes

1. Harriet Werley and Norma Lang, eds., *Identification of the Nursing Minimum Data Set* (New York: Springer, 1988).

2. Harriet Werley Papers, unprocessed, University of Wisconsin–Milwaukee, Manuscript Collection (hereafter HWP); Norma Lang Papers, unprocessed, University of Wisconsin–Milwaukee, Manuscript Collection (hereafter NLP); Irma Lou Hirsch Papers, Private Collection, Author (hereafter ILH).

3. The nurses involved with the NMDS believed there were many instances where nursing practice needed to be "defended." Distinguishing the difference between nursing care and medical care was particularly important to nurses because of attempts by the American Medical Association to interfere with decisions regarding nursing education and nursing scope of practice. See Julie Fairman, *Making Room in the Clinic: Nurse Practitioners and the Evolution of Modern Health Care* (New Brunswick, N.J.: Rutgers University Press, 2008).

4. For an in-depth treatment of the economic issues surrounding health care during the twentieth century, see Rosemary Stevens, *In Sickness and in Wealth: American Hospitals in the Twentieth Century* (Baltimore: Johns Hopkins University Press, 1999).

5. See Nancy Tomes, "Patients or Health-Care Consumers? Why the History of Contested Terms Matters," in *History and Health Policy in the United States: Putting the Past Back In*, ed. Rosemary Stevens, Charles E. Rosenberg, and Lawton Burns (New Brunswick, N.J.: Rutgers University Press, 2006).

6. See Lawrence Weed, *Medical Records, Medical Education, and Patient Care: The Problem-Oriented Record as a Basic Tool* (Cleveland: Case Western Reserve University Press, 1969). For a brief overview on nursing care planning (ADPIE), see Virginia Henderson, "On Nursing Care Plans and Their History," *Nursing Outlook* 21, no. 6 (1973): 378–79.

7. Patricia D'Antonio and Julie Fairman, "Organizing Practice: Nursing, the Medical Model, and Two Case Studies in Historical Time," *Canadian Bulletin of Medical History* 21, no. 2 (2004): 411–29.

8. In the 1970–1990 nursing literature there was a general sense that if the actions nurses took on behalf of patients were captured, the ability to bill for those services would follow.

9. The APA was designing a data set, PSRO was developing quality screens, and AHA was developing a discharge data set in cooperation with DHHS.

10. Nancy Pearce, Statistician, Office of Program Planning, DHHS, to Harriet Werley, 11 June 1985, HWP.

11. Department of Health and Human Services, *Criteria of Minimum Data Sets* (Washington, D.C.: Department of Health and Human Services, 1978).

12. Sherrill L. Leifer and Laurie K. Glass, "Planning for Mass Disaster in the 1950s: Harriet Werley and Nursing Research," *Nursing Research* 57, no. 4 (2008): 237–44; Harriet Werley and Norma Lang, Preface, in Werley and Lang, eds., *Identification of the Nursing Minimum Data Se*, xvii.

13. Norma Lang CV, 1986, NLP. For information about PSRO see Michael J. Goran, *The Evolution of the PSRO Hospital Review System* (Philadelphia: Lippincott, 1979).

14. Minutes, Local Data Base Group, 19 May, 27 June, 11 July, 25 July, 7 September, 12 October, 17 October, 21 November, 21 December 1983, HWP.

15. Jo Eleanor Elliot, Director, Division of Nursing, DHHS, to Harriet H. Werley, 17 August 1983, HWP; Minutes, Local Data Base Group, 27 June, 7 September 1983, HWP.

16. Minutes, Local Data Base Group, 11 July, 25 July, 17 October 1983, HWP.

17. Minutes, Local Data Base Group, 11 July 1983, HWP.

18. Minutes, Local Data Base Group, 17 October 1983, HWP.

19. Minutes, Local Data Base Group, 25 April 1985, HWP.

20. Portions of the nursing workforce were by this time (1985) recognized independently within health care organizations inasmuch as they were able to bill and generate revenue. These workers were NPs.

152   Jennifer Hobbs

21. Minutes, Local Data Base Group, 19 January 1984, HWP. Paper authors were not identified consistently in the archive material reviewed.

22. Draft, Minimum Variables in Cost Effectiveness of the NMDS, 1984, HWP.

23. Draft, Minimum Variables in Costing Out Nursing Care, 1984, HWP.

24. Minutes, Local Data Base Group, 19 January 1984, HWP.

25. Minutes, Local Data Base Group, 19 May, 27 June, 11 July, 25 July 1983, HWP.

26. Minutes, Local Data Base Group, 7 September 1983, HWP.

27. According to the information Werley had, the APA database was abandoned because of lack of funding for provider-specific data sets. However, it was probably because the APA was in the midst of a revision of the Diagnostic Statistical Manual. This was one of the more controversial revisions and took a great deal of the organization's resources. See Stuart Kirk and Herb Kutchins, *The Selling of the DSM: The Rhetoric of Science in Psychiatry* (New York: Aldine de Gruyter, 1992). Werley's information was obtained from Minutes, Local Data Base Group, 21 November 1983, HWP.

28. Minutes, Local Data Base Group, 21 November 1983, HWP.

29. Minutes, Local Data Base Group, 19 January 1984, HWP.

30. Stevens, *In Sickness and in Wealth*.

31. Elements in the public data set include *International Classification of Diseases, Ninth Revision, Clinical Manual* (known as ICD-9-CM) diagnosis and procedures codes, gender, date of birth, admission date, discharge date, admission priority, length of stay, discharge status, total charges (based on specific items such as prescriptions), admission source, payer source, and country of origin.

32. Minutes, Local Data Base Group, 31 May, 24 August 1984, HWP; Edward N. Brandt, Jr., Assistant Secretary for Health, Chairperson, DHHS Health Information Policy Council, to the Secretary, 25 July 1984, HWP; 1984 Revision of the Uniform Hospital Discharge Data Set, U.S. DHHS Health Information Policy Council, July 1984, HWP.

33. Minutes, Local Data Base Group, 31 May, 24 August 1984, HWP.

34. Ibid.

35. Ibid.

36. HCA financing was $103,000. Minutes, Local Data Base Group, 6 December 1984, HWP; Transmittal Form for Extramural Support, NMDS Conference, 21 February 1984, HWP.

37. NMDS Conference Group, *Nursing Minimum Data Set Conference Schedule, 15–17 May 1985* (Milwaukee: NMDS, 1985); List, Task Force Groups, NMDS Conference, n.d., HWP.

38. Ibid.

39. Harriet Werley, Opening Remarks, NMDS Conference, Milwaukee, 15 May 1985, HWP.

40. Norma Lang, Opening Remarks, 15 May 1985, NLP.

41. Jennifer Hobbs, "Defining Nursing Practice: The ANA Social Policy Statement, 1980–1983," *Advances in Nursing Science* 32, no. 1 (2009): 3–18.

42. Norma Lang, Opening Remarks, 15 May 1985, NLP.

43. Minutes, Local Planning Committee, 25 April, 29 May, 2 July, 11 July, 26 July, 6 September, 14 October 1984, HWP.

44. List, Task Force Groups, NMDS Conference, n.d., HWP.

45. Report, Demographic Task Force, 16 May 1985, HWP; Demographic Task Force Consensus Statement, Session 3, 17 May 1985, HWP; Minutes of Task Force on Demographics, Session 1, 17 May 1985, HWP.

46. Ibid.

47. Minutes of Task Force on Demographics, 10 June 1985, HWP.

48. Nursing Assessment Group Consensus Statement, 17 May 1985, HWP.

49. Nursing Assessment Task Force Report, 17 May 1985, HWP.

50. For example, the general categories for assessment were biophysical health and ten "problems." The ten problem categories were as follows: nutritional, elimination, sensory function, neurological, circulatory, respiratory, emotional, social, cognitive, and health management. Concern was raised over how these categories would apply to a typical medical-surgical patient, and the group suggested adding stress, anxiety, fear, and depression as categories. This addition of other areas continued through ambulatory care, home health, and so forth.

51. Nursing Assessment Task Force Report, 17 May 1985, HWP.

52. Nursing Diagnosis Task Force Report, 17 May 1985, HWP; see also J. L. Hobbs, "Defining Nursing Practice: The ANA Social Policy Statement, 1980–1983," *Advances in Nursing Science* 32, no. 1 (2009): 3–18.

53. The statement was discussed at the conference; the draft was sent to Werley about two weeks later. Nursing Diagnosis Task Force, Nursing Assessment Group Consensus Statement, 5 June 1985, HWP.

54. List, Task Force Groups, NMDS Conference, n.d., HWP.

55. Minutes, Session 3, 17 May 1985, HWP.

56. Intervention Task Force, Diagram of NMDS Contents, 17 May 1985; Intervention Task Force, Report on Nursing Intervention Task Force, Final, 17 May 1985, HWP.

57. Draft, Outcomes Task Force Consensus Statement, 17 May 1985, HWP; Final Report, Outcomes Task Force, NMDS Conference, 17 May 1985, HWP.

58. Ibid.

59. Nursing Acuity/Intensity Group Consensus Statements, 17 May 1985, HWP.

60. Ibid.

61. Author Tracking Form (1 of 6), Nursing Data Set Conference Proceedings Publication, May 1985, HWP.

62. Many of the participants went on to develop different parts of the data set and explicate the subsections. For example, the contingent from the University of Iowa worked on and eventually developed the Nursing Intervention Classification. Werley was supportive of these developments and focused on how the data set as a whole was being promoted. The requests to discuss and explain the data set were coming to both Werley and Lang, and Werley wanted more control. Comments accompanied the formal school memorandum communication between Werley and Lang, June 1985–October 1985, HWP.

63. Werley had multiple tracking forms and was continually writing the authors after just a few days beyond the set due date. Author Tracking Form (1 of 6). Comments accompanied the papers by Ozbolt, Gallant, Joel, Anderson-Stewart, Sovie, McCormick, Shultz, Saba, and Dowling, November 1985–April 1986, HWP.

64. An example of Werley's editorial style can be seen in Cecelia R. Zorn, M. C. Smith, and Harriet H. Werley, "Watch Your Language," *Nursing Outlook* (1991): 183–85.

65. Nursing Assessment Task Force Report Prepared by Suzanne Flaco, NMDS Conference, 2 August 1985, HWP; Nursing Diagnosis Task Force Report Prepared by Phyllis Kritek, NMDS Conference, 6 September 1985, HWP; Nursing Assessment and Nursing Diagnoses, Task Force Joint Report Prepared by Suzanne Falco, NMDS Conference 29 August 1985, HWP; NMDS Conference Report of Task Force on Intensity, 29 August 1985, HWP; Karen Rieder to Harriet Werley, Nursing Intervention Post Task Force Work, 19 August 1985, HWP.

66. A.M. Proceedings of Post-Conference Task Force Meeting, 16 September 1985, NLP.

67. The data set at this point was a series of categories with definitions, followed by subcategories. Some subcategories had checklists; others had references to larger data sources. For example, the ND category referred users to the NANDA taxonomy, the Omaha system, or some other framework for ND.

68. A.M. Proceedings of Post-Conference Task Force Meeting, 16 September 1985, NLP.

69. Ibid.

70. P.M. Proceedings of Post-Conference Task Force Meeting, 10 October 1985, NLP.

71. A.M. Proceedings of Post-Conference Task Force Meeting, 16 September 1985, NLP; P.M. Proceedings of Post-Conference Task Force Meeting, 10 October 1985, NLP.

72. The communication on the matter began prior to the post-conference. Handwritten notes by Werley to Lang were attached to formal school business communications, June 1985–October 1985, HWP. In the notes Werley began to question what activities Lang was engaged in surrounding the NMDS, particularly her presentation schedule. Werley requested that Lang clear presentation requests through her.

73. Note, September 1985, NLP.

74. Springer had committed to publishing the conference proceedings that were released in 1988; see note 1.

75. A.M. Proceedings of Post-Conference Task Force Meeting, 16 September 1985, NLP; P.M. Proceedings of Post-conference Task Force Meeting, 10 October 1985, NLP.

76. Proceedings of the Post-Conference Task Force Meeting on the NMDS, 16 September 1985; Lucille Joel to Harriet Werley, 30 October 1985, HWP; Carolyn Anderson-Stewart to Harriet Werley, 25 November 1985, HWP; Margaret Sovie, Professor of Nursing, University of Rochester, to Harriet Werley, 11 November 1985, HWP.

77. Harriet Werley to Norma Lang, 7 November 1988, NLP.

78. The correspondence surrounding the NMDS submission was routed through Kathleen McCormick. The first citation is a draft letter sent to Abdellah for review, and the second is the feedback. Harriet Werley and Norma Lang to James Mason, Acting Assistant Secretary for Health, and Chairman Health Information Policy Council, 1 October 1985, HWP; Kathleen McCormick, DHHS to Harriet Werley, 11 November 1985, HWP.

79. Harriet Werley and Norma Lang to James Mason, Acting Assistant Secretary for Health, and Chairman Health Information Policy Council, 6 August 1986, HWP; Ronald Blankenbaker, M. D., Chairman, National Committee of Vital and Health Statistics, to Robert E. Windom, M. D., Assistant Secretary for Health, 8 January 1987, HWP.

80. Letter routed to Irma Lou Hirsch from Jan Heinrich, Letter from Ronald Blankenbaker, Chairman, National Committee on Vital and Health Statistics, to Robert

Windom, Assistant Secretary for Health, DHHS, 8 January 1987, ILH; Robert E. Windom, M. D., Assistant Secretary for Health, to Harriet Werley, 3 April 1987, HWP.

81. Ibid.

82. Ronald Norby, Associate Chief of Staff, Associated Health Professions, VA San Diego Medical Center, to Harriet Werley, 20 April 1987, HWP.

83. Ron Norby, personal communication, 24 June 2007.

84. Harriet Werley to Vernice Ferguson, Director, VA Nursing Service, 2 July 1987, HWP.

85. Harriet Werley to Ida Cooney, Vice President, Foundation Hospital Corporation of America, 1 July 1985, HWP.

86. The story surrounding Werley's funding for the NMDS is commonly understood as coming primarily from the NIH, but there was no evidence to support that claim. Werley had moneys from the Healthcare Corporation of America Foundation and the Blanke Foundation, a foundation that funds University of Wisconsin–Milwaukee faculty projects. She did receive approval of her NIH application, but there was no evidence the project was funded. Ada Sue Hinshaw, Director, National Center for Nursing Research, to Harriet Werley, 29 September 1988, HWP.

87. Note, September 1985, NLP.

88. Harriet Werley to Ursula Springer and Ruth Chasek, 6 August 1986, HWP.

89. Harriet Werley to Norma Lang, 23 June 1986, HWP.

90. Note, September 1985, NLP.

REPORT FROM THE NURSING HISTORY SECTION AT THE 2009 INTERNATIONAL COUNCIL OF NURSES, DURBAN, SOUTH AFRICA

Guest Editors' Notes

In June 2009, the inaugural Nursing History Section was held at the International Council of Nurses (ICN) Congress in Durban, South Africa. It provided an important opportunity for an audience of scholars, leaders, and nursing pioneers to come together to start the conversation on how nursing has been critical to the evolution of health care. Much of what we recognize as nursing history has been shaped by a number of dominant narratives: the Nightingale story of nursing reform in the second half of the nineteenth century, and colonialism—be it nineteenth- or twentieth-century colonialism under the British Empire or American, French, Dutch, German, Portuguese, or Spanish rule. In addition to this political and military colonialism, nursing history is also dominated by English-language scholarship on the subject. This dominance is partly a reflection of the more plentiful support for nursing education and scholarship in English-language countries as a whole, and also an artifact of the bias in all science and scholarship toward the English language. One of the goals for future ICN Nursing History Section meetings is to counter these dominant forces in history and scholarship and to foster multiple voices and multiple perspectives in the development of a nursing narrative that reflects more closely the stories of nurses around the world.

The struggles to develop appropriate education for nursing, the challenges to establish regulatory frameworks, and the professionalization of the field have played out quite differently around the world in ways that have subsequently shaped both the nursing profession and the health care system. This section reminds us that nursing is a profession of multiple histories, histories that have been vital to the development of health care around the world. Reading this brief collection stimulates a plenitude of ideas for future studies: What would a comparison of education between different countries look like? What were other key relationships between countries that were critical to the professionalization of nursing in a region? What are the interrelations between the countries, such as the import or export of labor, money, and ideas? How have these interrelations led to similar and different experiences? What does a global history of nursing include?

In bringing different voices to light that have rarely been heard before, we center this section on ICN reports from the some African countries as well as the Islamic Republic of Iran, Romania, and Turkey. At the ICN conference, Lucilia Nunes, president of the board of nursing in Portugal, provided a good summary of the importance of history. "An interest in history," she stated, "comes from the urge to know who we are and where we came from. This influences us to search for memory. . . . So it is necessary to preserve the event and to use narratives to help us make sense of events. Indeed, without the vision of the past and the paths we have walked, we cannot sustain a professional identity and look to the future."[1]

BARBRA MANN WALL
University of Pennsylvania
Associate Professor and Associate Director
Barbara Bates Center for the Study of the History of Nursing
418 Curie Blvd., Fagin Hall #2016
Philadelphia, PA 19104

SIOBAN NELSON
Dean and Professor
Lawrence S. Bloomberg Faculty of Nursing
University of Toronto
155 College Street, Suite 130
Toronto, ON M5T 1P8

Note

1. Lucilia Nunes, (Report presented at International Council of Nurses, Durban, South Africa, June 2009).

The History of Nursing in Ethiopia

Abdurahman Ali
Ethiopian Nurses Association

In 1909, the first hospital in Ethiopia, Menelik II Hospital, was established and staffed by Russian health personnel. Russia had established ties to Ethiopia during a major battle against an Italian invasion in 1896, after which modern Ethiopia emerged under Emperor Menelik II. Unlike many of the other African countries, the victory over Italy ensured Ethiopia's sovereignty and freedom from colonization. When Menelik II's daughter and successor died in 1930, his cousin, Tafari Makonnen, was crowned Emperor Haile Selassie I. Menelik II Hospital served as a training facility for auxiliary health personnel until another Italian invasion in 1936. In 1939, Princess Tsehai, Emperor Selassie's daughter, completed her training in child nursing and became the first national nurse in Ethiopia.

During World War II, Ethiopian nurses came from a variety of areas. In 1942, for example, after Ethiopia was liberated from Italian occupation, Sister Meheret Paulos graduated in Jerusalem. She worked with the first unit of the British Army in Egypt until 1945 and then returned home to serve in various hospitals in Ethiopia. In 1945, Swedish medical and nursing personnel were recruited to alleviate the health care workforce in Ethiopia. In addition, the World Health Organization (WHO) "Field Mission" sent a physician and nurse to help organize "dresser" courses, or courses in auxiliary nursing. Then in 1949, Sister Sambatu Gabru graduated from a school in Beirut and had additional teachers' training in Canada. She served as matron of Menelik II Hospital and Haile Selassie I Hospital.

Schools of nursing also developed after World War II that slowly built up an Ethiopian nurse workforce. In 1949 at Haile Selassie I Hospital, the Ethiopian Red Cross established the first school of nursing, a three-year course for women; and, since then, the director has always been a Swedish nurse. In 1950, sponsored by the WHO, five Ethiopian women went to the British Hospital in Uganda for nurses' training and graduated four years later. Also in 1950, the Zewditu School of Nursing was established that admitted both male and female students into a three-year program. Seventeen Ethiopian nurses graduated from these programs in 1953. Other schools began in 1951 at the Princess Tsehai Memorial Hospital for female students; and, under the auspices of Swedish missionaries, at Tafari Makonnen Hospital in Naqampte for both women and men. The Haile Selassie I Public Health College was established in 1954 in Gondar, where community nurses' training began. These nurses became important members of health teams composed of nurses, health officers, and sanitarians. Then in 1959, a post-basic nurse midwifery course started with four students, the first post-education program of its kind in the country.

Other important events in the 1950s saw the establishment of the Ethiopian Nurses Association (ENA) in 1952, which has been a member of the International Council of Nurses (ICN) since 1957. The ENA played a large role in the formation of a nursing council with self-regulatory duties during the Haile Selassie regime. Requirements for nursing education admission included a minimum of sixteen years of age for both men and women and completion of a sixth- to tenth-grade education. Training periods lasted three and a half years with English as the primary language of instruction. With the exception of Gondor College of Public Health that gave a baccalaureate degree, the highest nursing award outside the university setting was a diploma.

In 1974, the nursing council ended when a military junta, the "Dergue," came to power and deposed Emperor Selassie. During the Dergue Era from 1974 to 1991, admission standards to nursing schools increased, with requirements of eighteen years of age and completion of a twelfth-grade education. The duration of training decreased to two and a half years and the diploma was the main award.

After the Dergue Era ended in 1991, many public and private universities began nursing education programs that granted bachelor's of science in nursing (BScN) degrees. Today, thirteen public schools and nine private colleges offer baccalaureate degrees, with two master's of science in nursing (MScN) programs. Furthermore, many of the three-year diploma programs are moving to regional colleges that offer three to four years of education. Significantly, every region of the country has at least one junior college for diploma nurses' training, and thirty private colleges also offer diplomas in nursing. Entry to BScN programs requires successful completion of a pre-university education, while diploma schools require a tenth-grade education.

Currently, nurses are the largest health care workforce in Ethiopia. They work as clinicians, educators, managers, and researchers in hospitals (general and specialty units), universities, the health ministry, and nongovernmental organizations. Nurses have replaced physicians in primary care health centers, where they perform health promotion and prevention, cure, and rehabilitation services. Nurses are particularly active in the prevention and care of HIV/AIDS as counselors, supervisors of home-based services, and researchers.

Working with the HIV/AIDS program is one of the key goals of the ENA, along with nursing regulation and leadership. The ENA's challenges are many, however, including lack of standards for clinical practice, lack of self regulation, limited continuing education opportunities, inadequate numbers of academic faculty, and lack of integration of education and clinical practice. The opportunities and accomplishments, however, have been significant, including expansion of university education, the beginning of graduate programs in nursing, the desire for greater research in evidence-based practice, and greater influence at the national policy level.

ABDURAHMAN ALI
Chief Executive Officer
Ethiopian Nurses Association
Yehualawork Building, No. 31
Debrezeit Road
P.O. Box 467
Addis Ababa
Ethiopia

The History of Nursing in Tanzania

Gustav Moyo
Tanzania Nurses and Midwives Council
Gregory Mhamela

In what was to become the nation of Tanzania, women and men who provided nursing care learned by apprenticeship and taught others the traditional "hands-on" skills of care at the clan, home, or family setting. These providers were either traditional healers or traditional birth attendants. Adult males and females practicing traditional healing focused on the use of herbs and meat products that conferred protection or some form of luck to the sick. The skills of traditional healing and curing were handed over to carefully selected members in the family. Many also believed in the hidden protective powers of gods and in the powers of devils and evil spirits in causing illness and death. They worshiped and prayed to adorned images and idols.[1]

Traditional healers were men and women who were believed to possess the powers of magic to curse and bewitch other people in collusion with the evil spirits or devils. Since 1928, the practice of witchcraft was, and still is, prohibited by law. Traditional care of the sick based on the supernatural mode and belief in one God also gained prominence.

In the later nineteenth century, commercial profit and religion were motivating factors that drove Europeans into Africa. Missionaries were the most common health care practitioners in the early parts of colonial rule. Catholic sisters were particularly active in the care of the sick. In the 1890s, other religious societies spread to the country to establish hospitals and start schools of nursing, including Lutherans; Methodists; Evangelical Anglicans; and mission societies from Scotland, England, Germany, and Sweden.

Arrival of European Nurses

The practice of nursing in the East African colony during the German rule before World War I went hand in hand with the arrival and expansion of medical services. The first nursing sister to arrive was Bertha Wilke in 1888, from the Evangelical Lutheran Missionary Society and the German Women's Union for Care of the Sick in the Colonies. Between 1898 and 1907, the same group sent other nurses who had been trained in Germany, several of whom died from malaria and other illnesses. Thus, the German Colonial Government started a malarial control program for the nursing sisters in order to have human resources for the malaria eradication campaign in Dar es Salaam.

After the defeat of Germany in World War I, the German colony came under British rule. In 1922, the British changed the name from Dutch East Africa, which included Rwanda and Burundi, to Tanganyika. It was at this time that the Medical Services Department started to be staffed by professionally qualified British nationals. In the 1930s, to ensure organized nursing in its colonies, the British Colonial Government formulated regulations for its nurses and midwives appointed to work overseas. Administration was conducted through two main structures: Her Majesty Queen Elizabeth's Overseas Civil Service and the Unified Colonial Nursing Service under the Secretary of State.

In 1948, the British Colonial Government established a Territorial Nursing Board of Studies comprised of British women, with the main function of overseeing the training system of nursing and midwifery in Tanganyika. In 1952, legislation for the registration of nurses and midwives was enacted, and in March of the following year the first general meeting of the Tanganyika Nurses and Midwives Council was held.

In 1955, the Territorial Colonial Office issued a memorandum directing nurses to pass a native language examination, but few abided by it. They also had to attend courses on nursing skills related to the care of tropical diseases. Her Majesty Queen Elizabeth's Overseas Civil Service's primary objective was to advance the interests of the inhabitants and to help them toward eventual self-sufficiency. One member of the Tanganyika Nurses and Midwives Council argued that it was undesirable for British women to go into African's homes because of the poor state of hygiene and the undesirable forces at work by witch doctors. The council rejected her ideas, however, and stated that nurses would be required to care for the sick; and work in midwifery, in maternity and child welfare work, in health education, and in disease prevention in both towns and rural areas.

Nursing Education

In the 1880s, Sewa Hadji Paroo first aired a proposal for the establishment of a school of nursing, which came into being as the Dar es Salaam School of Nursing. Nursing education faced tremendous challenges. Some of the systems were a legacy of colonial rule. Showing the influence of religion on nursing, the Community of Sacred Passion missionaries established the Magila Mission Hospital in 1876 and was the first to start general nursing training in 1939. Nurses went on to do their midwifery training and graduated in February 1945. The British Colonial Rule started the second school of nursing in Dar es Salaam in 1946 under the direction of an English woman. Other training schools began in the 1950s, and in 1956 the Dar es Salaam school became the Princess Margareth Nursing School. (The school's name was later changed to the Muhimbili School of Nursing and has remained so to date). In 1960 and 1961, a three-year general nurse training program for both girls and boys was available, with additional one-year midwifery training for girls.

British rule ended in 1961, and the name of the country changed to Tanzania in 1964, following the union with Zanzibar. After independence, the government began upgrading the nursing schools because many of the foreign nurses were leaving the country, which caused an acute shortage of nurses trained at a higher level. In the 1970s, nursing specialty programs started in pediatrics, public health, operating theater management, psychiatric nursing, and ophthalmic nursing.

Earlier, the Tanganyika Nurses and Midwives Council had noted that in due time, carefully selected African candidates would be sent to the United Kingdom for their nurses' training as future leaders and teachers in their own countries, and that advanced training schools for teachers also would have to be set up in Tanganyika itself, which in fact occurred. In 1964, the council decided to start training African nurse tutors in Dar es Salaam. However, it was not until 1973 that the training of nursing teachers actually started, with collaboration between the Ministry of Health, the Ministry of Education, and the WHO.

In 1984, the Ministry of Health encouraged the development of a curriculum for a nursing degree program and also began the discussion for specialist and advanced nursing practice. Through collaboration between the Nursing Education Section of the Ministry of Health, Muhimbili Medical Centre, and the Dalhousie University School of Nursing Project, Tanzanian nurses eventually were able to obtain a bachelor of science in nursing degree and a master's degree in the 1990s. Some graduates eventually became nursing faculty at Muhimbili University College of Health Sciences as tutorial assistants to help run the bachelor's program. Under WHO sponsorship, other women studied at a university in Ireland. Eventually, private institutions established bachelor's programs in Tanzania. Pauline Peter Mella passed the Territorial Cambridge School Certificate in 1962 at Marian College, engineered and championed the establishment of a faculty of nursing, and was the first to be appointed dean from 1991 to 1997 when the Faculty of Nursing Studies at the Muhimbili University College of Health Sciences was established.

In December 2002, the National Nursing Task Force produced the "Nursing Practice Model" for use in Tanzania to address the issue of nursing care provision. Then in September 2007, responding to the recommendations on the activities of nursing practice by the WHO Expert Committee, the Tanzanian Nurses and Midwives Council issued a document detailing the "Standards of Proficiency for Nursing Education and Practice in Tanzania," which was also in line with its functions provided in the law regulating nursing and midwifery in the country. Tanzania joined the International Council of Nurses (ICN) in 1973 after having formed its national nursing association in 1972.

During the colonial period beginning in 1888, when missionary societies started their expeditions into the African continent, they brought their ideas of nursing based on Nightingale's principles of good nutrition, hygiene, and ventilation, along with the supernatural care of the sick and nursing procedures. These were influential in Tanganyika and later Tanzania when the national nurse training syllabi and curricula were being set by nursing regulatory authorities. Today, care of the sick consists of a mixture of the traditional care of the sick based on the supernatural mode and modern scientific-based care centered on the patient, procedures, and nursing theory. In 2002 Tanzania enacted the Traditional and Alternative Medicine Act to regulate the practice of traditional healing in the country.

Gustav Moyo
Registrar
Tanzania Nurses and Midwives Council
10th Floor, Extelcoms Bldg
Samora Avenue
P.O. Box 6632
Dar es Salaam
Tanzania

Gregory Mhamela
P.O. Box 6632
Dar es Salaam
Tanzania

Note

1. Gregory Mhamela in conjunction with the Tanzania Nurses and Midwives Council, draft of *The History of Nursing in Tanzania*.

The History of Nursing in the Republic of Mauritius

Krist Dhurmah
Nursing Association of Mauritius

The history of nursing in the Republic of Mauritius is strongly linked to the influences of a few powerful nations from Europe that successively colonized the islands because of its strategic geographical location for exploration and trade with countries such as India, China, and other eastern countries. The chronology of events in the history of nursing is as follows: (1) the Dutch occupation from 1598 to 1710; (2) the French occupation from 1735 to 1810; and (3) the British occupation from 1810 to 1958. Prior to 1904, there was no formal school or college for nursing or midwifery training in Mauritius.

During the French occupation, doctors carried out in-house training of nurses, although a few nurses received their training in Europe. Patient care was mostly based on a medical model that was quite predominant at this period of nursing history. Another important feature was that as the voice of Christianity became stronger on the island, the focus of care of the sick and needy changed direction from community care to institutionalized care within the framework of the monastic system. A few religious orders established themselves in convents, charitable hospitals, workhouse infirmaries, and asylums for the care of persons afflicted with tuberculosis, psychiatric disorders, and leprosy. Some of the private institutions continue to this day under the administration of religious sisters.

From 1807 to 1817, two nurses, Louise Seylsier and Lise Jones, were attached to the Civil Hospital in Port-Louis. In 1844, during the British Occupation, Laureae Boulle was the first qualified midwife who had trained in England and who worked in Port-Louis at the Civil Hospital. Recruitment of the first group of nursing students occurred in 1904. The entrance qualification was the primary school certificate. Training was for two years with an additional six months' training in midwifery for those who wished to become midwives. Beginning in 1908, they received a certificate of competency after successful completion of their training. The colonial government recommended payment of a stipend to nursing students in 1906, and this practice is still in force even today for nursing students recruited by the state. In 1913, midwives were being trained and sent to serve in sugar estate hospitals to reduce infant mortality rates and maternal deaths.

The year 1946 is a hallmark in the history of nursing in Mauritius, when a Matron Davies introduced the modern method of nursing education, with the nursing program extending to three years. Doctors and qualified nurses gave the lectures, and it was at this time that the medium of instruction was changed from French to English. A high sense of discipline was inculcated to students during their training. An urgent need for more nurses came with the outbreak of poliomyelitis in the period from 1949 to 1952. Red Cross nurses served as auxiliary nurses in the government health services.

In 1958 the Central School of Nursing was established by virtue of a Government Notice dated May 10, 1958. It required that: (1) students shall be holders of SC or GCE (High School Year 10) in five subjects; (2) the director of medical services shall have the power to select candidates; (3) the tutors who were all English eventually be replaced by Mauritians; and (4) the duration of the course needed to be three years for general nursing and two years for midwifery.

In the 1960s and 1970s, hundreds of students were recruited to train in the United Kingdom in general nursing, midwifery, and mental health. In turn, many came back with a rich experience to serve Mauritius. Mental health nursing had its own trajectory. Before 1964, nurses with general training cared for patients with psychiatric disorders. Then in 1964, Mauritian nurses who had trained in mental health nursing in the United Kingdom were recruited to care for patients with psychiatric disorders in Mauritius. In 2004, following an acute shortage of psychiatric nurses to care for patients with mental health disorders, a program for receiving a diploma in mental health nursing (specialized nursing) was developed at the Central School at Candos, and a group of general nurses with some years of experience were recruited to follow this program of study. The curriculum for mental health nursing was developed by a senior nurse educator, Gurudeo Gobin, who obtained his training in psychiatric nursing from the United Kingdom. At the request of the Mauritian government, a WHO consultant approved this curriculum.

Community health nursing was also under the care of general nurses until 1989, when the first cohort of nurses were recruited from general nursing for one additional year training in community health nursing. Subsequently, another cohort of community health nurses trained in 2005 following recommendation of the WHO.

The Nursing Council of Mauritius was established after an enactment in 1992 to regulate nursing as a professional discipline. There is a pressing need to have a new enactment to consider the recognition and registration of nurses with specialist qualifications. Today, the council recognizes the categories of general nurse, mental health nurse, and midwife. Since 1975, the government has recognized trade unions as the main voice of nurses in many socio-economic forums.

In 1999, a baccalaureate program graduated 150 nurses; and in 2008, the Nursing Association of Mauritius advocated for the introduction of a diploma in general nursing to replace the certificate program. After consultation with the Ministry of Health and Quality of Life, the Pay Research Bureau recommended this change. Nurses in Mauritius could then get the baseline qualification to go for further education and training in nursing. By August 2009, the Cabinet of Ministers agreed with the introduction of a Diploma in General Nursing as a major health policy measure. Nurses now look forward to the future introduction of courses in specialized nursing via bachelor and master degrees in nursing.

While nursing has increasingly become more standardized, challenges still exist. The practice of nursing is still task oriented and has undergone very little change. Furthermore, medical control over nursing practice is ever present and has prevented nursing's normal evolution. While the nursing workforce remains the backbone of the health care system, nurses need regular updating of their knowledge and skills in order to apply evidence-based care to patients. We have a long way to go to change a system that is mostly dominated by doctors and non-nursing technocrats; however, with the new vision of the Ministry of Health and Quality of Life, as noted above, many important changes are in the pipeline.

Krist Dhurmah
Nurses Centre
159 Royal Road
Beau-Bassin
Mauritius

The History of Nursing in the Togolese Republic

BASSAN LAMBONI
National Nursing Association of Togo

In 1884, Germany declared a protectorate over a stretch of land in Africa along the Atlantic coast and the Gulf of Guinea and gradually extended its control inland. In 1905, this became the German colony of Togoland.[1] As soon as Gustav Nachtigal, along with the chief Mlapa III of Togoville, established their signature on the German protectorate in 1884, German doctors took the necessary measures to protect the colony and Togolese native populations, which lived together in harmony. The first hospital, Nachtigal Hospital, began its work at Anecho (Aného) from 1885 to 1889. At this time, the indigenous people were treated in pavilions while the principal building of the hospital was situated 100 meters away. The pavilions also received seriously ill patients arriving from the Gold Coast (Ghana) and as far east as Cameroon.

As the conquest of the territory was taking place, the preoccupations of Germans for the health of the Togolese in the *Muster Kolonie* (model colony) found expression in the construction of hospital and community clinics in principal localities with both a fixed health service and a mobile service (in Aného, Lomé, Kpalimé, and Atakpamé) where a doctor of German nationality resided. Periodically, the German doctor made rounds at Sokodé and Bassari (Bassar). German doctors also formed a group for indigenous nurses, the *Deutsche Frauen Verein* (the German Women's Association), to help carry out vaccinations and medicals treatments. After the German defeat in World War I, German Togoland became two League of Nations mandates administered by the United Kingdom and France.[2]

French Colonial Period

The Togo of French expression had its first regulation of health services with Decree #85 of August 1921, which instituted "the indigenous nurse profession." Then on May 29, 1945, the first Togolese nursing school was created for a basic diploma certificate, the elementary certificate of primary studies (Certificat d'Etude Primaire Elementaire, or CEPE). Doctor/Commander Camboge managed the program, and from 1945 to 1946, for admission to nursing school, one had to be a French subject and between the ages of 17 and 24. The length of the program was six months at first and later expanded to one year. The diploma certificate received by graduates on completion of the program was the *Brevet d'aptitude*, or "Certificate of Aptitude," and was awarded by the superintendent of the republic.

In 1950, the length of the program increased to two years with basic diploma certificates at the elementary or "O" level (Brevet d'Etude du Premier Cycle, or BEPC),[3] with two categories of nurses: those in charge of medical cases, and nurses or hygiene assistants who practiced prevention and administered vaccinations.

Period after Independence

Togo (officially the Togolese Republic) gained its independence from France in 1960.[4] Thereafter, nursing standards were raised, which included increasing the number of years of study. On May 13, 1964, for example, the nursing school was transformed at the École National des Infermier and Infermières de Etat du Togo (ENIIET), or National School of State Nurses of Togo. The length of time for study was two years, and students who succeeded at their exams received a state nurse diploma certificate. If the student wanted to present him or herself for the admission exam, the candidate had to be a holder of the elementary certificate or "O" level. Candidates at the baccalaureate or "A" level were admitted on qualification. Then on March 2, 1965, the National School of State Nurses was transformed into a paramedical school of Togo in response to requirements of other groups such as state laboratory workers. On November 6, 1975, the paramedical school was transformed into École Nationale des Auxiliaries Médicaux (ENAM), or National School of Medical Auxiliaries, and was organized into departments. At that time, the length of the formation program expanded to three years, and candidates taking the examination had to hold a certificate of the second degree and teaching.

On August 30, 1976, laws for nurses and obstetricians were created within the ENAM. A Department of Health Assistants was formed and was based at Sokodé. The admission in that department required successful passing of an exam among the candidates who were holders of Certificat d'Etude Primaire Elémentaire (CEPE) or Certificat d'Etude du Premier Degré (CEPD), or Certificate of First Degree Studies. The Department of Health Assistants must prepare for one year for an aptitude certificate in order to be employed, but the length of the formation has now been increased to two years. Until 1996, ENAM was the only school where nurses and their auxiliaries were officially taught. That year, the state also recognized the private school of Saint-Jean de Dieu Afagnan, which provided a state nursing diploma certificate, with many of the health assistants coming from a Catholic religious order. Then in January 1999, the standard for the recruitment of nurses who wanted to apply for the state nursing diploma certificate was raised to the "A" level (High School Year 12). This increase in entrance standards for nursing in Togo finally placed nursing education at the same level of other professions.

Bassan Lamboni
Président National Association Nationale des Infirmiers/ères du Togo
Membre de la Croix Rouge Togolaise
Formateur, Ecole Nationale des Auxiliaires Médicaux de Lomé
Département des Infirmiers d'Etat
Bd de la Victoire
B.P.: 1271 Lomé TOGO

Notes

1. http://www.nationsonline.org/oneworld/togo.htm.
2. Ibid.
3. The general certificate of education or GCE is an academic qualification that is used in the United Kingdom and other. The GCE traditionally comprised two levels: the ordinary level (O Level) and the advanced level (A or baccalaureate).
4. http://www.nationsonline.org/oneworld/togo.htm.

The History of Nursing in the Islamic Republic of Iran

Maryam Hazrati
Shiraz University of Medical Sciences, Shiraz, Iran
G. Mirzabeigy
President of the Iran Nursing Organization, Tehran, Iran
Ahmad Nejatian
Vice President of the Iran Nursing Organization, Tehran, Iran

Since 1979 in Iran (officially the Islamic Republic of Iran), Islam has been a significant factor in nursing's development and continued progress in that country. As in other countries before 1915, women or servants in the home carried out nursing care in Iran, and untrained personnel also cared for hospitalized patients. Religious limitations for women, low cultural status, and lack of education hampered nursing's standing and recognition.[1] However, in 1915 the American Presbyterian Missionary Society (APMS) began the training of a few nurses in a small missionary hospital; and a year later a three-year nursing school was established in Tabriz. After 1916, nursing schools across the country expanded, leading to greater need for educated nursing faculty. The WHO assisted, and other teaching recruits came from England and United States.[2]

In 1943, Iranian nurses educated abroad formed the Iranian Nursing Association (INA). After the Second World War, nursing gained momentum as a profession with the establishment of the three-year Ashraf School of Nursing with nursing faculty from England. In 1952, the Ministry of Health established a nursing division, and for the first time nursing officially became a structure of the government. The first university bachelor of science in nursing (BSN) program began in 1967 at Shiraz University, followed by the associate degree of nursing (ADN) program in 1975. Although this created some role ambiguity, thereafter nursing education in Iran was on the move, adding a master of science in nursing (MSN) program with many different specialties. Today, master's graduates are offered positions in fields such as critical care

Nursing History Review 19 (2011): 171–174. A Publication of the American Association for the History of Nursing. Copyright © 2011 Springer Publishing Company.
DOI: 10.1891/1062–8061.19.171

nursing, psychiatric nursing, community health, pediatric nursing, management, and education nursing.[3]

In 1979 when the Islamic revolution took place, the government decided that nursing school admissions should be 50 percent males, with the understanding that men should care for men and that women must be kept separate from the men. Previously, the majority of nurses were females who had to care for both men and women, a situation which was unacceptable to the new regime. But other problems were occurring. Faculty members were insufficient in numbers, and institutions for clinical placement were few, resulting in physicians and inexperienced nurses doing the teaching. This mix changed philosophy and educational models to reflect a medical model. Nurses were taught to manage diseases and to follow physicians' orders without questioning. This educational model was not only oppressive but it also silenced the nurses. Thus the difficulty of teaching professional nurses to be assertive and in control of their own practice was exacerbated. This called for a new approach.[4]

For many years, Iranian nurses had wanted to set up guild organizations or institutes to defend their professional rights, and many non-state institutes of the nursing profession have formed in the last fifty years. Because of the limitation of the scope of their activities, however, they could not take important strides toward the promotion of nursing. But collective pursuance of some nursing students and professors during the 1990s led to Iran's legislature approving a law establishing the Nursing Organization of the Islamic Republic of Iran (INO) in 2000 and 2001. This organization is the largest non-state guild system in the country and has the legal responsibility to represent all nurses in all sectors of nursing. The goals are many, including improving the quality of patient care and developing standards for nursing practice.[5] Significantly, countrywide elections are held for the positions of eighty-five boards of directors, each consisting of nine members and thirty members on the Supreme Council. The INO is the only nursing organization in Iran and possibly one of the few in the world that has been established by a vote of nationwide representatives. Because of its strong support from many nurses, the INO has established relationships with all the official authorities of Iran.[6]

All the organizations, ministries, and state and non-state houses have bound themselves to cooperate with the INO, thus making it possible to bring about many achievements. At the same time, the government does not interfere in the organization's affairs. Important activities of the INO include preparation of by-laws by the Supreme Council, setting priorities for Iran's nursing issues, and purchasing a building for administration activities. Most important, the INO maintains positive relationships with Iran's Supreme Leader, the highest political and religious authority in Iran; the President of

Iran, the highest executive authority; and the Islamic Consultative Assembly, the highest legislative authority. The INO leaders and/or the Supreme Council meet with these individuals on a regular basis.[7]

Several obstacles such as vague or abstract job descriptions, work overload, and poor staffing in hospitals occurred, and there was a lack of continuing education for nurses. Recently, after daily contact with the Commission of Health and Treatment, under the Consultative Assembly, nurses in the INO were successful in getting the approval of four important laws affecting nursing: (1) to get 15,000 nurses within four years to help meet the nursing shortage; (2) to raise nurses' salaries by 50 percent; (3) to set prices for all services provided by the nurses in Iran, thereby allowing nurses to work as independent practitioners and stabilizing nurses' positions in hospitals; and (4) to decrease the work hours of nurses.

The INO also meets with the Ministry of Health, Treatment, and Medical Training, which is in charge of nurses' training in Iran. As a result of persistence lobbying from the INO, nurses now can keep up to date with knowledge though continuous education sessions. The INO has also been successful in providing paramedics opportunities to participate in baccalaureate nursing programs rather than working as nurses without diplomas. Thus, with respect to the advances of the Islamic Republic of Iran, keeping up with other countries has led to the development of many basic and specialized sciences. Nursing is vastly needed by the society today, such that there are 140,000 people currently studying nursing at various levels. Students are graduating at the levels of BS, MS, and PhD.[8]

MARYAM HAZRATI
Instructor, Department of Nursing and Midwifery
Shiraz University of Medical Sciences, Shiraz, Iran
and Member,
Supreme Council of the Iran Nursing Organization

G. MIRZABEIGY
President of the Iran Nursing Organization
Tehran, Iran

AHMAD NEJATIAN
Vice President of the Iran Nursing Organization
Tehran, Iran

Notes

1. *A Review about Nursing in Islamic Republic of Iran* (Tehran: Iranian Nurses Organization, n.d.), 19–28; M. Tafreshi and A. Davachi, *Law and Regulations: Ethics, History and Development of Nursing in Iran* (Tehran: Gazl Publication, 2000); G. Mirzabeigy, Maryam Hazrati, and Ahmad Nejatian, High Council of Nursing Organization, Iran (unpublished presentation).

2. *A Review about Nursing in Islamic Republic of Iran.*

3. See also Mahvash Salsali, "The Development of Nursing Education in Iran," *International History of Nursing Journal* 5, no. 3 (2000): 58–63; Mahvash Salsali, "Nursing and Nursing Education in Iran," *Image: The Journal of Nursing Scholarship* 31, no. 2 (1999): 190–93; and Mohsen Adib Hajbaghery and Mahvash Salsali, "A Model for Empowerment of Nursing in Iran," *BMC Health Services Research* 5, no. 24 (2005), http://www.biomedcentral.com/1472-6963/5/24.

4. *A Review about Nursing in Islamic Republic of Iran*; Salsali, "The Development of Nursing Education in Iran"; and Salsali, "Nursing and Nursing Education in Iran."

5. *A Review about Nursing in Islamic Republic of Iran*; and Hajbaghery and Salsali, "A Model for Empowerment."

6. Mirzabeigy, Hazrati, and Nejatian, unpublished presentation.

7. Ibid.

8. Ibid.

The History of Nursing in Romania

Ecaterina Gulie
Romanian Nursing Association

The history of nursing in Romania started in 1775. While over the years its history was marked by many changes in nursing education, there were three key periods of major change: before World War II, after the war, and after the Romanian Revolution in 1989.

Before World War II

The Rockefeller Foundation was responsible for the establishment of three-year nursing schools post high school in the early part of the twentieth century. However, Romanian nurses soon became active. In 1919 at Cluj, Iuliu Moldovan, a physician, opened a nursing school led by Lucia Bologa Puscariu. Other early schools were established in 1921 and 1925 that focused on public health nursing. In 1929, another Institute of Public Health Nurses was established in Iasi, with Eugenia Costres becoming the director in 1934. Instructors in these early programs received their education in the United States, Canada, France, and Vienna. Romanian students' first four months of courses included personal hygiene, ethics, some economics, and relationships with patients and colleagues. After four months, they had to pass an exam before they could continue in the nursing program. Both nursing students and their faculty members lived in the nursing school building.

More information is available on Eugenia Costres. She obtained her education at the Institute from Cluj in 1919 and 1920. While there, she followed the objectives of the school: to obtain knowledge and skills to care for mothers and children; to work with mentors who were teachers in the Obstetric/Gynecology Clinic, Infant Clinic, and Center for Child Protection; and to obtain training in moral ethics of nurses. Then in 1927 and 1928, Costres went to the University of Toronto to study at the Faculty of

Nursing. Her interest in public health grew after visiting agencies in Boston, New York, and Birmingham. When she returned to Romania, she established the Institute of Public Health in Iasi and organized activities all over the country to improve sanitary conditions for mothers and children. She was especially active in rural areas. Her continued interest in education came with her appointment as director of the Institute of Public Health Nurses in Iasi. In this role, she provided both theoretical training for students and collaborated with instructors from the Iasi Medical School. She arranged for students to work with mentors who modeled not only competency but also conscientiousness and passion for their work. She also organized hygiene and other health classes for teachers in primary and secondary schools; and in her work as a sanitary inspector, she organized classes on tuberculosis and care of pregnant women.

The Association of Public Health Nurses was established in 1935 with Maria Pertea as president. This association joined the International Council of Nurses (ICN) in 1937. Costres attended the 1937 Quadrennial Congress in London, where she spoke about the value of quality care and the prestige of the nursing profession. Indeed, Costres spoke at many international meetings, and she always talked about Romanian nurses' public health activities. During World War II, she collaborated with the Romanian Red Cross, and along with students at the institute in Iasi, cared for soldiers in hospitals.

After World War II

In 1947, Communists proclaimed Romania a People's Republic. In 1948, through Decree 178 concerning the reform of education to a Soviet model, the Institutes of Public Health ceased, and the National Association of Public Health Nurses disbanded. It was also during the Communist period that schools developed for nurses, midwives, and sanitary officials. In 1949, the Health Science Society was established, under which eventually all categories of health personnel, including nursing, came. Then in 1955, medical assistants were trained to work in clinics in a two- or three-year program. The first national seminar for medical assistants on health education occurred in 1966. A revue, *Medical Life*, also appeared during this time.

In 1971, the National Center for Continuing Education for Medical Assistants was established with the support of WHO-EURO, of which another nurse significant to the history of Romanian nursing, Gabriela Bocec, became deputy director. In 1973, she became vice-president of the Department Nursing Staff inside the Health Science Society. Indeed, historians of nursing in Romania credit Bocec for introducing nursing to the country.[1] In 1989, she organized a course called "Concepts in Nursing" that was taught across the country.

After the Romanian Revolution in 1989

The 1989 Romanian Revolution overthrew Communist leadership. During that time, nurses had struggled to improve their situation, but their wages had remained low and their educational standards were not well developed. In 1990, as Romania prepared to enter the European Union (EU), EU standards for nursing education were adopted; and that same year, the National Association of Medical Assistants was formed. It became the Romanian Nursing Association (RNA) in 1993 with Bocec as president. The RNA and the Ministry of Health worked together with international experts from Denmark in collaboration with the WHO to establish new nursing curricula. Then in 1993, a new revue called the *Journal of Nursing* developed with Bocec as chief editor. Specialty courses for management, education, community nursing, and mental health came about in 1996, followed by other courses such as nursing research. The RNA organized three national congresses along with other congresses with international participation. Then in 1997 at the International Congress of the ICN, the RNA again joined the organization.

Many nurses from Romania participated in the international conferences, and they also obtained scholarships and studied in different universities outside the country. Today, the RNA is a member of the ICN, of the European Forum of Nursing Associations and Midwifery (WHO), and of the European Federation of Nursing Associations.

Ecaterina Gulie
Romanian Nursing Association
Str. Maguricea Nr 1, Bl 3F
Parter App. 1
Sector 1

Bucharest
Romania

Note

1. Gabriela Bocec, "Eugenia Costres," *Medical Life* 26, no. 5 (May 1978): 119–21; Lucretia Glocotici, *Patient Care: Highlights Historical and Ethical* (Romanian Medical Life Publishing, 1996); and Ecaterina Suvaiala, "Nursing Tradition from Iasi," *Nursing Journal* (1997), 5–7.

The History of Nursing in Turkey

Fusun Terzioglu
Hacettepe University

The traditional roots of modern nursing in Turkey date back to the efforts of Florence Nightingale, who cared for wounded English and Turkish soldiers in Selimiye Barracks in Istanbul during the Crimean War (1854–1856).[1] Until then, care of the wounded and sick was the responsibility of informally trained women. After the Crimean War, eleven nurses came to Turkey from Germany with Nightingale's care principles in mind.[2]

The necessity for trained nurses in Turkey reached its peak, however, during the Balkan War (1912–1913) and World War I (1914–1918), which brought large numbers of wounded and sick soldiers and refugees to hospitals. While early efforts in nursing were influenced by nurses from Western Europe, it was a local Turkish physician, Besim Ömer Akalın Pasha, who first emphasized the need for special training in nursing education in Turkey.[3] With his efforts, the first formal six-month nursing education program started in 1911. In 1920, the American Bristol Health School began a two-and-a-half-year nursing education program to train nurses for the American Hospital, followed in 1925 with the two-year Society of Red Crescent Nursing School, established through the efforts of the famed Mustafa Kemal Atatürk, the founder of the Republic of Turkey. This school became a four-year program in 1958.[4] Kızılay Nursing School also began a nursing program in 1925 requiring twenty-seven months of study, and it set certain conditions for acceptance: being literate, in good physical condition, and morally educated. After 1946, this institution became the key school that sent graduates to other nursing schools as educators and administrators.[5]

Other nursing schools opened in the 1940s and 1950s, but not baccalaureate and post baccalaureate programs. The first bachelor-degree program opened in 1955, a master in nursing in 1968,[6] and the first nursing doctorate program in 1972 at Hacettepe University School of Nursing (HUSN).[7] Even though there are currently eighty-one schools of health with departments of nursing, each needs faculty who are well trained in the health professions. By 2006, there were only six universities that offered doctoral degrees in nursing.

Hence, graduates of the Haceteppe University program have provided the faculty needed to raise the qualifications of understaffed and underfunded universities in Turkey.

The professionalization of nursing in Turkey was enhanced in 1933 when the Turkish Nurses Association (TNA) was established. It became an active member of the International Council of Nurses (ICN) in 1949; and currently, with fifteen branch offices, the association has its own journal for 2,785 members nationwide.[8] In addition to the TNA, there are twenty-two nursing associations for specific specialties. The TNA has periodically sponsored a journal since 1959.

Despite its accomplishments in education and professional organizations, nursing in Turkey is still primarily a field for women; this leads to nurses' being neglected by decision makers at work.[9] Environments are entrenched in a steep hierarchy, and societal factors such as the nursing shortage have also contributed to the muting of nurses' voices, especially in the decision-making arena that drives the health care market and policy.

Nursing functions and roles are defined by law as well as other regulations and directives. The Nursing Law of 1954 cited very restricted roles, with nurses working primarily to assist other professionals. As such, it was not in accordance with twenty-first-century hospital and nursing practice realities. Nurses receive insufficient and inappropriate education related to the services they are supposed to give. Insufficient education along with the lack of legislation appropriate to changing conditions have created problems concerning the protection of nurses' rights, which lead to their neglect by decision makers.[10] In addition, there are few accepted standards for nursing services, and few continuing education and in-service training programs existed until 1993.[11] To correct these deficiencies, TNA nurses worked for more than fifteen years to update nursing laws, and their efforts were successful with the approval of a new law in April 2007. Although it will take five years for implementation, these new changes have given nurses many opportunities to acquire expertise, earn a training certificate, and obtain more men into nursing, along with the professional articulation of nursing roles and standardized nursing education at the university level.

Political forces have also affected the nursing profession in Turkey. To meet European Union requirements, nurses are trying to change the total number of hours of nursing education, including theory and clinical practice. They recently established a system of academic credits such as the European Credits Transfer System in order to promote student and educator mobility. Thus nurses and nurse educators are revising nursing practice and curricula to meet the ever-changing needs of society.

In summary, advances in technology, rising acuity of clients, and early discharge of clients from health care institutions require nurses to have up-to-date knowledge of nursing skills. Contradicting this is the low social position of women in medical facilities and Turkish society in general. Despite their gains, nurses are still frequently perceived as physicians' assistants rather than autonomous professionals in their own right. Nursing is commonly perceived as "lowly women's" work, thus undermining nurses' abilities to bring change.[12] With the 2007 change in nursing law allowing more men into schools of nursing, this could change. Yet the nursing shortage remains.

FUSUN TERZIOGLU
Associate Professor
Vice President of Nursing Department
Hacettepe University
Faculty of Health Science
Nursing Department
06100, Ankara, Turkey

Notes

1. N. Eren and G. Uyer, *Saglik Meslek Tarihi ve Ahlaki* [History and Deontology of Health Professionals], 4th ed. (Ankara: Hatiboglu Yayinevi, 1991); and S. Erhan, *Hemsirelik Tarihi* [History of Nursing] (Istanbul: Divan Matbaacilik Tesisleri, 1978).
2. There is a Florence Nightingale museum in Istanbul, Turkey. F. Ulusoy, "Nursing Education History in Turkey," *Cumhuriyet University Journal of School of Nursing* 2, no. 1 (1998):1–8; Ş. Özaydın, "Start of Nursing in Turkey and Samples from its Development in the Last Thirty Years," *T Klin J Med Ethics, Law and History* 10 (2002):258–62; and Z. Özaydın, "Upper Social Strata Women in Nursing in Turkey," *Nursing History Review* 14 (2006): 161–74.
3. Ulusoy, "Nursing Education History."
4. Ulusoy, "Nursing Education History," and L. Birol, *Red Crescent Nurses Serving to Human* (Ankara; Doğuş Publishing, 1975).
5. K. Kukulu, "Nursing in Turkey," *Nurse Educator* 30, no. 3 (2005):101–103.
6. F. Erdil and N. Bayraktar, "Hacettepe Üniversitesinde Hemşirelikte Lisans Üstü Eğitimin Gelişimi," in *1st International and 5th National Nursing Education Congress Book* (Nevşehir, Turkey, 2001), 199–202.
7. B. Yurugen, *Turkiye'de Hemsirelik ve Hemsirelik Egitimi Tarihi* [Nursing and History of Nursing Education in Turkey] (Gaziantep, Turkey: Yuksek Ogretim Kurumu, 2005); Turkish Council of Higher Education, "Turkey Health Manpower Situation Report, 2007," *Turkish Council of Higher Education,* http://www.yok.gov.tr; and The Council of

Higher Education of the Republic of Turkey, "Homepage," http://www.hemsirelersitesi.com/hemsitar.htm.

8. History of Turkish Nurses Association, "History," http://www.turkhemsirelerdernegi.org.tr/?page=page&cmd=show&lid=0&pid=10.

9. Kukulu, "Nursing in Turkey."

10. Ibid.

11. S. Aksayan and G. Cimete, "Nursing Education and Practice in Turkey," *Journal of Nursing Scholarship* 32, no. 2 (2000): 211–12.

12. Kukulu, "Nursing in Turkey."

NOTES AND DOCUMENTS

Networks of Identity: The Potential of Biographical Studies for Teaching Nursing Identity

Maria Itayra Padilha
Federal University of Santa Catarina/Brazil

Sioban Nelson
University of Toronto

Abstract. This article reviews the historiographical elements of the professional identity of nursing, focusing on what historians have denoted as the "history of the present." Professional identity interacts with elements of power, gender, politics, philosophy, and history, and its value is tied to the importance it assumes at any given time in any given society. The collective identity of the profession is elucidated by the construction of nursing history, linked to the history of women and gender relationships in professional care and educational, organizational, and class practice, and also by the biographies of individuals who have shaped this identity through their reputations and life stories. In this light, it is argued that biographies could help illuminate the elements of identity formation of interest to nursing scholars and further the development of the profession; they could also bring discussions of the past and present into the teaching–learning process for nursing students. The authority and significance of these identities will also be discussed.

Like other professions, nursing has constructed and deconstructed its history over time, at one moment freeing itself from archaic paradigms, at another adopting new ideas and paradigms in its effort to understand nursing as a practice, with its own political and social background, and as a maker of opinions. The position of nursing in society is influenced by the concepts, prejudices, and stereotypes that have formed its historical trajectory. This trajectory, even today, influences the idea of what nursing is, where it comes from, and its significance as a health care profession.

In Brazil's nursing education system, nursing history is a mandatory curricular requirement, although it is not necessarily taught by historians. This article emerged from discussions about the challenges of teaching nursing history in this context and about the relationship between professional identity and nursing history. It focuses on what historians denote as the "history of the present."[1] Historians of the present are concerned primarily with the relationship between the past and the present as an epistemological factor that determines the way a search for knowledge is constituted. For instance, history of the present sees the way one questions the past as indicative of contemporary concerns. Looking at the past through the lens of the present affects how we come to truth, how knowledge is produced, and the value of the knowledge produced.

History and Brazilian Nursing Education

Nursing history has been taught in Brazil since 1923, when the Nurses' School at the National Public Health Department (Departamento Nacional de Saúde Pública, DNSP), currently the Anna Nery Nursing School (Escola de Enfermagem Anna Nery), opened as the first formal nursing school in Brazil. American nurses, supported by the Rockefeller Foundation, founded the school as part of the foundation's highly influential geopolitical strategy of the period, in which Brazil played a major part. The foundation, directed by Ethel Parsons, an American nurse of the International Health Service, established a technical mission for the development of nursing in Brazil. The school adopted the North American model, which became the prototype for other nursing schools in the country. This model was based on what is taken in Brazil to be the Nightingale paradigm of scientific principles of hygiene and public health and a feminist perspective on political, regulatory, and economic concerns for the profession.[2]

As new nursing schools in Brazil opened, they continued to include the history of nursing in their curricula, considering it "a fundamental aspect of the formation of a professional identity for professors and students, in search for a better insertion of nursing in society and in the development of a lasting social commitment."[3] The history course has survived changes in the curriculum over time, and has been linked to other content considered to support the formation of a professional identity from an ethical and legal point of view. The overarching principles were that the formal education of the nurse demands a historical, ethical, and social base in the art of nursing. In 1931, the course was renamed Ethics and Nursing History, and until 1949 all schools of nursing were required to include nursing history in the professional formation component of the nursing curriculum.[4] A 1949 regulation preserved nursing history under this same course title. In 1962, history was reaffirmed as a core element of the basic nursing school curriculum and was extended to embrace ethics as a specific topic.

In 1972, following the university reforms of 1968, another curricular change introduced a class in history of nursing that included medical deontology and professional legislation and diminished the relative weight of nursing history in the overall curriculum.[5] This content continued to be taught in connection with the legal and ethical aspects of the profession, as it was considered important for how decisions about nursing as a profession were made. A new minimum curriculum following 1994 regulations (Portaria Ministerial 1721/94) incorporated guidelines and projects from the major organized movements, especially the Brazilian Nursing Association (Associação Brasileira de Enfermagem; ABEn). It was in the process of elaborating on the new directives that the ABEn obtained its greatest success in defense of its professional interests, in a form aligned with principles of the larger changes in education and health care. In 1997, the Brazilian National Curricular Directives set a route to what had been put in place under the 1996 Law for Directives and Bases of National Education (Lei de Diretrizes e Bases da Educação).[6]

These radical changes in the educational, political, and ideological spheres have flowed from pedagogy in nursing into nursing history. These 1997 curriculum eliminated pre-nursing courses like history, ethics, and basic sciences, including this content in the professional courses. Nursing history is now under the heading "Human and Social Sciences."[7]

Until recently the content of the nursing history course followed traditional historical pedagogy in that it was almost exclusively interested in individuals and institutions dominated by the elite. The curriculum focused on memorizing selected events, without sufficient discussion of the context behind these so-called facts or the debates concerning them.

Alongside these general curricular developments, the movement for rejuvenation of teaching and research in nursing history gained momentum during the 1980s, when the Anna Nery Nursing School held the Third National Meeting of Fundamental Nursing, which included a discussion of scholarly historical work. In 1993, the year of the school's 70th anniversary, the school founded the country's largest Documentation Center (Centro de Documentação), while simultaneously creating the first research group in the history of Brazilian nursing, the Research Group for Historical Studies in Brazilian Nursing (Núcleo de Pesquisa de História da Enfermagem Brasileira; NUPHEBRAS).[8]

Another important scholarly activity that has strengthened methodological approaches to teaching nursing history has been an increase in research groups in history of nursing associated with graduate programs in nursing across the country. Since 1995, 16 groups have been created and registered in the Directory of Research Groups of the National Council for Scientific and Technological Development (Conselho Nacional de Pesquisa; CNPq),[9] the national research and scholarly council. The council recognizes history of nursing as one of its formal research areas. Nursing history is thus considered a full-fledged area of research and scholarship in Brazil.

Revising the Historical Canon

The 1980s and 1990s proved to be amazing decades of revision and critique of the nursing historical narrative tradition around the world. Celia Davies, in *Rewriting Nursing History*, brought together intellectuals, several with nursing credentials, to look at aspects of British nursing in light of new trends in social history. Janet Wilson James, in her essay "Writing and Rewriting Nursing History: A Review Essay," reviewed the history of nursing using documentary analysis of relevant themes in women's history. Patricia D'Antonio, in "Revisiting and Rethinking the Rewriting of Nursing History," reread previous texts, especially Davies and James, to reconsider nursing history by thinking about the women who were nurses. Sioban Nelson, in "Reading Nursing History," examined nursing history from the traditional professional celebrations of the first half of the twentieth century to the sociologically influenced studies of the 1960s and the feminist and critical revisions of the 1980s and 1990s. In another essay, "The Fork in the Road: Nursing History Versus the History of Nursing," Nelson discussed the state of nursing scholarship and offered a critique of its uneasy fit with historical scholarship. All these authors have been widely cited in papers discussing nursing history from a critical perspective, and their opinions have become key elements in this field of study.[10]

Similar revisions and critiques were occurring among scholars of the history of nursing in Brazil. Raimunda Germano, in *Education and Ideology in Brazilian Nursing*, critiqued the Nightingale model of nursing education and the manner in which nursing faculty used classroom spaces. Denise Pires, in *Medical Hegemony in Health Care and Nursing: Brazil, 1500–1930*, used a historical perspective to discuss the changes in the knowledge and practice of Brazilian Indian society; this work explored colonization and the nurse/physician power relationships, and traced a counterpoint between Brazilian and international nursing. Maria Cecilia Puntel de Almeida, in *Nursing Knowledge and Its Practical Dimension*, studied the relationship between knowledge and nursing practice since Nightingale, along with the historical transformations of practice. Cristina Loyola in *The Risk and the Embroidery: A Study on Formation of Professional Identity* discusses the construction of professional identity in nursing from Charles Dickens on, singling out a comparison of Sairey Gamp and Florence Nightingale.[11]

In books on nursing history in general, nurse-historians Waleska Paixão and Taka Oguisso present histories of nursing from its religious origins to its professionalization. They show the pioneers of profession and the principal events that have influenced nursing practice. A third book on nursing history, by Valeria Lunardi, is a summary of the history of nursing, focusing on the Nightingale era.[12]

Teaching Nursing History in Brazil: Biographies

Biographies offer a subjective interpretation of the trajectory of a person's life. They include not only events and their locations, but also the person's opinions, motives, and plans for the future, as well as his or her perceptions and interpretations of the past. Biographies are always selective, one consequence of which is that in the end product we have more than a biography.[13] While Michel Foucault does not deal with biography in of itself, he offers a new perspective on the dialectic between individuals and the context that surrounds them. The individual as a historical person is observed within a complex network, that involves friendship ties, social conditions, membership in philosophical-religious groups, and the context and area in which the person acted, among other factors.[14] The appropriation of biographies becomes possible then in a general fashion, within historical discourse, given that *lives* are not interpreted as an end in themselves, but in relation to the context that contributed to their construction.

Biographies, or life trajectories of nurses, have been used in nursing education to demonstrate activity in various areas—development of a specific professional area, creation of nursing schools and professional associations, development of nursing theories, and social and political advances for the profession. Within the discipline of the history of nursing these biographies have been used to contextualize a specific period and relate it to the development of nursing as a profession and to form collective identities. Some nursing historians use biographic studies as to discuss the profession and the importance of the history of nursing and construction of its identity with their students.[15] Others revisit and revise methodological aspects in the use of biographic methods in nursing history.[16] We use biography to help students think about issues of professional identity.

Biographies and Professional Identity

Identity may be conceptualized as the individual and collective, subjective and objective, biographical and structural processes that conjunctively construct individuals and define institutions. Work, employment, and professional education are pertinent areas of social identification for individuals themselves (products of the secondary socialization process). But social identities are not limited to these: from infancy one meets sexual, ethnic, and class identity. The child lives the experience of initial social identity (the product of the primary socialization process) through the categorization conferred by others, via the ethnic, political, religious, professional, and cultural belongings of one's country, and also through scholastic performance. From this duality (identity for the other to confer and for you to construct), but also from inherited social identity, all identity strategies are originated, among which are those concerning presentation of one's self, which may have great importance for future development of professional life.[17]

The daily practices, images, and speech produced in social interaction support the idea that identity is a producer of subjectivity. Thus, identity produces new subjects with new behaviors linked to the reality that produced them. In Foucault's concept of identity, reality serves as an instrument for control, for coercion, but it may also be reused to work as an element of change and transformation. Individuals are able to approximate the reflection surrounding identity with techniques or technologies of self—they develop a set of reflective practices through which they are led to recognize themselves as subjects, in which they not only fix on behavioral rules, but also seek to transform themselves, modify themselves in their singularity, making their lives an endeavor that carries ethical and aesthetic values that respond to certain criteria.[18]

By applying this notion of reflection in the field of nursing, we can understand that our professional identity has been constructed from various sources, among them the relationship between our professional identity and society in respect to our care-based, educational, scientific, social, and political roles. Professional identity also varies with time, place, and custom. Biographies show nurses participating in a shared identity, building an imagined community.[19] However, that community was part of a wider one. Parsons, for example, hesitated to use the word "enfermeira" (feminine nurse), and not "enfermeiro" (masculine nurse), in light of the negative connotation the feminine form carried. Instead, she used the English word "nurse" in order to differentiate the professionals formally educated under her supervision from the other nurses in Brazilian society at that time.[20] However, the term did not catch on, and terms such as "nurse of the highest quality," or public health, or simply "graduated" prevailed, indicating that a new category had been created.[21]

Biographies help illuminate the elements of identity formation of interest to nursing scholars and further the development of the profession; they can also bring discussions of the past and present into the teaching–learning process for nursing students. Biographies help students and professionals understand what to expect from a nurse. The question is whether these life stories provide a sense of the professional identity and values of nursing for large numbers of people, or reach merely nurse historians or nurses who are interested in history. Biographies deal with the individual, the trajectory of a given life. They are specific and concrete. From an epistemological point of view, how are we to be cautious about generalizing? How are we to navigate the intersection between the individual pathway and the society to which that person belongs?

The responses to these questions will depend on the validity of the biography as an educational tool in history of nursing or clinical courses. We are conscious that nursing history must be clearly articulated in curricula in the same way as methods and strategies. As Janie Brown and Patricia D'Antonio affirm, "The teaching of our history imparts to our students and colleagues not only a broader understanding of the origins of our current successes and dilemmas, but also provides an analytical approach to complex clinical and professional issues that defy simplistic explanations."[22]

Celia Davies in "Rewriting Nursing History—Again?" proposes a new agenda for the future in terms of five key areas in the history of nursing. One of them is *the internationalization of nursing history*. Davies points out the importance of opening frontiers of knowledge in the history of nursing through participation in international conferences for nursing historians and those interested in history whose first language is not English.[23] We agree with Davies, and we want to further this discussion, proposing that essential books and articles for international discussion and reflection about the history of nursing be translated into languages beyond those of the publishing author, to at least reduce, if not eliminate existing barriers to knowledge.

Another form of socialization and internationalization of already produced knowledge in history made available to the public are articles in online periodicals on a myriad of sites, as well as the articles published in *Nursing History Review*, the first periodical created especially to promote studies related to the history of nursing, and *Nursing Inquiry*, which aims to dedicate one issue per year to historical research. We would also like to add a point regarding the political agenda of the history of nursing: especially in countries in which the subject is mandatory, such as Brazil, the history of nursing is frequently taught (and administered) by nonhistorians who have not concentrated in the history of nursing.

One of the great contributions of the history of nursing is the critical-reflective formal education of its professionals, who are capable of thinking about nursing within a field of dynamic and contradictory forces, past, present, and future. Through the study of history using biographies, students have the opportunity to develop insights and a greater understanding of the nursing profession, as well as of how to extend the multiple educational requirements of a thorough curriculum.[24] The study of history promotes student development of critical abilities concerning historical events and questions, and reveals how these events may have altered the profession. Historical biography makes mediation between the past and the present possible, while offering students the opportunity to situate themselves in a clearer reality of the present.

We are reminded that school is still a privileged institution for the transmission of culture. In the scholastic environment, the teacher is the principal actor who transmits culture. In a sense, the professor is the faithful guardian of culture, the heir. But he or she does not simply receive culture. As an intellectual he or she is capable of establishing links between the diverse areas of knowledge of the world, comprehending how the different interpretations of the world were constructed, and knowing the students, situated in their sociohistorical context. It is important to finish with the critical aspect that characterizes the professor's interpretations of culture, for it leads the students to observe the cultural panorama without the professor's interpretations being imposed upon them. Rather, the professor provides the incentive and instruments for the students to follow their own itineraries, in a search for the construction of their own knowledge.

Maria Itayra Padilha
Professor of Nursing
Leader, History of Nursing Knowledge Research Group (GEHCE)
Federal University of Santa Catarina/Brazil (UFSC)
Rod. Amaro Antônio Vieira, 2371/818. Ed. Paris. Itacorubi.
Florianópolis, Santa Catarina, Brasil CEP 88034–10

Sioban Nelson
Dean and Professor
Lawrence S. Bloomberg Faculty of Nursing
University of Toronto
55 College Street
Toronto M5T 1P8 Ontario
Canada

Acknowledgments

Maria Itayra Padilha would like to thank the National Council for Scientific and Technological Development (CNPq) for scientific support, and friends of Research Group in Nursing History at Federal University of Santa Catarina for data collection.

Notes

1. The New History movement began in France with the journal *Annales d'histoire économique et sociale* in 1929. Thenceforth there has been greater comprehension of historical change and the value of documents and memory, clothing, and everything that can be considered remembrance. Some of the principal authors from that period are Marc Bloch, François Simiand, Henri Hauser, Jacques Le Goff, and Lucien Febvre. See, e.g., Jacques Le Goff, Roger Chartier, and Jacques Revel, *La nouvelle histoire* (Paris: Retz-C-EPL, 1978); Michel de Certeau, *L'écriture d'histoire* [The Writing of History] (New York: Columbia University Press, 1988); Peter Burke, *The French Historical Revolution: The Annales School, 1929–1989* (Stanford, Calif.: Stanford University Press, 1991).

2. Eloita Neves and Maria Ivone, "Nursing in Brazil: Trajectory, Conquests, and Challenges," *Online Journal of Issues in Nursing* 5 (2000): 325–40.

3. Ieda de Alencar Barreira et al., "Renovação do ensino e pesquisa em história da enfermgem," *Revista Enfermagem da UERJ* 5, no. 2 (1997): 487–94.

4. Taka Oguisso and Genival Fernandes de Freitas, "História da Enfermagem: O ensinar e o pesquisar na Escola de Enfermagem da Universidade de São Paulo," *Revista de Pesquisa: Cuidado é fundamental* 9 (2007): 79–91.

5. Brasil Ministério da Saúde, *Enfermagem: Legislação e assuntos correlatos* (Rio de Janeiro: Fundação Serviços de Saúde Pública, 1974).

6. Ana Estela Haddad et al., *A trajetória dos cursos de graduação na saúde: 1991–2004* (Brasília: INEP, 2006).

7. Brasil Ministério da Educação, Lei 9.394, de 20 de dezembro, Diretrizes e Bases da Educação Nacional, *Diário Oficial da União* (Brasília) 1 (1996): 833–44.

8. Maria Itayra Padilha and Sioban Nelson, "Teaching Nursing History: The Santa Catarina, Brazil, Experience," *Nursing Inquiry* 16, no. 2 (June 2009): 171–80.

9. There are 301 nursing research groups in Brazil.

10. These texts help us understand the professional identity of nursing from the point of view of women's history, social history, and work history. See Celia Davies, *Rewriting Nursing History* (Totowa, N.J.: Croom Helm, 1980); Janet Wilson James, "Writing and Rewriting Nursing History: A Review Essay," *Bulletin of the History of Medicine* 58, no. 4 (1984): 568–84; Patricia D'Antonio, "Revisiting and Rethinking the Rewriting of Nursing History," *Bulletin of the History of Medicine* 73, no. 2 (1999): 268–90; Sioban Nelson, "Reading Nursing History," *Nursing Inquiry* 4, no. 4 (1997): 229–36; Sioban Nelson, "The Fork in the Road: Nursing History Versus the History of Nursing," *Nursing History Review* 10 (2002): 175–88.

11. These books are the result of master's theses and doctoral dissertations and have influenced other researchers in the historical perspective. Raimunda Germano, *Educação e ideologia da enfermagem no Brasil* (São Paulo: Cortez, 1984); Denise Pires, *Hegemonia médica na saúde e a enfermagem: Brasil, 1500 a 1930* (São Paulo: Cortez, 1989); Maria Cecília Puntel de Almeida, *O saber de enfermagem e sua dimensão prática* (São Paulo: Cortez, 1986); Cristina Maria Loyola Miranda, *O risco e o bordado: Um estudo sobre a formação da identidade profissional* (Rio de Janeiro: Escola de Enfermagem Anna Nery/UFRJ, 1998).

12. Waleska Paixão, *História da enfermagem* (Rio de Janeiro: Júlio C. Reis, 1951); Taka Oguisso, *Trajetória histórica e legal da enfermagem*, 2nd ed., Série Enfermagem (São Paulo: Manole, 2006); Valeria Lunardi, *História da enfermagem: Rupturas e continuidades* (Pelotas: Autor, 1999).

13. Helga Kruger and Bernd Baldus, "Work, Gender and the Life Course: Social Construction and Individual Experience," *Canadian Journal of Sociology* 24, no. 3 (1999): 355–79; Christopher Maggs, "A History of Nursing: A History of Caring?" *Journal of Advanced Nursing* 23, no. 3 (1996): 630–35; Sonya Grypma. "Critical Issues in the Use of Biographic Methods in Nursing History," *Nursing History Review* 13 (2005): 171–87.

14. Particularly Michel Foucault, *L'archéologie du savoir* [The Archaeology of Knowledge] (New York: Pantheon, 1995), 62–70. Foucault shows a new way of deep discursive analysis of biographical records in a historical perspective.

15. These experts have indicated new ways to teach nursing history in undergraduate and graduate nursing programs in Brazil, Canada, and the United States. Ieda de Alencar Barreira, Jussara Sauthier, Suely de Souza Baptista, Lucia Helena Silva Corrêa Lourenço, and Tânia Cristina Franco Santos, "Renovação no ensino e na pesquisa de história da enfermagem brasileira," *Revista Enfermagem da Universidado do Estado do Rio de Janeiro* 5, no. 2 (1997): 487–94; Stephanie Kirby, "Teaching Nursing History: The Redwood Experience," *Nurse Education Today* 18, no. 4 (1998): 310–16; Margareth Lait, "The Place

of Nursing History in an Undergraduate Curriculum," *Nurse Education Today* 20, no. 5 (2000): 395–400; Sandra Lewenson, "Integrating Nursing History into the Curriculum," *Journal of Professional Nursing* 20, no. 6 (2004): 374–80; Maria Itayra Padilha, "O ensino da história da Enfermagem nos Cursos de Graduação em Enfermagem em Santa Catarina, Brasil," *Trabalho, Educação e Saúde* 4, no. 2 (2006): 325–36; Meryn Stuart, "Teaching in Graduate Programs" (paper presented at the Pre-Conference of the American Association for the History of Nursing Annual Conference, Rochester, Minnesota, 2006).

16. Sonya Grypma, "Critical Issues in the Use of Biographic Methods in Nursing History," *Nursing History Review* 13 (2005): 171–87; Natalie Riegler, "Some Issues to Be Considered in the Writing of Biography," *Canadian Bulletin of Medical History* 11 (1994): 219–20.

17. Among publications about collective memory that show associations between the political, social, and individual are Cathy Caruth, *Unclaimed Experience: Trauma, Narrative, and History* (Baltimore: Johns Hopkins University Press, 1996); John Gillis, "Commemorations: The Politics of National Identity," in *The Invention of Tradition*, ed. Eric Hobsbawm and Terence Ranger (Cambridge: Cambridge University Press, 1983); Ulric Neisser, "What Is Ordinary Memory the Memory Of?" in *Remembering Reconsidered: Ecological and Traditional Approaches to the Study of Memory*, ed. Ulric Neisser and Eugene Winograd (Cambridge: Cambridge University Press, 1990), 356; Pierre Nora, "Entre mémoire et histoire," in *Les lieux de mémoire*, ed. Pierre Nora (Paris: Gallimard, 1984); Claude Dubar, *La socialisation: Construction des identités sociales et professionnelles* (Paris: Broche, 1991).

18. Foucault's discussion about identity is linked to two other themes: power and sexuality. In the case of power, Foucault justifies the importance of this study because it permits the creation of history in different ways in our culture, in which human beings have been subjects. Michel Foucault, "The Subject and Power," in *Michel Foucault, Beyond Structuralism and Hermeneutics*, 2nd ed., ed. Paul Rabinow and Richard Dreyfus (Chicago: University of Chicago Press, 1995), 234–53; Michel Foucault, *History of Sexuality*, vol. 2, *The Use of Pleasure* (New York: Vintage, 1988).

19. See Joan Lynaugh, "Introduction, Section 2: Identity: The Meaning of Nursing," in *Enduring Issues in American Nursing,* ed. Ellen Baer, Patricia D'Antonio, Sylvia Rinker, and Joan Lynaugh (New York: Springer, 2002).

20. Brazilian nurses of that era were mostly poor, black, and freed slaves. This model does not fit with the new model of nurses. The other model was the Sisters of Charity, who worked at the hospitals as servants of God. Maria Itayra Padilha, *A mística do silêncio: A prática de enfermagem na Santa Casa de Misericórdia do Rio de Janeiro no século XIX* (Pelotas: UFPel, 1998).

21. The expression "high level nurse" is still used in many hospitals to differentiate undergraduate nurses from other members of the nursing group (nursing assistant, nursing technician). Glete de Alcântara, *A enfermagem moderna como categoria profissional: Obstáculos à sua expansão na sociedade brasileira* (Ribeirão Preto: Escola de Enfermagem de Ribeirão Preto, Universidade de São Paulo, 1966), 20.

22. Janie Brown and Patricia D'Antonio, "Nursing History and Scholarship: Critical Issues for the Discipline," *Journal of Professional Nursing* 6, no. 6 (1990): 319.

23. Celia Davies, "Rewriting Nursing History—Again?" *Nursing History Review* 15 (2007): 21–24. The other four points of Davies's agenda are nursing, health policy, and the state; not professionalization but professional identity?; nursing practice, nursing knowledge, and caring; and living lives as nurses.

24. Lewenson, "Integrating Nursing History into the Curriculum," 376.

IN MEMORIAM

Karen Buhler-Wilkerson, 19 May 1944–13 February 2010: Spreading the Contagion of History

Karen Buhler-Wilkerson, who was always a public and community health nurse first, will be remembered for the contagion for history she spread through the inhaling of archival dust, the fevers and pain of writing it all down, and the multiplying of historical cells to create a new entity. No one could have quite predicted that she would become historian extraordinaire when she took up the accordion as a teenager, followed in her family's footsteps into the health care business, and sought to live her life always on her own terms. It is perhaps her lasting legacy that we all live and do our work as honestly as possible—regardless if the histories we write ruffle professional respectability and regardless if our choices for where we live and who and how we love challenge simple binaries.

Karen's life was above all, as her life partner Neville Strumpf put it so eloquently at her funeral, "fully lived." Fittingly somehow, her life began and ended in the Philadelphia that she loved, although there was also the cabin she rebuilt in the Poconos, and the vacations to Charleston, Blue Mountain Lake in the Adirondacks, and the south of France. Karen was part of a peripatetic natal family: her mother, the ever committed nurse, and her father, the dentist turned dean of several dental schools, moved Karen and her brother John to Buffalo, then Atlanta, and then Charleston. Karen trained at Emory University and worked first as a home care coordinator in a retirement community, beginning her life-long commitment to home care and the chronically ill.

Brought to the University of Pennsylvania in 1972 to teach community health nursing (sight unseen by the then dean with only her CV and reputation preceding her); yet often in part-time and adjunct positions, she found herself drawn more and more to history. While still teaching, working in home care, raising her two young sons, and rehabbing a Center City town house, she enrolled in Penn's Department of City Planning with a focus on health care history and policy for her PhD.

Perhaps a nurse who respected aging, who understood the gifts of knowledge that we gain over time, and who never shied away from the detritus we all shed, would in fact understand the nuances of history. She believed in the importance of the tidbits found in archival work that can create a body of scholarly understanding. Two serendipities made all of this happen: Karen worked with the ever generous medical and policy historians Charles Rosenberg and Rosemary Stevens, and Dean Claire Fagin brought Joan Lynaugh to Penn, herself a nurse-turned-historian. Joined by Ellen Baer, these "founders" of Penn's nursing history powerhouse had vision, historical training, and unmatched political skills nurtured by Fagin's intention to put nursing at the center of health care and university hierarchies.

Too well trained to believe in either preventive or hagiographic historical writing, Karen and her history comrades dug in and wrote historical truths. They also knew how to build the infrastructure, get the grants, and organize the supports that would renew nursing history. Karen learned to be an archivist and then directed the Center for the Study of the History of Nursing at Penn after Joan retired. The fact that I (a non-nurse historian) write this now in the *Nursing History Review*, edited by one of Karen's former students, is testament to the field she helped to revive and prosper, and the wide embrace of historians of every kind she made possible.

Karen loved the archives. One summer, she took the train every day from Philadelphia up to New York to wallow in Lillian Wald's papers, tracked down missing data at Henry Street, and spent weeks in her beloved Charleston searching through the history of the Ladies Benevolent Society. "You wouldn't believe what I am finding," she would call to say after rummaging through boxes and boxes, her characteristic charm and laughter coming through the phone line. "I love Lavina Dock," I confessed to her right after we first met, even though we both knew she must have been difficult to work with. It was the kind of historical love affair Karen deeply understood. She never lost what historians call "archive fever" and the funny kind of love that comes from, as one of my colleagues so bluntly put it, "reading dead people's mail."

Karen thought that mail actually meant something. The historian's task, she believed to the depth of her enormous soul, meant we had to confront contradictions in the historical figures we fell in love with and make peace continually with what we could never know. She thought history should be serviceable to policy (as witnessed by her two books on the history of public health nursing and on home care, as well as her major policy article that concluded that after two centuries of trying there would always be "the unavoidable tensions between fiscal reality and legitimate need" in home care). She thought racism should be named and fought, and she always tried to make sure the diversity of experience shown through her work. Her scholarship was recognized again and again by numerous major awards (including the President's Award from the American Association for the History of Nursing) and her election to the American Academy of Nursing.

Karen's sense of the fulsomeness of life never kept her just in history land. She was always in the community, setting up new programs whether it was with Bayada Home Care specialists or Penn's Living Independently for Elders nursing practice. She also loved art, food, cats, dogs, fast sports cars (who else buys a 1986 Porsche 911 when life is getting shorter?), and anything funky and fun. Her homes were always models of what an imagination could do, mixing colors of enormous vibrancy with the elegance of family memorabilia. Her artistic sensibility came through the organizing she did of major exhibitions of the RN uniform and of prints on nursing at the Philadelphia Museum of Art.

Karen was the first "Southern lady" I ever knew who owned two complete sterling silver tea sets and who had been taught to pour properly by her mother. She could also cook grits and shrimp, belt back scotch, and just be amazing fun. She was determined to find every barbeque joint at whatever professional meeting we attended, especially in the South. Sometimes we drove to parts of towns I would normally avoid, but we were always having a good time and in the company of as many as could fit in the cars.

Karen retreated to write alone when she had to. She set high standards for herself, often going to her mountain cabin or someone's seashore home to write away from the every day. She worried whether her writing was elegant enough or said the right things, surely a sign of someone who took her tasks seriously. Mostly, however, she thought our field had to grow. She encouraged all of us to do the best history we could and to live our lives as fully as possible.

Karen was ever the teacher, the public health nurse historian who would use experience and sober examination of data to create new history or policy. With Neville, she wrote an unbelievably moving article on her five-year sometimes just plain awful story of living with the ovarian cancer that finally ended her earthly days. At her funeral, more than 300 of us crowded that church to pay her tribute—and then ate really good food. She would have wanted to be at that party we said to ourselves as the missing her began to set in. She will, in what she taught us and built, always be there.

SUSAN M. REVERBY, PhD
Marion Butler McLean Professor in the History of Ideas and Professor of
Women's and Gender Studies
Wellesley College
Wellesley, MA 02481

MEDIA REVIEWS

Cultures of Health: A Historical Anthology. 2009. Sponsored by Canadian Foundation for Innovation; Ontario Research Fund; University of Windsor and its Department of History and the Canada Research Chair (CRC) in the History of International Health at the University of Windsor, Canada. Editor: Stephen Palmer. Design: Gerry Porter. http://hih.uwindsor.ca/wordpress/

Cultures of Health: A Historical Anthology is a Web site designed to showcase and make available to the public research carried out in the history of international health. The work of the site is performed under the auspices of the Canada Research Chair with room for expansion to include the work of other contributors. Although the primary agenda is identified as international or global health related to Latin America from 1800 to the present, as an "experimental" and "ecumenical" site it tacitly acknowledges the value of leaving geographical and temporal boundaries more broadly defined. The Web site promotes itself as a venue for students and established researchers to present and discuss ideas and sources that are not yet worked into the complex, finished "whole" of paper, article, thesis, or book. Designed to be especially suited for the presentation and discussion of research "fragments," its aim is to attract an eclectic mix of sources into an electronic repository of sorts, to stimulate historical conversations about the cultural dimensions of disease, health, and medicine. And eclectic it is.

The homepage is comprised of a feature "Latest Article" (when accessed it was Palmer and Malone's superbly written, "Border City Medicine: Windsor's History of Innovative Health Practice"); a series of intriguing "Asides," which are links to newly released books; history of medicine and nursing live and online exhibits, podcasts and blogs; and a compilation of vaguely defined "Recent Posts" plus links to archives of each of these features. The right-hand column is one of the strongest features of the Web site. Comprised of links categorized under the headings of "Languages" (English, Spanish, French, and Portuguese), "Categories" (with a drop list that includes "Nursing"), "Cultures of Health Collections," "Related Sites," "Libraries and Collections," "Journals," and "Organizations and Associations," this feature acts as a convenient "favorite bookmarks" of sorts for researchers and students. It includes sites of particular interest to nurse historians, such as the AMS Nursing History Research Unit (Ottawa), the Barbara Bates Center for the Study of the History of Nursing, the *Canadian Bulletin for the History of Medicine*, *Nursing History Review*, and the American Association for the History of Nursing. I trust that the absence of links to the Canadian Association for the History of Nursing and the University of Virginia Center for Nursing Historical Inquiry are oversights that will be remedied. Although I found the Web site to be user-friendly overall, I was puzzled about its purpose until I found the mission statement tab. A textbox with a brief explanation of the Web site's aim displayed on the homepage would quite easily resolve any potential confusion.

The Search toolbar at the top of the Web page is a helpful way to search the contents, and will be invaluable as the volume of material grows. The search term "nurs" brought up links to five e-articles focusing on history of medicine, and four links to nursing archival projects, including the Nova Scotia Nursing History digitalization project Web site, the nursing cap exhibit at the Canadian Museum of Civilization, and an exemplar from the Barbara Bates Center for the Study of the History of Nursing. Here the value of digitalization over print publications becomes clear; the visual images of primary sources are stunning.

Each posted article or Web page includes a section for readers to post comments. Such opportunity for conversation between authors and readers is where *Cultures of Health* best meets its mandate as a venue for researchers and students to discuss and share their ideas related to health history, including nursing history.

Authors who are interested in contributing articles to *Cultures of Health* are required to provide a proposal to the editorial team and sign an academic hosting agreement. There is no peer review process; the idea is that the authors use this venue to invite feedback to their works-in-progress. Conforming to the Creative Commons mode of licensing electronic publications, authors retain copyright and are free to publish elsewhere. Although this idea fits well with the push towards open access, authors may be reluctant to present unpolished written work. On the other hand, if posting an article to *Cultures of Health* is viewed in a similar light to presenting an unpublished paper at a conference, authors might find it quite appealing.

To live up to its potential, this Web site must be seen as more than a source of information or links to other useful sites; it must engage readers to actively participate. Its relevance to students and researchers of nursing history will depend on the degree to which they themselves contribute to and engage with the material posted. Bookmark this site. Better yet, contribute to it. It promises to be a source for some lively interaction.

Sonya Grypma, PhD, RN
Associate Professor
School of Nursing
Adjunct Associate Professor
Department of History
Trinity Western University
7600 Glover Road
Langley BC V2Y 1Y1
Canada

Brought to Life: Exploring the History of Medicine. The Science Museum. Supported by the Welcome Trust. Project Manager: Simon Chambers. http://www.sciencemuseum.org.uk/broughttolife.aspx

The Science Museum in London, founded in 1857 with objects that were displayed at the Great Exhibition, contains thousands of objects from various fields of science, including medical science. The *Brought to Life* Web site is a complementary adjunct to the Science Museum's collections, providing online access to images of the artifacts contained in its medical collections and comprehensive textual information on a wide range of topics associated with the history of medicine. Designed to be informative and educational, the Web site is aimed at "teachers and students working on the history of medicine, and related subjects, in schools and universities."

While no particular historiographic framework is evident, much of the material is written in the idiom of social history. The material is largely descriptive, with little critique of the history of medicine as a social practice or scientific medicine's role in society. Instead, the content and tone appear to be partly responsive to the general public's abiding fascination with medical science and with all things gory and gruesome. Nevertheless, some serious and controversial issues are addressed, such as medical ethics, including the legal acceptance of brain death and changing views on organ transplantation. Other topics associated with the social history of medicine include travel and faith healing, disease and deformity as spectacle and curiosity, and women in medicine. The patient's experiences of hospitalization and the history of the use of dead bodies in medical training are also addressed in articles.

The Web site is built around five major sections, namely "Topics and Themes," "People," "Objects," "Technology and Technique," and "Timeline." Each major section contains subfolders containing a range of articles presented in multiple formats, including static text, photographs, short video clips, and interactive cartoons. All textual material is clearly and concisely written and easily downloadable. The "Themes and Topics" section is one of the major elements of the Web site, bringing the user to ten subthemes that include "Diseases and Epidemics," "Hospitals," "Public Health," and "War and Medicine." Each subtheme contains multiple articles aimed at second-level students and undergraduate students studying history. Although largely descriptive, the material is nevertheless informative, containing a chronology of major events, dates, and associated images.

The "Technologies and Techniques" link takes the visitor to over 100 short articles, from anesthesia to war surgery, and the "People" section is presented as an interactive timeline that features key individuals in the history of medicine. Numerous digital images accompany each article or are otherwise contained under the major section "Object." For example, a variety of surgical instruments, including a bullet locator from World War I and a bullet extractor from an earlier period are presented. A number of interactive components are incorporated, including an interactive timeline of key milestones in the history of medicine. One interactive section features the iron lung and contains real patient histories of dependency on an iron lung.

Navigation is simple and vertical scroll bars are available where textual material exceeds the available screen space. While the content is generally well organized, a number of the design elements might be improved. For example, link and scrolling techniques are not used consistently throughout. The "Topics and Themes" pages are organized vertically around link tabs presented as text boxes to the left of the screen, while the links to each of the "Techniques and Technologies" topics (from "amputation" to "wet nursing") are presented as photographic icons, displayed alphabetically and searched by scrolling horizontally or by clicking a topic name in a drop-down menu. The interactive timeline element is rather difficult to navigate and requires reloading each time the user returns to the main tab. Audio and sign language versions of the textual material are available for some but not all sections. There are numerous links to relevant external Web sites, such as the Wellcome Library, but few direct links to digitized primary sources. One notable exception is a link to a digitized version of Florence Nightingale's *Notes on Nursing*.

The major section "Techniques and Technologies" contains a short article on nursing, which is referred to as "one of the oldest medical occupations." The text contains just five short paragraphs and a link to Nightingale is provided, with copy here also cursory. For each textual article a short bibliography is provided. In the case of nursing, three outdated references are listed, namely Brian Abel-Smith's *History of the Nursing Profession* and two books by Christopher Maggs.

Derived from the Science Museum's collection related to medical history, the *Brought to Life* Web site is in essence a resource for the lay user and for secondary school teachers and students, and while it offers important facts for a novice of medical history, it offers little depth material for the scholar of the topic or related topics. Nevertheless, it is an important medium for public engagement with the history of science, and as such, is a valuable resource.

Gerard M. Fealy, RGN, PhD
Associate Professor/Director
UCD Irish Centre for Nursing & Midwifery History
UCD School of Nursing, Midwifery & Health Systems
University College Dublin
Ireland

Canada's Role in Fighting Tuberculosis. Produced under contract to Canada's Digital Collections (CDC) Program, Industry Canada, by a CDC team at the Saskatchewan Lung Association. Gordan Holtslander (team leader), Darrel Lagasse (multimedia assistant), Verma Loewen (multimedia assistant), Scott Rutherford (project manager). http://www.lung.ca/tb/credit.html

Three pictorial symbols of tuberculosis (TB) introduce *Canada's Role in Fighting Tuberculosis*, a Web site developed by a collaborative team from the Saskatchewan Lung Association and the Canadian Lung Association to serve as a resource for those with a general interest in TB. Images of the tubercle bacilli, a TB sanatorium, and several isoniazid tablets set out the Web site's purpose, which is to provide users with an overview of the broad historical arc occurring between the early Canadian TB epidemics of the late nineteenth century up to the contemporary resurgence of multidrug resistant TB. The involvement of Canada's Digital Collection (CDC) in the development of the Web site positions it as a resource geared toward a wide audience of individuals.

Users of *Canada's Role in Fighting Tuberculosis* will find a functioning Web site that is easy to navigate though several value-added features such as a site map or search engine would be helpful. The home page provides links to three topical themes, a list of supplementary materials ("Glossary," "Teacher's Guide," "Works Cited"), and three community of interest categories ("Index,"

"Site Credits," "Search/Index") all located at the left side of the page. The first theme, "About TB" is located in the top center of the home page and provides users with broad topical links such as, "What Is Tuberculosis," "How Does Pulmonary Tuberculosis Develop," and "Do I Have Tuberculosis." While the content is of some value to those unfamiliar with TB, it reads like information that one might find on a typical Centers for Disease Control or Web MD site. Annotated links, provided to the right of the text, offer further explanations on the cause, spread, and treatment of TB. The downside to these offerings is that at least two of the links have either expired or are absent of actual content. The section ends with links for interactive games including "Hangman" and a "Matching Game" to test the user's knowledge of TB. The games are arguably intended to engage the user; yet, they largely fail to promote critical thinking or allow opportunities for learners to interact with the site in a meaningful way.

The second theme, "TB History," traces the trajectory of TB in Canada beginning in 1867. Here the site combines a range of mostly secondary sources and a small number of primary sources. Much of the text is taken from George Jasper Wherrett's *The Miracle of the Empty Beds: A History of Tuberculosis in Canada* (1977), which according to the Web site developers "is the most comprehensive account of TB in Canada."[1] A time line of important dates is presented, though it does little to include intersecting moments in history or the relationship between the medical occurrences surrounding the anti-TB crusade and Canada's social, cultural, and political currents. A section on the prevention of TB includes an overview of preventoriums and BCG vaccination, but does not contain adequate citations. The most glaring omission in this section is the absence of an interpretative voice. The developer's association with the CDC may have limited their ability to take a particular point of view. The absence, however, leaves the Web site user with a great deal of secondary source information but limited synthesis or analysis and very little additional historical sources or Web sites.

The third theme, "TB Today," offers users an overview of TB treatment beginning with the development of antimicrobials in 1948 and the initiation of direct observation therapy (DOT) in 1990. The main purpose of this section is to caution users that "TB is still killing people in Canada, and remains one of the biggest killers of humans in other parts of the world."[2] This section presents several graphs that depict the current prevalence and incidence of the infectious disease.

The developers of *Canada's Role in Fighting Tuberculosis* have included a broad range of photographic visual representations. The site allows users to slightly enlarge images; many of the images, however, are not accompanied source credits. Reference citations for the photos are located under the "Image Catalog" section of the Works Cited page, which is located in a completely different area of the site. Despite its ill placement, the Image Catalogue provides useful information, including descriptions of the images used throughout the site along with abbreviated citations. The weakness of the Image Catalogue is the absence of a reference key to locate collections where the images were found. Also missing is an explanation for the selection of particular documents. Further, the developers fail to account for copyright issues for materials listed on the site, limiting the ability for image copying and reproduction.

As with any other historical artifact, information found on the Web must be held to a standard—judged on the validity and reliability of the information presented. Users of *Canada's Role in Fighting Tuberculosis* should expect information pertaining to the natural course of illness in TB, peppered with a historical overview of Canada's efforts to eradicate it. The historical section suffers from severe technical and methodological challenges so for those interested in serious history, this Web site fails to deliver.

J. MARGO BROOKS CARTHON, PHD, APRN
Post Doctoral Fellow
Barbara Bates Center for the Study of the History of Nursing Center for Health Outcomes and Policy Research University of Pennsylvania School of Nursing
Philadelphia, PA 19104

Notes

1. George Jasper Wherrett, *The Miracle of the Empty Beds: A History of Tuberculosis in Canada* (Toronto: University of Toronto Press, 1977).
2. Canada's Digital Collections Program, "Canada's Role in Fighting Tuberculosis," http://www.lung.ca/tb/credit.html

Classic Nursing Films 1927–1945. 2007. Quality Information Publishers. (Production detail listed with each film below.) 441 N. Louisiana Avenue, Suite P; Asheville, NC 28806. $11.99. http://www.qualityinformationpublishers.com/. Three films comprise this DVD: (1) *The Army Nurse* (1945) a seventeen-minute official film of the U.S. War Department, produced by the Army Pictorial Service of the Signal Corps for the Motion Pictures and Special Events Division of the War Finance Division of the U.S. Treasury Department; (2) *Your Life Work: Nursing* (1942) an eleven-minute film produced by Vocational Guidance Films, Inc.; manuscript by Arthur P. Twogood, associate professor of vocational education at Iowa State College; and (3) *Artificial Respiration* (1927) an eleven-minute film produced by Loucks and Norling, Inc., New York.

Set in the summer of 1945 and therefore at the closing of the European theater of war, the early part of the first film, *The Army Nurse.* sounds initially as if it were directed toward enlisted men to describe the progression of their care from field and evacuation hospitals to general hospitals in the war theater and finally to a U.S. general hospital, with descriptions of hospital trains, planes, and ships as modes of transportation. But midway into the film, the nurse-focused detail comes into focus. At the end of the film, the superintendent of the Army Nurse Corp, Florence A. Blanchfield, makes an appeal for viewers to "buy a bond," explaining that 57,000 nurses have served in the Medical Department of the Army to date, that nurses are still being sent overseas to replace those who have served, and that 300,000 veterans are recovering in U.S. general hospitals, and will be for some time to come.

There is little glamour and lots of hardship portrayed in *The Army Nurse*. Also shown is the recognition of nurses' key roles. The narrator says at one point, "she is a nurse first, woman second, and officer third." The film as a whole accents the professional role, though there is more reference to the nurse as symbol of safety, comfort, home, and feminine nurturance than might be expected, and only one reference to nurses' officer status. Taken as a whole, I speculate that this was intended as a short pre-film to precede theater newsreels to which the music and visuals are comparable. This would hardly be classified as entertainment now. If presented with an introduction, it could hold undergraduate attention, and it is rich enough to be used in a number of ways with graduate nursing history students. Certainly nurses who served in World War II or the Korean War would find it interesting, if only by comparison and contrast to their individual experiences.

The second film on the DVD *Your Life Work: Nursing* was designed to inform high school students about the field of nursing. No sources for its information are identified, but it clearly reflects characteristics the National League of Nursing Education wished were true throughout the country (e.g., nursing school applicants who had taken college preparatory courses and were in the top one-third to one-half of their high school graduating classes; nursing curricula rich in the basic sciences; and post-graduate work or college degrees for public health and leadership positions). Communicable disease nursing shows up as a major experience in the curriculum; and in keeping with its idealized depictions of nursing, the film mentions mental illness nursing and public health as student experiences.

The film describes the major types of registered nurse employment. Private duty nursing, the field in which so many graduate nurses were actually employed in 1942, gets first but briefest mention. Within public health nursing, various subareas such as factory first aid nursing, along with psychiatric nursing and prison nursing (to attract increasing numbers of men), school nursing, and home nursing are depicted. The various fields of government service such as enrolled Red Cross, military, Indian Health Service, U.S. Public Health Service, and Veterans Administration nursing are highlighted. Finally the film addresses institutional nursing, including staff nursing and the administrative and educational fields. The viewer needs to be interested in the information presented, or what it says about nursing practice and education in 1941–1942, to endure the dull didacticism of the narration. But, if one can get past that, the film provides focus for discussion of the organized nursing version of nursing and nursing education on the eve of World War II.

Artificial Respiration, the last film on the DVD, is a silent film, as would be expected from its date (1927). It instructs viewers in the prone pressure method of artificial respiration or resuscitation, useful to re-start breathing after drowning, "gas asphyxiation" (dramatized by a white-shirted man with bow tie lying under a tail pipe emitting exhaust, repairing the car, when the garage door blows shut), and electric shock (occasioned when a man grasps a downed electric wire).

This is purely artificial respiration accomplished by applying lower rib cage pressure at a rate of twelve to fifteen times per minute. At one point the instruction is to continue until rigor mortis sets in; at another it asserts that people have survived after three to four hours receiving the treatment. The film advises that once the victim revives, rescuers should not allow him sit up and should keep him warm. In the case of "gas asphyxiation" a physician or "the gas company" should be called. The physician in the picture brings a small tank of air containing a 95 percent oxygen and 5 percent carbon dioxide mix and a mask. Otherwise there is no mention of ambulance, first aid, or other supplementary or subsequent measures. The only woman in the otherwise all-male cast brings a glass of liquid to the emergency scene and is waved off, with the instruction that unconscious people should not have fluids.

I would classify this as a first aid film meant for non-medical persons rather than a nursing film. Although the level of knowledge about human physiology among the general population was less in the late 1920s than it is now, still I would rate this film's medical knowledge as equal to that of a middle schooler of that era. Current viewers, even with healthy historical curiosity, may find themselves impatient with its slow, repetitive pace.

MARILYN E. FLOOD, PhD, RN
Associate Dean Emeritus
School of Nursing
University of California San Francisco
San Francisco, CA 94143–0604

Opening Doors: Contemporary African American Academic Surgeons. 2007. National Library of Medicine and the Reginald F. Lewis Museum of Maryland African American History and Culture, Bethesda, Maryland. Curated by Margaret A. Hutto and Jill L. Newmark. Exhibition design by RCW Communications, Inc. Exhibition fabrication by Adler Display, Inc., and CSI. http://www.nlm.nih.gov/hmd/about/exhibition/travelingexhibitions/openingbanner.html

Who are today's most accomplished African American surgeons and educators? What are the historical antecedents to their practice and teaching? These are the questions that *Opening Doors: Contemporary African American Academic Surgeons,* a traveling exhibit and its accompanying Web site, strive to answer as they honor historical and contemporary African American academic surgeons.

The Web site is organized logically in four, easily navigated sections. The first section, "Pioneers," profiles six hospitals and schools that made important contributions to the training of black surgeons and to the advancement of the careers of African American academic surgeons. Included in this section are images of primary documents such as hospital reports and photographs of surgeons, hospitals, and operating rooms. All of the images are linked to well-reproduced, high-quality JPEG (Joint Photographic Experts Group) images that allow for close inspection of their many details. Most images have a caption that gives the viewer further insight into the image's historical context.

The second section, "Contemporary Pioneers," provides an in-depth look at four contemporary individuals who have made major contributions to academic surgery. The page for each of the four surgeons begins with a present-day photograph and a quote exemplifying that individual's philosophical approach to life and medical practice. A biographical sketch and career highlights follow. Each page contains engaging images intended to bring this person to life, such as photographs of the individual in earlier years of practice, family photographs, and images of their publications. A page that is especially effective in captivating the audience is that of Alexa I. Canady, MD, pediatric neurosurgeon. This portion includes illustrations of Canady's practice in the form of three vivid crayon drawings drawn by elementary students complete with poignant captions.

The third section, "New Frontiers," presents seventeen African American surgeons who currently hold prestigious positions in academic surgery. Each of these surgeons is featured in two or three paragraphs, which highlight their training locations, major career achievements, and current position. The fourth section, "History," briefly describes medical education of African Americans from around the time of the Civil War through the twentieth century. Historical context is explored in a section on racial inequities in health care, including several images of floor plans of segregated hospital wards, and an 1811 medical manual detailing special considerations for medical care of slaves. Interestingly, the history section is placed in the far-right position on the exhibit's home page, making it likely to be the last portion of the site to be visited, instead of the first. However, the placement is likely a reflection of the exhibit designers hope that even viewers who are not usually interested in history would become drawn into the stories of the featured individuals and want to learn about the historical antecedents to their practice.

As minorities continue to be underrepresented in medicine, and particularly in academic medicine, encouraging young African Americans to pursue a career in medicine or surgery was without doubt a compelling reason for the development of this exhibit. The exhibit will certainly spark interest among young people who will find at least one, if not many, of the featured surgeons appealing as a role model. Moreover, the exhibit will also serve to intrigue young African American women; the exhibit features a nearly equal number of female and male surgeons.

Viewers should be aware that the Web site and traveling exhibit do not provide a comprehensive view of the topic of African Americans in academic surgery. Rather, the exhibit approaches the topic in a case study format, designed to use the power of the appeal of individual people to capture interest. An exhibit of a broader purpose and scope would benefit from exploring the lives and work of more African American surgeons and a more thorough examination of historical contexts of racial issues in society and medicine.

I was disappointed at the limited nature of the traveling exhibit. It consisted of six standard exhibit panels of approximately three-by-eight-feet each, and included only highlights of the same materials available on the Web site. Moreover, the traveling exhibit displayed is in only a two-dimensional, noninteractive format. As multimedia exhibits have become more commonplace, many viewers have come to expect a high level of interactivity. Also, as the exhibit itinerary includes many university medical libraries full of undergraduate and medical students, it seems unfortunate that the exhibit does not contain more engaging materials to draw in members of the very group the exhibit is intended to reach. However, despite these minor critiques, this exhibit and Web site provide a valuable service in raising awareness of the important contributions of African American academic surgeons.

ANNE Z. COCKERHAM, PHD, CNM, WHNP-BC
Course Coordinator
Frontier School of Midwifery and Family Nursing
25853 Spring Farm Circle
Chantilly, VA 20152

REVIEW ESSAY: WOMEN AND WAR

Mobilizing Minerva: American Women
in the First World War
By Kimberly Jensen
(Urbana: University of Illinois Press, 2008) ($30.00 paper)

World War II Front Line Nurse
By Mildred A. MacGregor
(Ann Arbor: University of Michigan Press, 2008) ($26.95 paper)

Until the twentieth century, the position of women in wartime had been an anomalous one. Subjected as civilians to the threats posed by advancing armies, yet restrained, as women, from active involvement in conflict, their positioning on the home front had made them, at best, the passive observers of warfare and, at worst, its victims. When they broke free of the societal constraints that had placed them in such passively ambivalent roles—to become "camp-followers," to engage personally in warfare, and to offer support and nursing care to armies—they were universally derided as women of low reputation and questionable morals.

At the end of the nineteenth century, seismic social forces were already creating massive changes in the behavior and perceptions of women, such that, by the second decade of the twentieth century significant numbers believed they were ready to demonstrate how important their contributions could be in time of war. Kimberly Jensen begins her perceptive analysis of these changes with a description of the Washington, D.C., Suffrage Parade of 1913. In doing so, she illustrates both the courage and determination of those women (and men) who marched publicly to advertise their adherence to the principle of woman suffrage, and the strength and bitterness of opposition to them within sections of the American population. From this prelude, Jensen moves rapidly into a careful analysis of the relationship between women's claims to citizenship (including the vote and the right to full civic involvement) and their contributions to the war effort during the First World War. Focusing on the period from United States' entry into the war in April 1917 to the end of the war in November 1918 and then into the first years of the postwar period, Jensen offers us a clear insight into how women's increasing claims to full citizenship were given form and substance by their involvement in war. She demonstrates how women found many ways of overturning the accepted order of society in which traditional gender roles of women as "protected" and men as "protectors," had left women powerless and vulnerable in time of war.

Nursing History Review 19 (2011): 210–213. A Publication of the American Association for the History of Nursing. Copyright © 2011 Springer Publishing Company.
DOI: 10.1891/1062–8061.19.210

Meticulously researched and written in a thoughtful and precise style, *Mobilizing Minerva* offers the reader an insight into the ways in which three distinct groups of American women positioned themselves as participants in—rather than observers or victims of—the First World War. She considers the work of female physicians, looking, in particular, at the ways in which they mobilized their efforts in the support of women and children who had suffered from the violence of war. She also considers women as the "bearers of arms," examining the way in which early feminists drew on the popular social motif of the American pioneer woman, who was capable of wielding a fire-arm to protect herself and her family, instead of relying upon a man to. In doing so, she draws on other examples—particularly the Russian Women's Battalion of Death, the news of which created both fascination and consternation among Americans. She offers her readers a clear insight into just how subversive the arguments for women's independence and self-protection were.

It is, however, Jensen's third group—that of military nurses—that was perhaps the most radical in its demands. In their drive for recognition and acceptance as war-participants, nurses went further than any other group by campaigning for equal status with men of similar position and responsibility. They demanded nothing less than officer status.

When America entered the war in April 1917, many nurses were already members of Nursing Reserves having offered their services, through the Red Cross, to the nascent base hospital units, which were attached to well-established university hospitals throughout the United States. When their country declared war, many travelled overseas with their units under the auspices of the Army Nurse Corps. Unfortunately, none had officer status, and this put them in an ambivalent position vis-à-vis both medical officers, some of whom appear to have treated them with contempt, and enlisted men, untrained individuals taken on shortly before the units left the United States to work as orderlies. Responsible as they were for the day-to-day care and treatment of their patients, nurses could only work effectively if enlisted men were willing to accept their training and follow their orders. But, as Jensen illustrates, there is evidence that, in a number of cases, medical officers disrupted their efforts, countermanded their orders, and engaged in what modern society would label "workplace harassment." Jensen does not offer us a clear indication of the size and scope of the problem, though she does present some very compelling cases in which senior nurses were harassed by medical officers and then labeled "sick" and removed from duty after protesting against their treatment.

The dilemma of the nursing profession is captured in Jensen's arresting narrative, as is the conflict between those such as Daisy Urch, herself a victim of harassment, who argued for officer status, and Julia Stimson, whose meteoric rise to the position of superintendent of the Army Nurse Corps was probably due in part to her formidable social skills. Stimson argued that officer status would not protect nurses. Their role could only be supported and their position secured by an ability to present themselves as genteel ladies, who could mobilize the gallantry of the medical officer colleagues. Stimson was not alone in believing that the status of the nursing profession must rest on the social caliber of its members, and it is probably because of this fragmentation in the views of the service that members of the Army Nurse Corps were only awarded "relative rank" under the Jones-Raker Bill in June 1920.

Jensen's intense and compelling analysis of the difficulties faced by the members of the U.S. Army Nurse Corps during the First World War makes, at times, for disturbing reading, and it was partly for this reason that I found Mildred MacGregor's *World War II*

Front Line Nurse—a personal account of her experience as an American military nurse during the Second World War—such an immense lift to the spirits. Reading both books offers an extraordinary insight into how much the lives of women—and specifically of military nurses—had changed between the Armistice of November 1918, and the entry of the United States into the Second World War in 1941. The styles of writing in these two books has a significant impact on the way in which the reader's impressions are formed and the two worlds depicted are viewed. Jensen's analysis is a strong and forthright scholarly interpretation of the grim struggle for women's rights in the early twentieth century. MacGregor's narrative is an exciting and high-spirited gallop through the personal adventures of an independent professional woman of the 1940s. Yet those worlds—the world of the First World War Base Hospital and that of the Second World War Third Auxiliary Surgical Unit—seem so different that it is difficult to believe that they were separated by a period of only 25 years.

First Lieutenant Mildred Radawiec embarked for Europe in December 1942, enduring some of the worst mid-Atlantic storms of the century to arrive in England and a posting in Oxford just before Christmas. Mildred's narrative is redolent of a sense of freedom and independence as she—a spirited but inexperienced young woman from Michigan—discovers the hardships and adventures of a war-torn, bleak, and rain-swept England. Soon finding herself posted to North Africa, she experiences the heady excitements of some hair-raising journeys through the Atlas Mountains, the adventure of "sleeping rough" in tents and the romance of a war experienced vicariously through the stories of her Air Force boyfriends. One of the most striking elements of MacGregor's narrative is the sense of sexual liberation (bounded and controlled by deliberate and determined personal "moral standards") that it exudes. Although engaged to a doctor "back home," the author dates and "flirts" with a number of fellow servicemen, always, however, managing to keep them at a safe distance that will permit her the freedom she desires. Her recounting of her feelings towards these "friends" is one of the most touching elements of her account, as she recognizes the strains endured by those who have to enter combat on a regular basis and their need for light-hearted romance to offer them comfort and relief. One of the most entertaining sections of the book is that in which the author dons a silver lamé evening gown to ride to a party in the back of an Army wagon. Upon arrival, she is immediately approached by an Air Force lieutenant, who becomes the focus of a romantic attachment for the remainder of the war.

In 1944, the scene darkens as Mildred's unit is detailed for service in Northern France. Landing on Omaha Beach sixteen days after D-Day, she experiences the horror of modern warfare, as she nurses severely mutilated and dying soldiers just behind the Allies' advancing front lines. Through her compelling narrative, we gain an insight into the intensity of the struggle endured by the Allied forces and the relentlessness of the work experienced by those who cared for their injured. The text is interspersed by accounts of the progress of the war itself, and by narratives taken directly from *Front Line Surgeons* (recounting the experiences of those male members of the Auxiliary Surgical Units who operated directly on the front line).[1] For the reader, these accounts make MacGregor's book something more than a narrative of one nurse's experiences. We are offered a history of the last two years of the war in Western Europe from many angles—that of the nurse herself, embroiled in one small "sector," experiencing the intensity of day-to-day experience; that of other surgical workers; and, in addition, a bird's-eye view of what was happening across a broad and complex front.

Many accounts have been written of nurses' experiences in the two world wars. Kimberly Jensen's *Mobilizing Minerva* and Mildred MacGregor's *World War II Front Line Nurse* provide us with two very different accounts, both highly original and both deeply compelling. The status, role, and position of female nurses in the highly masculine environment of war continued to be a difficult and ambiguous one until the late-1940s. As Jensen points out, it was not until the Army-Navy Nurses Act of 1947 and the Women's Armed Services Integration Act of 1948 that American military nurses were given full officer status.

CHRISTINE E. HALLETT
Reader in Nursing History
The School of Nursing, Midwifery and Social Work
Jean McFarlane Building
The University of Manchester
Oxford Road, Manchester, M13 9PL, UK

Note

1. Clifford L. Graves, *Front Line Surgeons* (San Diego, Calif.: Frye and Smith, 1950).

REVIEW ESSAY:
NURSING IN NEWFOUNDLAND

From the Voices of Nurses: An Oral History of Newfoundland Nurses who Graduated Prior to 1950
By Marilyn Beaton and Jeanette Walsh
(St. John's, Newfoundland: Jesperson Publishing, 2004)
(154 pages, $14.95 CAN)

A Life of Caring: 16 Newfoundland Nurses Tell Their Stories
By Marilyn Marsh, Jeanette Walsh, and Marilyn Beaton
(St. John's, Newfoundland: Breakwater Books Ltd., 2008)
(202 pages, $17.50 CAN)

After listening to an elderly nurse share her nursing stories with younger nurses at a dinner hosted by their professional association, authors Marilyn Beaton and Jeanette Walsh were inspired to record the experiences of older Newfoundland nurses lest their stories be lost. *From the Voices of Nurses* and the later *A Life of Caring* do just that. Based on oral interviews of 33 and 16 nurses respectively, these books effectively capture the memories of nurses who trained and worked in disparate, often remote practice settings in Newfoundland during the 1920s to 1940s. Taken together, their narratives expose the key role nurses played in the delivery of health care to the small country of Newfoundland prior to its entry into the Canadian confederacy in 1949.

While both books deal with the subject of nurses who graduated from Newfoundland between 1920 and 1949, they are organized differently. The earlier *From the Voices of Nurses* is organized around four themes: nursing education, practice after graduation, environmental influences (e.g., war), past and present nursing practices. *A Life of Caring*, co-authored with Marilyn Marsh, is organized into sixteen chapters, each representing one nurse who graduated in Newfoundland between 1920 and 1949. The central theme in both books is that nursing in pre-Confederation Newfoundland, while underresourced and even "unsophisticated," creatively addressed some of the most profound health care needs of a predominantly poor and isolated population.

Both books contain abridged stories as told by the nurses themselves. And it is the stories that fascinate.

From the Voices of Nurses explores the reasons these women entered nursing, the type of education they received, and their provision of nursing services after graduation. Prior to Confederation, three schools of nursing existed in Newfoundland, and students' experiences varied depending on which institution they attended. Many of the stories reveal a high level of resiliency, adaptability, creativity . . . and mischievousness. For example, as part of their training as "ladies," Lillian Moakler reported that nursing students at the General Hospital were required to wear hats and gloves when they were out in the daytime. Instead of abiding by this rule, the students would leave their hats and gloves hanging in the trees just outside the hospital and then collect them once they returned.

One of the most fascinating parts of the book was how the nurses' stories exemplify the interaction between history and geography—the sea in particular. All three nursing schools were located in St. John's, and students who came from isolated areas had to journey there by boat or train. Mary House recalled that she arrived at Grace Hospital two months prior to the start date of her program as she had to travel by boat before the water froze. Outport nurses (those nursing in isolated small-port settings), as well as nurses who worked in nursing stations and cottage hospitals, provided health care to isolated areas of Newfoundland with limited resources. They were often the sole health care provider in the area, and their care was significantly impacted by the lack of roads. Not only did nurses adapt their practice to the situations that they found themselves in, but they also experienced greater autonomy and self-reliance due to their isolation from St. John's.

In *A Life of Caring* the reader is able to get a good sense of who each nurse was. Although the authors offer no analysis of these women's experiences or nursing practice, it does offer a fascinating glimpse into the lives of a group of women who practiced as much by their wits as by training. It complements *From the Voices of Nurses* well by illustrating the creativity and fortitude required by nurses (and their patients) dealing with illness, injury, and childbirth along the rugged coastlines of the isolated nation of Newfoundland.

The oral record in both books supports the authors' main thesis, that these nurses made a vital contribution to the health of Newfoundlanders, often as the sole provider in a region. Less clear is evidence to support Beaton and Walsh's contention that nursing in Newfoundland was different pre- and post-Confederation, since indicators such as poverty, difficulty accessing health care, and barriers to care remained well into the 1960s. Neither book claims to be, nor should be seen as, providing a scholarly or critical analysis of the period. Written in the tradition of compiled nursing memoirs exemplified by three popular Northern Nursing books (edited by J. Karen Scott & Joan E Kieser, 2002, 2005, 2009; published by Kokum Publications), these books' appeal lies in the nature of the stories themselves.[1]

For scholars who are interested in oral history, early twentieth-century nursing education, the development of professional nursing in the Maritimes, or the notion of "place" in nursing in isolated settings, both *From the Voices of Nurses* and *A Life of Caring* should be seen as valuable primary sources to inform academic studies. For those simply interested in firsthand accounts of early twentieth-century nursing Newfoundland ports and outports, the stories will not disappoint.

LYDIA WYTENBROEK, BN, BA, RN
Master of Arts in Interdisciplinary Humanities (History) Student
2009–10 Social Sciences & Humanities Research Council of Canada Graduate Scholarship Recipient
Trinity Western University
Langley, British Columbia, Canada

SONYA GRYPMA, PhD, RN
Associate Professor, School of Nursing
Adjunct Associate Professor, Department of History
Trinity Western University
Langley, British Columbia, Canada

Note

1. J. Karen Scott and Joan E. Kieser, eds., *Northern Nurses: True Nursing Adventures from Canada's North* (Oakville, Ontario: Kokum, 2002); J. Karen Scott and Joan E. Kieser. Eds., *Northern Nurses II: More True Nursing Adventures from Canada's North* (Oakville, Ontario: Kokum, 2005); and J. Karen Scott and Joan E. Kieser, eds., *Northern Nurses III: Belcher Islands & Northern Quebec—the 1960s: Memoirs of Kathleen Mary Jo Lutley and Heather J. Duncan Clayton* (Oakville, O, Ontario: Kokum, 2009).

REVIEW ESSAY: PHARMACEUTICALS, HISTORY, AND AMERICAN SOCIETY

Prescribing by Numbers:
Drugs and the Definition of Disease
By Jeremy A. Greene
(Baltimore: The Johns Hopkins University Press, 2008)
(336 pages; $49.95 hardcover; $25.00 softcover)

Medical Research for Hire: The Political
Economy of Pharmaceutical Clinical Trials
By Jill A. Fisher
(New Brunswick: Rutgers University Press, 2009)
(256 pages; $65 hardcover; $22.35 paper)

As this reviewer sat down at a computer to write her review of these two books, she realized that she had taken notes and drafted her impressions using a pen distributed at a recent conference. What caught her eye this time, however, was that this particular pen advertised a new medication. Much has been written about the "pharmaceuticalization" of American health care in recent years, and the presence of a writing implement on one nurse's desk was a reminder of the ubiquity of therapeutic medicinal chemistry in twenty-first-century American society.

Interestingly, despite their influence on nursing and medical practice, pharmaceuticals have received relatively little scholarly attention from historians of health care. There are signs, however, that this may be changing. Two recent books, *Prescribing by Numbers* and *Medical Research for Hire*, examine different facets of the way in which knowledge about pharmaceuticals shapes the knowledge base that drives medical and nursing practice, perceptions of risk, diagnostic categories, and even the experience of illness. These works join a small, but growing, body of vibrant scholarship on the history of pharmaceuticals.

As physician and historian Jeremy A. Greene, author of *Prescribing by Numbers*, observes, studying pharmaceutical history is a valuable and underused tool through which the forces undergirding contemporary health politics and policy generation can be examined. Greene's nuanced and lucid research yields new insight into the mechanisms that linked specific medications to the management of particular chronic diseases in the postwar era. Greene convincingly argues that pharmaceuticals played an active role in the construction of risk and disease prevention, evolution of diagnostic criteria, and the design of new therapeutic modalities.

Prescribing by Numbers explicates three case studies. Greene's first exemplar focuses on Diuril between 1957 and 1977. The agent is viewed through the lens of the research laboratories and marketing departments at corporate giant Merck, Sharp, and Dohme. Although the drug soon became associated with treating hypertension, it did not originate as an antihypertensive. Greene traces the way in which promotional strategies and advertising campaigns intersected with research agendas and medical practice in ways that gave the drug a new identity, while also redefining hypertension itself. The second section of the book analyzes Orinase, the first oral antidiabetic, in the years between 1960 and 1980. Shifting definitions of coronary heart disease and its risk factors between 1970 and 2000 is the theme surrounding the third and final case study, which looks at the history of the anticholesterol agent Mevacor. Greene's magisterial conclusion unites the three cases through a discussion of a provocative early twenty-first-century suggestions for the creation of a "polypill," a proposed combination agent engineered to treat multiple conditions and predisease states at the same time.

Medical Research for Hire addresses a different facet of pharmaceuticals and American society, that of the drug clinical trial industry. Jill A. Fisher asks two questions: How did pharmaceutical clinical trials become an industry alternative to standard medical care? And what are the implications for doctor-patient relationships when physicians recruit their own patients into drug studies (p. 4)? Fisher answers the second question more comprehensively than she does the first one. Her approach is ethnographic and not historical, which makes it hard for her to address a historical question. In order to fully consider the rise of the randomized clinical trial (RCT) and its impact on clinical practice and pharmaceutical research, for example, a detailed explication of the evolution of those Food and Drug Administration practices and regulatory structures that led to the RCT becoming the accepted standard for drug efficacy would be necessary.

Fisher's examination of the second question is what makes this work novel, worthwhile reading, and a solid scholarly contribution. Of particular interest to nurses and nurse historians is the many ways in which nurses pervade the work. Much of *Medical Research for Hire* addresses not just the physician-patient relationship, but also that of the nurse and patient. Fisher employs all of ethnography's advantages; a major strength of this book is hearing the voices of the many actors involved in clinical trials research. The volume is organized around the various roles of those who participate in the drug trials industry such as physicians (usually the investigators), research coordinators and monitors (often nurses), and, of course, subjects. Fisher sees the work of these individuals largely through the lens of class and gender. Her argument regarding nurses, that they play much the same role (invisible, undervalued) in clinical trials that they do in health care delivery is interesting, but at times her conclusions appear to overreach, or at least are not fully supported by the data she presents. For example, on page 71 Fisher concludes that male research coordinators seem to have a higher status than that of women in the same job. Her evidence is derived from one male research coordinator's comment, but we do not know if physician-investigators or pharmaceutical industry representatives, those who accord that status, necessarily agree.

Nonetheless, the focus on nurses and Fisher's explication of the role conflict that some nurse research coordinators experience, as well as the potential ethical challenges faced by nurses who practice in this arena, are richly detailed and very thought provoking. Fisher addresses the many ethical dilemmas raised by the for-profit clinical trial industry and she sees the issues surrounding pharmaceuticals more dichotomously than Greene. According to Fisher, it is money that drives the political economy of clinical trials: payments to physicians looking to restore funding to their practices that managed care has eroded; subjects who enroll in trials because they are unemployed and need the money; and the uninsured who participate in the hope of getting an effective treatment they could not otherwise afford. She is not wrong that money pollutes the entire enterprise; she does, however, downplay the many other reasons for the proliferation of RCTs that Greene explores, such as changes over time in the policies surrounding biomedical research, pharmaceutical regulation, and advertising.

The growing body of historical scholarship pertaining to pharmaceuticals stands to make an important contribution to scholarship surrounding health and illness over time in the United States. Pharmaceutical history also represents a rich new analytical vein for historians of nursing. We know little about the way in which pharmaceuticals influenced nurses and their work over time, for example.[1] Historical studies of nurses and pharmaceuticals stand to forge a richer understanding of the full breadth and depth of nursing practice across settings and over time by tracing the intellectual processes, psychomotor skills, technical aptitude, and creativity necessary to get medications into patients without psychological or physical harm.

Cynthia A. Connolly, PhD, RN
Associate Professor
University of Pennsylvania School of Nursing
418 Curie Blvd.
Philadelphia, PA 19104

Note

1. One recent book that does begin to address the paucity of historical scholarship on nurses and pharmaceuticals is Arlene Keeling, *Nursing and the Privilege of Prescription, 1893–2000* (Columbus: Ohio State University, 2007).

BOOK REVIEWS

Mary Putnam Jacobi and the Politics of Medicine in Nineteenth-Century America
By Carla Bittel
(Chapel Hill: University of North Carolina Press, 2009) (328 pages, $40.00 cloth)

In *Mary Putnam Jacobi and the Politics of Medicine in Nineteenth-Century America*, Carla Bittel explores the life of one of the foremost physicians of the period. Born into the publishing family of George Putnam, Jacobi (1842–1906) was initially drawn to a career of writing, publishing her first piece at the age of seventeen. Yet, after attending medical lectures and dissections at the New York Medical College, she turned her attention to science. She studied at the New York Infirmary with Elizabeth Blackwell; attended the New York College of Pharmacy, graduating in 1863; and traveled to Civil War battle fields to aid in soldiers' hospitals, a shocking mission for a middle-class woman in that time. Unwilling to return to her life in New York, she found a teaching position with the Freedman's Bureau in Virginia. These experiences reinforced her commitment to address the needs of those less fortunate. Intent on obtaining a medical degree, Jacobi entered the Female Medical College of Pennsylvania, one of two women's medical colleges of the day. Her thesis on the spleen, written in Latin as was the custom then, clearly reflected her view about the centrality of laboratory science to contemporary medicine, a view that Bittel traces through the rest of her life.

Dissatisfied with her education, Jacobi traveled to France in 1866. After spending more than a year attending clinics and laboratories, she was admitted the prestigious École de Médecine as the school's first female student. French radicalism sharpened Jacobi's political philosophy and French laboratories honed her interests in science, strengthening her positivist worldview heavily influenced by the philosopher Auguste Comte. Drawing on personal correspondence and the letters, essays, and short stories Jacobi sent from France for publication in U.S. magazines, Bittel astutely traces how these political and medical ideals served to reinforce Jacobi's feminist outlook.

Jacobi returned to New York in 1871, determined to forge a medical career that would foster the equality of women in medicine and in society. Over the next several decades, she gained membership in previously all-male medical societies, pursued a research career with extensive publications, maintained a medical practice, and taught a rigorous scientific curriculum at a time when women's advanced education was controversial. Edward Clarke published his now infamous *Sex in Education; or, A Fair Chance for the Girls* in 1873, employing a series of case studies to argue that too much education, too much mental exertion, especially during menstruation, would shatter the health of young women. Feminists quickly denounced his claims. In *The Question of Rest for Women during Menstruation*, which won Harvard University's Boylston Prize in 1876, Jacobi presented statistical and experimental evidence that physical and mental activities were beneficial; she demonstrated the physiological equality of women and men. This work and the subsequent book of the same title firmly fixed Jacobi's scientific reputation.

Bittel employs the term "politics of medicine" in two distinct ways. First, she analyzes Jacobi's life through the lens of gender politics. Both the content and the organization of nineteenth-century U.S. medicine denigrated women, asserting that biologically women were less than men and were unsuitable doctors, claims that Jacobi argued against her entire career. Second, Jacobi vigorously advocated for science *in* medicine. Medicine and medical education were in transition. Jacobi exemplified the younger generation of doctors who insisted on the critical role of scientific training and investigation. This stress on science put her in opposition to many physicians who were less convinced of the pivotal role of science. It also put her in opposition to many, such as Elizabeth Blackwell, who championed the entrance of women into medicine for their supposed female quality of sympathy. Jacobi preferred the physician as an unemotional authority, with nurses conducting caring duties. Jacobi wedded these two aspects of the politics of medicine, employing science to demonstrate gender equality.

Bittel has produced a comprehensive intellectual biography of a critical nineteenth-century thinker. We learn much about the development of Jacobi's medicine and politics but little about the results of these and little about how the structure of medical practice was changing in these times. Bittel claims pivotal roles for Jacobi in the social reform and educational movements of the time. Chapter 6 details much of Jacobi's reform and suffrage work but provides little context on the Progressive era. Still, for those who want to know more about how an independent, nineteenth-century woman created a professional life despite societal constraints, this is a highly informative read.

RIMA D. APPLE, PHD
Professor Emerita
University of Wisconsin–Madison
Madison, WI 53706

Health and Medicine in the circum-Caribbean, 1800–1968
Edited by Juanita De Barros, Steven Palmer, and David Wright
(New York: Routledge, 2009) (309 pages, $103.00 cloth)

Health and Medicine in the circum-Caribbean, 1800–1968 is a collection of essays that traces the history of health and medicine in the nineteenth and twentieth centuries in the French, Spanish, British, Danish, and Dutch Caribbean. The editors relate the history of formally educated and informally trained providers of medicine and the clients who sought their medical expertise. The essays document the diverse individuals that called the Caribbean home and the varied medical traditions on which they relied.

Unlike previous studies of health in the Caribbean, this volume does an excellent job in investigating the varied areas of the Caribbean. Chapters about the British Caribbean include essays that focus on midwifery, the treatment of venereal disease, and infant health. One essay considers health in the French Antilles in the World War I era. The Dutch Caribbean is looked at in a chapter on hookworm eradication. The essay on the Danish West Indies considers midwifery. Finally, several essays reflect on areas once held by Spain. These articles investigate medicine in Cuba; biomedicine in Yucatan, Mexico; prostitution in the Dominican Republic; and medical professionalization in Puerto Rico. The British Caribbean and the Spanish Caribbean dominate the volume, but the inclusion of essays that stretch across the circum-Caribbean is admirable. Similarly, the essays consider varied historical periods, including slavery, emancipation, colonialism, and independence.

The volume editors did a fine job selecting essays that treat practitioners of professional medicine as well as folk healers. A particularly strong chapter that investigates professional medical workers is Denise Challenger's "A Benign Place of Healing? The Contagious Diseases Hospital and Medical Discipline in Post-Slavery Barbados." Challenger documents how "the Contagious Diseases legislation entangled medical doctors, matrons, and nurses as mediators of freedom. The medical practitioners of the CDH [Contagious Diseases Hospital] were central to shaping the autonomy that Afro-Barbadian women could experience in the newly freed society" (p. 99). Similarly, Niklas Thode Jensen does a superb job analyzing midwifery on St. Croix. His essay, " 'For the benefit of the planters and the benefit of Mankind': The Struggle to Control Midwives and Obstetrics on St. Croix, Danish West Indies, 1800–1848," is a well-written, well-organized, and interesting analysis of folk medical and spiritual practices. Debbie McCollin's excellent "World War II to Independence: Health, Services, and Women in Trinidad and Tobago, 1939–1962" bridges the gap between formal and informal medical providers by looking at "the traditional role of women as health care providers and their subsequent role in the formal health structure of the colony" (p. 227).

The book also excels in choosing essays that showcase the diverse populations that called the Caribbean home. One essay that succeeds in this regard is April J. Mayes's "Tolerating Sex: Prostitution, Gender, and Governance in the Dominican Republic, 1880s–1924." This multilayered analysis of public health takes into account Dominican authorities, American naval personnel, and Afro-Antillean residents. The chapter highlights the "multi-ethnic, multi-national, and multi-racial population" of the Dominican Republic in the late nineteenth century and early twentieth century (p. 123).

Health and Medicine in the circum-Caribbean, 1800–1968 will appeal to a variety of readers. Historians of the Caribbean will discover a wide-ranging analysis of the region. Historians of medicine will find a fine collection of essays about professional medicine, public health, and folk healing. Nurses will appreciate several essays that illustrate the history of nursing in the Caribbean and how nurses navigated between physicians and their patients.

Karol K. Weaver, PhD
Associate Professor, History
Susquehanna University
514 University Avenue
Selinsgrove, PA 17870

Rural District Nursing in Gloucestershire, 1880–1925
By Carrie Howse
(Cheltenham, Gloucestershire: Reardon Publishing, 2008)
(208 pages, $50.00 paper)

Rural life in the United Kingdom at the turn of the century was difficult and became worse if one was sick. Fearful of institutions, the rural people depended on wealthy ladies to bring them warm broth and cheerful news until scientific advances led to nursing involvement. Carrie Howse's book gives us a close-up view of women's work in many levels of society in a rural area at the turn of the twentieth century. She shows how charity care changed to trained nursing care under the guidance of women to better the lives of the poor. District nursing also bettered the lives of the nurses and the women supervisors.

Rural district nursing began in Gloucestershire under the headship of Elizabeth Malleson, a woman who moved from the intellectual circles of London to Gloucestershire with her husband. In Gloucestershire, she pursued the idea of bettering the lives of the rural poor. Her ideas began with a reading room for the local men and progressed to other social issues including care of the sick. Malleson is credited with forming the Rural Nursing Association, which coincided with the formation of the Queen Victoria's Jubilee Institute for Nurses (QVJIN). The QVJIN started an urban district nursing program, guided by Florence Nightingale, which then supported the rural movement. Malleson's story gives the view of the lady administrators and what they came up against while promoting health in rural populations. She shows how charity care changed to trained nursing care and what it took to bring it about.

This book presents new-found primary sources that provide evidence about the lives of the rural district nurses, their lady supervisors, and their patients at the turn-of-the-century. Utilizing a combined framework including social and women's history, Howse brings to our view a part of nursing that has not been explored yet is important for understanding rural life, illness among the poor, and independent nursing work. The opening chapters explain the history of district nursing and rural district nursing and place them in the context of the times (chapters 1, 2, and 3). The book quotes women of all classes with chapters covering the professional status of nurses (chapter 4), the working life of the rural nurses (chapters 5 and 6), and the reproductive lives of the women they cared for in the villages (chapter 7). Howse offers a wonderful amount of details regarding salaries, living quarters, duties, training, and a well-documented discussion of the views of patients regarding sex, birth, and birth control. The reader has a good understanding of their prudish society, which did not allow the exchange of reproductive information between mothers and daughters, a restraint that seems implausible given that living on a farm provides abundant evidence of the reproductive activities of animals.

Howse's book encompasses the trends in professional nursing between 1880 and 1925 giving rich details of nursing work and the obstacles nurses had to overcome to deliver care. The sections on midwifery practice give the reader an understanding of birthing practices and moral values of the times and show us how little attitudes have changed about the distribution of welfare, and funding for health care and nursing work. One can see the same dilemmas occurring in this British nursing history as in public health nursing history in the United States: whether to do bedside care or prevention education; how to finance nurse visits; and how to supervise nurses. Those interested in nursing, public health, midwifery, rural life, and women in society will find enjoyment in reading this book.

Jeannine Uribe, PhD, RN
Assistant Clinical Professor
Drexel University
College of Nursing and Health Professions
Bellet Bldg. 1237
1505 Race Street
Philadelphia, PA 19102

Containing Trauma: Nursing Work in the First World War
By Christine E. Hallett
(Manchester, UK, and New York: University of Manchester Press, 2009)
(288 pages, $95.00/£60.00 cloth)

As Christine Hallett points out in the opening pages of *Containing Trauma: Nursing Work in the First World War*, the First World War nurse was once and still remains an iconic figure inhabiting the imaginations of her generation and of those thereafter. History has not treated her well. Certainly, as Anne Summers has argued, military service remained the most significant way in which a woman could assert the prerogatives of citizenship.[1] But as the sense of the "Great" war's futility, destructiveness, and mindlessness grew in the minds of contemporaries and historians, the figure of the nurse emerged as one enmeshed in the political callousness and the military propaganda that destroyed a generation of young British men.

Yet, as Hallett argues, the voice of the nurse herself has remained silent. Hallet's initial intent, in her long-awaited book on nursing in the First World War, was to uncover what nurses' themselves wrote about their service. To this end, she mines an impressive array of letters, diaries, oral histories, autobiographies, and published articles found among holdings in Great Britain, Australia, New Zealand, Canada, South Africa, and the United States. She does succeed in what she describes as filling a space in the historical record and that, in and of itself, would be a signal accomplishment. But Hallett takes her nurses and their voices further. She seriously considers that which has been too often marginalized in nursing's history: the actual work of nurses as they cleaned patients, irrigated wounds, and changed dressings. She metaphorically wraps this work with her book's title: what nurses did, she argues, was not about outcomes but about the process of containing physiological and psychological trauma. And she leaves her readers with a stunning paradigmatic shift in understanding the work and worth of nurses—both in the past and, perhaps, in the present. The older tropes of passivity and victimization now yield to one of active engagement.

In *Containing Trauma,* Hallett argues that nurses gave meaning to their work—across different treatment scenarios and in many different geographical locations—by constructing it as a process of creating safe boundaries within which healing could take place

(p. 16). She turns first to their work on the Western Front, that constantly bombarded line of trenches and barbed wire stretching from the North Sea to the Swiss border. German soldiers fought on the East; those from France, the United Kingdom, and, later, the United States on the West. All the soldiers, no matter from which country they came, faced overwhelming casualties in the face of the new tools of modern warfare, which included the machine gun and toxic gasses. Hallett focuses on the nurses' work of containing physical trauma. She writes of their rapid evaluations of and aggressive responses to signs of shock, or physiological collapse, in their soldiers: they quickly (and sometimes simultaneously) replaced fluids, restored circulatory functions, administered stimulating medications, controlled hemorrhages, cleaned raw wounds to prevent sepsis and gas gangrene, and provided the oxygen and baths that "contained" the suffering of those exposed to mustard and other gasses. Most compelling, however, is their work with their dying soldiers. Certainly, Hallett points out, death was what they worked to prevent. But when death seemed inevitable, they offered themselves as a "containing presence" as they sat with the dying men offering comfort and aggressive pain relief (p. 68).

Hallett then turns to nurses' work in their patients' recovery. Here she concentrates on their work of containing a clean environment as they struggled with preventing pressure ulcers, treating the "trench foot" that had developed among soldiers standing for days in the freezing waters, battling disease-bearing lice, and making difficult decisions when facing the dilemma of controlling a soldier's pain or limiting the dangerous respiratory effects of opiates. Nourishing food takes on special importance: it was critically important to provide the fuel that would generate the tissue that would contain the body's rupture. As does massage and other forms of physiotherapy, the nurses' work not only repaired a damaged body but also a soldier's sense of self.

Of course, nothing challenged this sense of self as much as the psychological trauma of slaughter and suffering. Hallett's nurses provided the "psychic containment" that enabled soldiers to "hold themselves together" while they began to heal from devastating physical and emotional injuries (p. 158). In ways that echo current practice, she talks of the process of being with the young men as they came to terms with their terror and their fear. But her strongest analysis comes in a vignette describing a motherly nurse holding a sobbing soldier to her breast saying, "Face it now, Sonny, and get over it." Far from being heartless, the enjoinder to "face it" was valued as a means to regain self-respect in an Edwardian culture that valued the "stiff upper lip"; yet it came from a mother-like figure that could both contain a child-like regression and provide a needed push in the process of assimilating loss (pp. 164–165). This process, however, came at an enormous cost to the nurses themselves. They practiced a "self-containment" in which they subordinated their own emotional and physical needs not to the medical establishment, as has been the standard interpretation, but to those of their patients. Certainly, Hallett acknowledges, this controlled, disciplined persona left nurses vulnerable to charges of coldness and callousness by both their contemporaries and later historians. But given their uncomfortable and often dangerous living and working conditions, as well as the toll of daily encounters with physically and psychologically traumatized patients, nurses themselves needed to be as contained as the work they did.

Hallett forthrightly acknowledges what some might see as problematic: that her perspective as both a nurse and a historian has shaped a text that might be seen as polemical or a work of advocacy (p. xii). *Containing Trauma* does focus on exemplar practices, carefully chosen descriptions, and deliberately constructed memories, and it gives a particular voice to many who had difficulty articulating the exact nature of what they did in ways that may or may not have seemed familiar.

Yet, Hallett's ability to draw on her very carefully considered stance is her strength and also the strength of her book. She creates meaning in the seemingly mundane. She stays true to her data, yet also critiques and contextualizes the data in ways that yield a new way of thinking about the work of war-time nurses. As with any work that breaks new theoretical ground, *Containing Trauma* raises as many questions as it answers. What of the care of soldiers with infectious diseases—diseases as deadly in war time as those from bullets and gasses? Hallett briefly considers the treatment of infectious diseases when she turns to the nurses in the eastern Mediterranean, but she also leaves tantalizing clues that these illnesses did not hold the same drama as those attending wounds. And what of references to the fact that soldiers and volunteers sometimes resented the containing work of nurses? Hallett's paradigm suggests we might re-read writings from the First World War with a new perspective. And, in the end, one of the greatest strengths of *Containing Trauma* is that it suggests a new research paradigm for nursing history scholars.

PATRICIA D'ANTONIO, RN, PhD, FAAN
Associate Professor of Nursing and
Associate Director, Barbara Bates Center for the Study of the History of Nursing
University of Pennsylvania School of Nursing
2017 Claire M. Fagin Hall
418 Curie Boulevard
Philadelphia, PA 19104

Note

1. Anne Summers, *Angels and Citizens: British Women as Military Nurses, 1854–1914* (London: Routledge & Kegan Paul, 1988).

Place and Practice in Canadian Nursing History

Edited by Jayne Elliott, Meryn Stuart, and Cynthia Toman
(Vancouver, Toronto: University of British Columbia Press, 2008) (232 pages, $98.00 USD/$85.00 CAD cloth; $34.95 USD/$29.95 CAD paper).

In June 2005, a group of academic and clinical historians convened in Ottawa for the first Hannah Conference on Canadian Nursing History. Sponsored by Canada's Associated Medical Service, a nonprofit organization that supports research in the history of medicine and health, the conference marked the establishment of the Nursing History Research Unit (NHRC) at the University of Ottawa's School of Nursing. *Place and Practice in Canadian Nursing History* is the material result of that meeting and the NHRC's first publication. If this collection is an indicator of the unit's future contributions, then the history of Canadian nursing is in good hands.

The last decade has seen the history of Canadian nursing elevated to new levels of rigor and sophistication. Asking novel questions, employing new categories of analysis, and undertaking research in untapped archives, historians have enlivened their field. Moreover, they have incorporated the history of Canadian nursing more firmly into the history of medicine and more general social and political histories. This volume is a clear part of that historiographical trajectory. Its three editors, all contributors as well, are each NHRC affiliates: Stuart, its director; Toman, its associate director; and Elliott, a research facilitator and administrator. The six other authors represent a mix of established and emerging scholars, all faculty at schools of nursing or history departments throughout Canada. Together, these nine authors constitute a new generation of historians of Canadian nursing who are eager to expand and enrich their discipline.

The editors are keenly aware of the vibrant state of their field and see this collection as an effort to develop it further. They position the essays as a complement to the sweeping general survey *On All Frontiers: Four Centuries of Canadian Nursing*. Whereas the editors of that book promised "a broad, rather than deep, treatment" of various themes in Canadian nursing history,[1] *Place and Practice* develops some of its central but less explored themes. Chronologically, this volume is less wide-ranging than *On All Frontiers*, spanning the late nineteenth century to the 1970s. The result is a more focused, more detailed, and more analytical consideration of nursing history in the era of modern professional nursing.

The twin themes of practice and place, as the book's title suggests, supply the collection's overarching organizing framework. In regards to practice, the essays seek to disrupt the idea of "'nurse' as a universal category of identity" (p. 1). "Nursing," here, is not limited to professional graduate nurses who worked in hospitals or training schools. Rather, it includes individuals who undertook nursing work in both formal and informal settings. Covering experiences in the military, in community health projects, and in rural and outpost regions, the essays collectively ask who counted as a nurse and what constituted "nursing" at various points throughout this period. The authors show that scholarly treatment of the practice of nursing work must be more inclusive and must consider a range of professional and voluntary health and healing activities.

Place, as both a geographical and a cultural concept, provides further conceptual unity to essays that cover diverse periods and subjects. Place denotes the physical sites in which a nurse worked, and here includes war zones, urban health centers, remote settler colonies, and First Nations communities. The essays show that location was a determining factor in what a nurse could accomplish. Working outside traditional hospital settings sometimes offered greater individual freedom, but other times constrained agency and options. Place also refers to social position. Whether a nurse was working class or middle class, Anglophone or Francophone, native or immigrant, proved a determining factor in her power as a reformer, a healer, and a professional. Place, the editors assert, must therefore be treated as a fundamental unit of analysis, as important to understanding the history of nursing as gender, race, class, or religion. Together, the essays beautifully support that contention.

Individually, the nine essays in *Place and Practice* contribute to our understanding about variety of topics in twentieth-century Canadian nursing. They will be of particular interest to historians interested in points of contact between nurses of different ethnic and regional backgrounds, in the development of the nursing profession and other forms of nurse work, and in shifting and competing identities of nurses and other healers. The collection, though, is truly greater than the sum of its parts. An indicator of a vital moment in the field of Canadian nursing history, it offers an array of new analytical approaches and poses important new questions that are sure to enhance further scholarship in this burgeoning field.

JULIA F. IRWIN, PHD
Assistant Professor
Department of History SOC 107
University of South Florida
4202 E. Fowler Ave
Tampa, FL 33620

Note

1. Christina Bates, Dianne Dodd, and Nicole Rousseau, *On All Frontiers: Four Centuries of Canadian Nursing* (Ottawa: University of Ottawa Press, 2005), 2.

Power, Politics and the History of Nursing in New Jersey
By Frances Ward
(New Brunswick, NJ: Rutgers University Press, 2009) (310 pages, $39.95 cloth)

This history is the culmination of years of research and writing by Frances Ward while she was dean of the Rutgers School of Nursing. It is the story of the development of nursing in New Jersey from 1882 through the early years of the twenty-first century. The author lays out her ideas about the evolution of nursing in New Jersey in the introduction. She posits that American nursing, including nursing in New Jersey, was influenced by Christian monasticism dating back to the third century B.C.E. and that influence persists in permeating nursing to the present day.

Six of the seven chapters present the history of nursing in New Jersey chronologically. Threaded throughout each chapter is the idea that despite the work of nursing leaders, the nursing profession was restrained from developing into its full potential because of its subservience to and control by politicians, medicine, and hospital administration. In chapter 7, Ward adds helpful clarity to this history. She recaps the major developments in nursing and ties them together succinctly and clearly.

Chapter 1 is particularly helpful in setting the stage for what was occurring in New Jersey during the 1880s. Nursing began with the industrialization and urbanization of the northeastern section of the state. There were different manufacturing sites in Newark, Orange, Paterson, and Elizabeth. These industrial centers required hospitals to care for their workers, and they required schools of nursing to produce nurses to staff the hospitals. The first of these was Newark City Hospital, which opened in 1882. It would have been helpful if the author described the geography of the rest of New Jersey and what was going on with nurses in those areas.

The usual pieces of the nursing history puzzle are traced in subsequent chapters. There is the formation of the New Jersey State Nurses' Association and then the enactment of legislation to license nurses. We learn of the nursing leaders who worked tirelessly to advance nursing. They were assisted by regional and national nursing leaders as they tried to gain control over licensure, nursing education, and the work and practice of nurses. It would have enriched the story if the stories of these leaders were fleshed out more.

The life of the student nurse during the early days of modern nursing in New Jersey, including a strict adherence to order and discipline, was not much different from that experienced by other student nurses of the time. There were continuous contentious discussions and studies about nursing education and how it should define nursing practice. There were the persistent episodic shortages and oversupply of nurses with ensuing state and national entities and commissions studying and making recommendations to remedy the problems. Even though the names of these entities were initially spelled out when their abbreviations were used, it became difficult to keep them straight and interfered with the flow of the story. Ward explores how war, specialization, and economic security impacted the nursing profession. We find scant information about how race affected nurses and nursing in New Jersey, especially in the early years of its development. Furthermore, it is a stretch for the author to suggest that nursing faced the same set of circumstances experienced by African Americans as they struggled for their civil rights.

The nursing profession will never be completely free of those wanting to control it; however, nurses in New Jersey were not passive actors, and by the early twenty-first century they had achieved the level of professionalism through legislation that allowed them to practice in autonomous roles. The history of nursing in New Jersey provides a good benchmark from which to examine the history of nursing in other states. The author ends her well-researched book with a reflection on her personal experiences as a nurse practitioner and her freedom to be able to practice as an autonomous nursing professional.

For many travelers to the Northeastern United States, New Jersey is a place to drive through to get to New York City and then further up into New England. Until the publication of this book, it was the same for nursing history. This book fills an important gap in the history of nursing and enlarges the interconnectedness of nursing in the Northeast and in the United States.

CARLA SCHISSEL, RN, PhD
Nurse Practitioner
1886 Windemere Drive
Atlanta, GA 30324

When Sister Ruled: The Nursing Sister

By Peter Arden
(London: Robert Hale, 2005) (256 pages, $17.95, paper)

Where the matron was the head of the hospital, the sister was her faithful lieutenant. First addressed by Peter Arden in *When Matron Ruled*,[1] the story of British nursing hierarchy is continued in *When Sister Ruled: The Nursing Sister*, an exploration of the development and role of the nursing sister. After matron, the next level of nursing hierarchy was that of nursing sister, equivalent to the more familiar title of head nurse in the United States. However, a nursing sister had more responsibilities than a head nurse. Sister was the authority on the ward who directed, ran, and ensured that those under her jurisdiction functioned to her specifications, including both nurses and patients. Arden traces the development of the sister from its religious origins to those select women of the Victorian era of higher birth and social status. Those with lower status remained nurses and would not rise to the rank of sister.

Sister operated as the head of a department. Duty was paramount, and sisters were selfless and devoted in their role. Within the hospital hierarchy, in addition to the specific ward, the rank of sister included those in charge of laundry, diet, and surgery. And while each sister had a name, she was known more for her function: Sister Casualty, Sister Laundry, Sister Kitchen, and so forth. Sister Tutor had nursing students under her purview, and many a student owed her success to the diligent efforts expended by this sister. Home Sister oversaw those living in the nurses' residence, and strictly maintained the standards of behavior and decorum that were expected of the nurses under her care. As time progressed, promotion to sister came through merit and not social status, and men were able to achieve this promotion and title.

Arden sets the theme for each chapter by its title, and provides the background for each theme. Interspersed with this historical documentation are the first-person accounts of the many nurses, students, and the sisters themselves, whose stories underscore each chapter's theme and content. Throughout the book these first-person accounts reveal the pride and satisfaction in the role of sister and its importance to the successful supervision of care and patient outcomes. Arden has provided a thorough detailing of the wide influence that the nursing sister provided, from the hospital ward to the military nurse and those who provided nursing care beyond the British homeland. Those not familiar with the role and function of sister will discover Arden's narrative dispels the quaint image of British nurses as prim girls in starched veils and blue uniforms.

The nursing sister was the leader of the nursing team who held it to high standards of care and, in doing so, created camaraderie among the nurses and motivated her staff to meet her standards and not let her down. *When Sister Ruled: The Nursing Sister* is a compelling documentation of dedication, duty, and respect for authority, always underscored by the responsibility to provide the best care to the patient. Those interested in tracing evolution of roles in nursing and women's authority will find this book an appealing addition to their library.

TERESA M. O'NEILL, RNC, PHD
Professor
Our Lady of Holy Cross College
4123 Woodland Drive
New Orleans, LA 70131

Note

1. Peter Arden, *When Matron Ruled* (London: Robert Hale, 2002).

Student Bodies: The Influence of Student Health Services in American Society and Medicine

By Heather Munro Prescott

(Ann Arbor: The University of Michigan Press, 2007) (234 pages, $50.00 cloth)

In an era when more and more adult children are moving back home to live with their parents, historian Heather Munro Prescott's book offers important insights into how the very definition of adolescence—especially from the medical perspective—hinges more on the social and cultural than on the biological. It used to be that "adolescent" was just another term for "teenager." Today, however, certain medical experts argue that thirty-year-olds are adolescents, too. Pushing the age limit upward is a reflection of the fact "that the period of semidependency usually associated with adolescence has been extended because of longer periods of education, preparation for careers, and/or economic dependence on parents" (p. 3). This may sound like a medically imprecise way to define a category of patients, but college health, as Prescott deftly shows us, has always been as much about molding and shaping behavior as it has been about treating disease.

The first third of *Student Bodies* is dedicated to the history of physical education, a story that spans the mid-nineteenth century to 1920, when the physicians who were members of the newly established American College Health Association began to distance themselves from non-physician physical educators and coaches. Before 1920, the practice of college medicine occurred in the gym, not in the clinic. Here physician physical educators measured and manipulated student bodies, making them stronger so that they would not succumb to the ill effects of book learning. This was the age of doctors William Hammond, Edward Clarke, S. Weir Mitchell, and G. Stanley Hall, all of whom claimed that an intellectual life put undo strain on the nervous system, leading to increase incidences of neurasthenia (a vague anxiety disorder), tuberculosis, and other infectious diseases. "Physicians argued," Prescott writes, "that the ravages of TB gave young men effeminate, pigeon-chested bodies that exposed sufferers to ridicule by their more 'manly' classmates" (p. 112). Women were seen as particularly unsuited to receive a college education. This is why the origins of college health—which Prescott details with careful and industrious archival work—are found in all-women schools such as Vassar and Radcliffe. In order to keep white middle-class women strong and breeding (a special concern for eugenicists), brain work was accompanied by calisthenics, weight lifting, and posture exercises in order to prevent feminine frailty.

It was not until the second decade of the twentieth century that the college health clinic as we know it today would supplant the gymnasium as the locus of medical science. One of the earliest attempts of institutionalizing student health in a clinic setting was at Cornell University. Prescott tells us that Cornell built an infirmary because "most [dormitory] housekeepers did not want the bother of caring for sick students, nor would they accept the disruption to household routine caused by the presence of private nurses" (p. 70). Among the greatest disruptions were epidemics. Indeed, Prescott demonstrates that the biggest boon to the college health clinic was the influenza epidemic of 1918–1919. In the face of infectious disease, college administrators began to think of student medical care as a necessity to a well-functioning, densely populated place of higher education. At the University of Michigan, for instance, President Marion

LeRoy Burton convinced the trustees to allot $5,000 of university money in order to create an student infirmary in 1918, with students contributing $3 a semester. In many ways, the college infirmary was one of the first sites of socialized medicine in the United States, predating the Veterans Administration's system of universal health care for all those who serve in the military.

While American universities may have been progressive in terms of health care delivery, they were woefully backward when it came to, as Prescott puts it, letting "outsiders in." College medicine, more than anything else, helped to legitimate the exclusion of women, Jews, blacks, and homosexuals from elite institutions. Focusing on Yale in the 1950s, she demonstrates how school psychiatrists readily breeched the doctrine of doctor-patient confidentiality if a student admitted to having homosexual desires—a practice that would not change until after countrywide student protests in the 1960s.

Student Bodies touches on many important facets of social history in medicine, from the treatment of African Americans at all-black colleges to how women gained access to elite all-male institutions by tearing down entrenched gender assumptions concerning health and higher education. While more attention to how nurses helped shape college medicine would have made Prescott's gender analysis even stronger, *Student Bodies* is a welcome addition to the history of medicine, for it offers a window into the highly complex, yet little-studied world of student health, a practice largely born from middle-class fears about teenage children flying the coop.

BETH LINKER, PHD
Assistant Professor
History and Sociology of Science
University of Pennsylvania
365 Cohen Hall
249 S. 36th Street
Philadelphia, PA 19104–6304

Caring and Curing: A History of the Indian Health Service

By James P. Rife and Capt. Alan J. Dellapenna, Jr.
(Landover, MD: PHS Commissioner Officers Foundation for the Advancement of Public Health, 2009) (170 pages, $34.95 cloth)

In 1955, the Indian Health Service (IHS) was transferred from the Department of Interior to the U.S. Public Health Service. After much reorganization, this was one step closer on the historical journey of the IHS to carry out its congressionally legislated mission to elevate the health status of American Indians and Alaska Natives to a level comparable with the rest of the nation. The third book published by the PHS Commissioner Officers Foundation for the Advancement of Public Health, *Caring and Curing* is the culmination of a project by the Indian Health Service History Project to document the fifty years of work since the transfer. The authors, James P. Rife, a senior historian with

History Associates and Capt. Alan J. Dellapenna, Jr., of the IHS, collected a vast amount of historic documents, photos, and oral histories from the National Archives, the Library of Congress, the National Library of Medicine, and Indian health-related records from university archives. Additionally, they actively sought out documents and accounts from people who worked in the IHS.

In this thoroughly researched book, Rife and Dellapenna endeavor to inform the reader, the public, and those professionally connected with IHS of the struggles and successes of caring for Native Americans from the vantage point of the physicians employed by the IHS. By charting the historical trials and triumphs of the IHS, this book focuses on the shifting political and socioeconomic climate that affected health care for American Indian and Alaskan Natives since its inception. While the authors' main purpose is to provide a historical context for the story of the successes of the IHS, it honestly addresses the failures of Indian health care, acknowledging that there is remaining work to be done by the agency and continued need for collaboration with the Native America population.

The chapters are logically organized starting in the late 1700s with the initial responsibility of the federal government in "dealing with and protecting all Indians living in the territory outside of the original thirteen colonies" (p. 1). With limited federal funds, efforts were initially placed on protecting soldiers from infectious disease within the native population. In 1824 health care for Native Americans was moved under the Office of Indian Affairs (OIA) within the War Department. When the OIA was transferred again to the Interior Department in 1849, a corps of civilian field physicians was developed to provide a new round of inoculations. Rife and Dellapenna describe the various inadequate efforts to control and treat infectious disease among the native population during the late 1800s and into the early 1900s as a "national disgrace" (p. 4). They describe the years between 1936 and 1962 as a new beginning for Indian health, starting with the initial attempts of transferring Indian health care to the U.S. Public Health Service in 1936. The remainder of the book focuses on the events following the transfer in 1955, especially through the succession of directors of the IHS and collaboration with Indian tribal leaders. This book illustrates the improvements in Indian health care through building health care facilities on reservations and promoting preventative health, despite growing pains and controversy. Throughout this account, Rife and Dellapenna demonstrate the cultural barriers between white providers and native populations and how this affected progress in improving care.

It is evident that Rife and Dellapenna have a passion for history. Their historical account is rich in primary sources, especially government documents and oral histories of IHS physicians. The hundreds of historical photographs provide a vivid illustration of how care for Native Americans has progressed during the past two decades. Of particular interest to the nurse reader are the striking photos of the destitute living conditions of Native Americans and the strikingly modern health care facilities built later to provide care. For quick reference, the appendix includes a useful list of chronological events in U.S. Indian health and organizational development of the IHS.

Caring and Curing provides a very detailed history of Native American health care from the physician's viewpoint and leadership. A particularly fascinating part of the book is the history of the Native American physicians, such as the first female Native American physician, Dr. Susan LaFlesche Picotte. But the historical contribution of nurses, nurses' aides, and other health care professionals is noticeably absent. While there is some mention of nurses and "field matrons" as the "good Samaritans of the Indian Service" (p. 5), the authors do not describe their experience or duties in any detail. While the training and contribution of Indian nurses is highlighted on one page (p. 36), the nurse reader wishes the authors would have incorporated more input and historical perspective from Native American health care providers and their community. Oral histories from nurses would have added tremendously valuable information to round out the history of Native American health care.

This book is written for and valuable for staff connected to the Native American health care system. It provides a detailed account of the political and organizational struggles in providing care for Native Americans and can be a springboard to providing a more nursing-relevant account of the events.

CHRISTINE BREWER, BSN, MSW, MSN CANDIDATE
University of Pennsylvania
804 S. 49th St., 2R
Philadelphia, PA 19143

Examining Tuskegee: The Infamous Syphilis Study and Its Legacy
By Susan M. Reverby
(Chapel Hill: University of North Carolina Press, 2009) (416 pages, $30.00 cloth)

In my undergraduate research course, I remember the professor noting how unwise it would be to design a prospective study on humans where the results would not be known until the participants died, as human life span was so long, the investigator might be dead before the subjects. This was in the late 1960s, before public knowledge broke that the United States Public Health Service (PHS) had done just that: carried out a study that went on for so many years that several of the participants outlived the originators of the study. Yet, conducting an incredibly poorly designed study was not the only error perpetrated by the PHS, which also committed numerous ethical failures and unjust acts. In *Examining Tuskegee: The Infamous Syphilis Study and its Legacy,* Susan M. Reverby provides a masterful and comprehensive historical analysis of an egregious example of medical research malfeasance carried out by an arm of the United States government. Reverby brings to this account excellent scholarship and tremendous abilities as a historian, allowing the complex narrative involving issues of race, racism, sex, poverty, medical power, and widely held stereotypical images of African American men and manhood, to unfold in a compelling and thought provoking manner.

The book, divided into three sections, begins with one entitled "Testimony." This section provides an exhaustive recording of the events known to have happened. In 1932, the PHS initiated a study to observe the effects of untreated late latent syphilis on African American men in Macon County, Alabama. The men were subjected to blood draws, spinal taps, and autopsies upon death. Physicians responsible for the study misinformed the men about its nature and engaged in active lying and deception regarding so-called treatment administered, which consisted merely vitamins and tonics. In the 1940s, when penicillin became available, physicians failed to inform the men about this new treatment and in many cases actively prevented them from receiving it. The study continued for 40 years. A few individuals questioned the study's ethics but it was not until 1972, after an Associated Press investigative reporter broke the news in the national press, that the study received the scrutiny it deserved. The resulting outcry effectively ended the study and was followed by a federal investigation, Senate hearings, a lawsuit, and eventually a monetary settlement awarded to the men and their families.

The book's second section, entitled "Testifying," elucidates the viewpoints of those involved in the study. In what I found to be the book's most moving chapter, Reverby analyzes the men participants' experiences using medical records, the men's words, and the words of their families. She eloquently emphasizes their dismay at finding out the deceptions to which they were subjected at the hands of their government as well as the dignity with which the men survived the experience. A chapter on the white physicians who carried out the study explores how their mindset, much of it callous, all of it suffused with racism, allowed them to turn a blind eye to the effects of their actions. A subsequent chapter focusing on Dr. Eugene H. Dibble, Jr., the African American physician responsible for the study's affiliation with the Tuskegee Institute, delves into the complex motivations leading to the institute's association with the study. The final chapter in this section centers on the role of public health nurse Eunice Rivers Laurie, who was charged with ensuring the cooperation and participation of the men. Rivers, also African American, remains a controversial figure, viewed in some cases as powerless to act against dominant white physicians and alternatively as the men's protector surreptitiously helping them to obtain penicillin treatment. Rivers remained circumspect about her activities during her years with the study, and Reverby treats her reticence to reveal her full story with respect; Reverby concludes that Rivers felt pride, not shame, in the work that comprised the bulk of her professional career.

In the book's last section, called "Traveling," Reverby examines the years after the study ended and places the study within the cultural lore of American life. The study gave rise to a plethora of myths; was the subject of numerous documentaries and fictional plays and film; and led to the institution of bioethical safeguards designed to protect human subjects in research studies. Reverby documents the events leading up to the 1997 public apology rendered to the surviving men and their families by President Clinton and returns us to those most important to remember, the men.

This is a powerful story told in a powerful way. Reverby skillfully bridges the divisions between the facts as known and the mythology that sprang up once knowledge of the study entered the public domain. A massive amount of historical documentation exists on the study worthy of Reverby's prodigious expertise as a historian to capably examine, analyze, and draw conclusions. One of the strengths of this work is her meticulous handling of the data. As an example of how to do and present historical research, this is a gem.

Yet, the importance of this work goes well behind its usefulness as a historical case study. The Tuskegee story is an American tragedy. *Examining Tuskegee: The Infamous Syphilis Study and its Legacy* cogently illuminates the many narratives comprising this horrific chapter in our country's history. It is an examination of the difficult and politically charged areas of race and racism in America, situating them as the core issues in how the study came to be conceptualized, carried out, and continued for 40 years. This book, impressive in its scope and depth, contributes greatly to our understanding of not just the events described but also of racial and social injustice in general.

Jean C. Whelan, PhD, RN
Assistant Adjunct Professor of Nursing
University of Pennsylvania School of Nursing
Philadelphia, PA 19096

Make Room for Daddy: The Journey from Waiting Room to Birthing Room
By Judith Walzer Leavitt
(Chapel Hill: University of North Carolina Press, 2009) (385 pages, $35.00 cloth)

Judith Walzer Leavitt, accomplished childbirth and women's historian, credits an alert archivist, Susan Sacharski of Chicago's Northwestern Memorial Hospital, with the discovery of a large set of "Fathers' Books" that spurred her latest research. The thick notebooks, written from the 1940s to the 1980s, hold fathers' thoughts and feelings as they awaited the birth of their children in hospitals and provide insight into men's birthing experiences as they moved from their exile in waiting rooms, through their gradual admission to labor rooms, then to delivery rooms, and finally into today's birthing rooms. Supporting her focus on "place," the author has organized the book along the four chronologically sequential spaces that defined men's participation in hospital-based births: the waiting room in the 1940s and 1950s, the labor room in the 1960s, and ultimately the delivery and birthing rooms of the 1970s and 1980s. As she began to explore the experience of childbirth from the viewpoint of the previously largely ignored fathers, Leavitt discovered new insights into the themes of privilege, place, and power.

Birth occurred primarily in hospitals during the period of this book, and because "place defines," the very structure and the geography of the hospital itself, contributed significantly to the early intimidation of fathers, who eventually learned to make the spaces less alien and more accommodating (p. 11). The "privilege counts" tenet permeating medical care throughout the ages has traditionally resulted in segregation by both class and race. In the history of childbirth, reform in hospitals was a movement of the privileged, primarily white, middle- or upper-class men; thus this history is limited to them (p. 13). This story also reveals "power shifts." Leavitt has found that the authority that mothers-to-be and their female friends initially held over birth shifted to male physicians in mid-twentieth century. However, the growing presence of fathers led to "a gendered, masculine bonding between male physicians and fathers-to-be" that eventually resulted in decision making becoming more of a shared process, to include the mothers-to-be (p.13). The author concludes that while supporting the mothers who gave birth, fathers also created and defined a historically new domestic role for men.

Leavitt has used multiple examples from popular TV shows of the era, such as *I Love Lucy* in the 1950s and *Happy Days* in the 1980s; articles in women's magazines; and samples from fathers' and mothers' own words to create a highly engaging, readable history, richly illustrated with photographs and cartoons. While the use of popular culture as evidence is entertaining, it is important to remember that the point of entertainment, and of TV sitcoms in particular, is to entertain, and thus the fictional situations surrounding birth in mid-century were often, as they are today, grossly exaggerated. Other sources, such as hospital reports, medical and nursing obstetric texts, journal articles, parents' responses to the author's query, and various oral histories provide a balanced view of the experience of men in childbirth in the twentieth century. While men eventually earned a place at their partners' bedsides for birth, Leavitt recognizes that in the twenty-first century men continue to experience ambivalence when it comes to defining their roles at birth. Her hope is that this research will spur further analysis for a more complete understanding of what it is that women and men and health care providers want out of the birthing experience, and that further analysis will improve the birth outcomes for all.

As a biological and cultural event, childbirth affects and is affected by all involved. The history of childbirth is a study in changing medical practices, but it is also a study of changes in family and social history. Perhaps the greatest contribution of this book is a renewed awareness of the importance of the kinds of questions asked in the pursuit of historical insights. Juxtaposed with prior histories of childbirth, this book is a telling example of the value of questioning previously hidden or ignored aspects of a topic. As Leavitt notes, "the very framing of the questions changes how we tell history and the meaning derived from the historical record" (p. 7).

This book will obviously appeal to those interested in the history of childbirth. It also will be useful to women's historians, social and cultural historians, as well as educators and scholars interested in the process of developing and asking questions of the historical records of the past. Even those involved in the current policy debates about health care reform could be interested in looking at all the stakeholders involved in the care of the family, based on the outcomes revealed through history. The history of childbirth has been examined from midwives', physicians', and women's points of view, but this is the first to address specifically the fathers' experience. This book restores the father to his legitimate place in the story of reproduction in American society.

Sylvia Rinker, RN, PhD
Professor Emerita
Lynchburg College
3641 Ridgecroft Drive
Lynchburg, VA 24503

Under the Radar: Cancer and the Cold War
By Ellen Leopold
(New Brunswick, NJ: Rutgers University Press, 2009) (284 pages, $25.95 cloth)

For Americans, the spirit of hope following the end of the Second World War was followed almost immediately by the advent of the so-called cold war between the two super powers. As tensions escalated, the United States and the Soviet Union worked diligently to further enhance their nuclear arsenals. Fortuitously for the United States, a therapeutic use for nuclear power emerged during these postwar years. Cobalt radiation, developed in the 1950s, was found to be highly effective in controlling cancerous growths, particularly deep-seated tumors. The medical and scientific communities rapidly embraced this new science, which supported the image of American scientific and medical prowess. Through the intersection of the scientific might of nuclear therapy and the helplessness of the people exposed to it, Ellen Leopold delves into the back stories. She pursues the relationship between military and medical nuclear technology—and uncovers a deeply unsettling link between cancer, the cold war, and radiation therapy. This link, Leopold argues, affects the way society thinks about cancer today. Critical understanding of this link is central to framing our current conceptualization of cancer therapeutics, our fear of cancer, and the guilt a cancer diagnosis may produce.

Through a social historiographical framework, Leopold describes how the nuclear scientific community faced a substantial loss of weapons' development funding after the close of the wartime hostilities. Nuclear scientists involved in weapons research then turned to the expanding medical industry to finance their research agenda. Leopold asserts that the medical community, unskilled in nuclear physics yet anxious to be part of the social cachet surrounding all things scientific, were pleased to cooperate. Physicians ventured into the field of cancer radiation therapy without appreciating the science. Treatments were nonuniform, with minimal data on acceptable dose levels. Operators were unevenly trained and machines of were of various strengths. Physicians essentially allowed their patients to become guinea pigs in radiation exposure experiments, without explanation or patients' consent.

Leopold's story was inspired by a young housewife, Irma Natanson, who was diagnosed with breast cancer in 1955. Natanson was one of the first patients treated with cobalt radiation and was left with horrendous burns. In the years that followed, after great suffering as well as significant emotional and financial costs, Natanson sued her radiologist and the hospital. A testament to her strength was that she spoke out at a time when patients, particularly female patients, were invariably intimidated into silence by the powerful mid-century medical establishment.

The argument for linking radiation therapy and the cold war is deftly woven. Leopold explains how private research and development funds were essential in maintaining nuclear research under the guise of treating cancer. Frighteningly, the military's need for human experiments with radiation, although morally unacceptable, could be translated into irradiating terminally ill cancer patients. Since medical authority was unquestioned and patients had little influence over their treatment, the field was wide open for what was, in reality, human radiation experiments. Leopold analyzes the issue of informed consent, as the desperate and the helpless were among those subjected to radiation. This so soon after the Nuremburg trials renders the United States' actions more chilling. She traces the rapid ascendency of radioactive cobalt therapy over radium and X-rays, which exemplified the postwar message of "good" uses for atomic power. Then she describes the awakening of public concern about nuclear safety—which makes for fascinating reading. Typically, the American public of the 1950s trusted their government. The press, too, followed the line of unquestioning support of government ingrained by the war effort and the cold war insularity. The American Medical Association and the American Cancer Society were essentially silent, and cancer patients themselves had no voice. Finally, the Atomic Energy Commission, not the medical establishment, called for reasonable standards of radiation safety.

This highly readable book, thoroughly contextualized in the era of the cold war, covers key material in understanding the scientific and military roles in the evolution of radiation therapy since mid century. Leopold's arguments are well reasoned and supported by extensive notes. Since radiation's discovery just over a hundred years ago, the social effects of radiation therapy have not been analyzed adequately, especially when one appreciates its overarching presence in everyday life and its potential for great harm. This book makes a significant contribution to our understanding of radiation, cancer radiation therapies of mid-twentieth century, and medicine at the height of its paternalistic power. It also introduces us to a powerful heroine, Irma Natanson. This book will serve multiple audiences in the fields of science and the humanities, as well as lay readers interested in understanding the back stories of our society.

Brigid Lusk, PhD, RN
Professor and Chair, School of Nursing and Health Studies
Northern Illinois University
1240 Normal Road
DeKalb, IL 60115

Officer, Nurse, Woman: The Army Nurse Corps in the Vietnam War

By Kara Dixon Vuic
(Baltimore: The Johns Hopkins University Press, 2010) (271 pages, $50.00 hardcover)

Utilizing a feminist paradigm, Kara Dixon Vuic's evocative and unique dissection of the collective gender experiences of Army Nurse Corps officers in the Vietnam War and its aftermath breaks new ground in the history of military nursing. The volume's scholarship, insight, and objectivity were paradoxically both troubling and awe inspiring to me on a personal level. Although I did not serve in the combat theater of the Vietnam War, my period of service did include the Vietnam era. My memories of this tumultuous chapter in our history formed the basis for my subtle sense of unease that soon was mitigated by Vuic's extraordinary level of research and erudition.

The stated purpose of Vuic's opus is to examine the interplay between the U.S. Army's campaign in Vietnam and the ascendant women's movement that occurred almost simultaneously in the late 1960s and early 1970s. The analysis revolves around the philosophical meanings and the conjectural conflict that existed among three different belief systems about Army nurses' roles in that combat theater. The first view characterizing Army Nurse Corps officers' function was that idealized by the Army. The second model of Army nurses' participation was that promoted by feminist theory. And the third, a blend of the first two, was the mixed perception held by those Army nurses who took an active part in the war. The three camps demonstrated substantial discrepancies in outlook with only few points of accord.

Vuic's organization of this treatise coherently explicates the book's thesis. The first chapter focuses on the Army's efforts in this timeframe to recruit nurses using femininity and patriotic duty as key features of the marketing campaign. The second chapter accurately describes Army nurses' career indoctrination, the integration of males and racial minorities into the profession and the Army Nurse Corps, and the milestone achieved when Anna Mae Hays was promoted to brigadier general, a first for an Army nurse. The third chapter highlights education and practice and discusses the rationale for educating Army nurses at the baccalaureate level, namely to support their expanded scope of practice and leadership skills in combat and to facilitate parity with other officers. Chapter 4 draws attention to the part played by femininity and types of uniforms to boost soldiers' morale and to serve as bargaining chips to obtain scarce supplies and equipment. It also elucidates the propagated belief that female nurses upheld nursing and personal hygiene standards in a military unit. Chapter 5 deals with all aspects of marriage, pregnancy, abortion, and contraception in the theater in Southeast Asia. Next, chapter 6 scrutinizes other implications of sexuality in the war zone, studying the novelty of females in combat, the accordance of special treatment for women, the prevalence of sexual harassment, and the crime of rape. One of the only facets of sexuality not covered in this section is the topic of sexually transmitted diseases. Chapter 7 outlines the fundamentally opposing opinions of the nurses' combat participation as articulated by many Vietnam War nurse veterans versus those views presented in Lynda Van Devanter's autobiographical volume, *Home Before Morning: The Story of an Army Nurse in Vietnam*,[1] and ABC television's fictionalized production *China Beach*. These works provoked passionate debate and fiery polemics, and the differing views of the nature of Army nurses' participation reminds us of the validity of the axiom that truth has many facets. The book's final section presents Vuic's summary interpretation of the historical data and reaffirms the expansive significance of the study. The end portions of the publication offer copious notes documenting the researcher's evidence, an interesting essay on her sources, and an ample index.

By far, the positive aspects of Vuic's discourse surpass its flaws. The book offers a solid, coherent case that fully supports the author's thesis. Vuic's scholarship and research are impressive. She demonstrates a remarkable ability to navigate through difficult, highly complicated archives and synthesize the gathered data into meaningful patterns of information. Minor factual errors inevitably crept into the work, such as her reference to Camp Bullis as "Fort Bullis" and the incorrect titling of Spurgeon Neel as the surgeon general. In truth, Neel did serve later as deputy surgeon general but never was nominated to the position of surgeon general. During his first tour in the Vietnam War, he was the United States Military Assistance Command, Vietnam, Surgeon, and senior advisor to General Westmoreland. In his second Vietnam tour, Neel was the commanding general of the 44th Medical Battalion and Surgeon, United States Army, Vietnam. In no way, however, do such small inaccuracies seriously detract from Vuic's scholarly body of research-based knowledge. I found *Officer, Nurse, Woman* quite intriguing. I can unreservedly recommend it as a valuable addition to the literature documenting nurse participation in the Vietnam War.

Mary T. Sarnecky, DNSc, RN
Colonel, Army Nurse Corps (Retired)
Contract Historian
United States Army
Office of the Surgeon General
2856 Cacatua Street
Carlsbad, CA 92009

Note

1. Lynda Van Devanter with Christopher Morgan, *Home Before Morning: The Story of an Army Nurse in Vietnam* (New York: Beaufort Books, 1983).

Moments of Truth in Genetic Medicine
By Susan Lindee
(Baltimore: Johns Hopkins University Press, 2005) (270 pages, $25.00)

The purpose of this excellent book is to "explore . . . the institutions, disciplines, practices and ideas that began to reconfigure human disease in genetic terms" (p. 1) during the years between 1955 and 1975. Calling human cytogenetics a "sleepy subspecialty" (p. 1) in the late 1950s, author Susan Lindee notes the intense interest in the topic a mere ten years later: "by 1966, most U.S. states had elaborate neonatal testing programs created by legislators intrigued by . . . [some tests] and clamoring for more" (p. 1). Using substantial primary and secondary sources, the book is "a study of a period of transformation in one of the most high-profile biomedical fields of the late twentieth century. . . . At another level, it is a study of the realization of an idea. The idea is that all human disease is a genetic phenomenon subject to technological control" (p. 2). And, finally, it is "a study of the patchwork qualities of knowing" (p. 2), as the title, *Moments of Truth*, also suggests.

After a thorough and fascinating introductory chapter, Lindee presents five chapters, each representing critical steps in the rise of genetic medicine, or case studies, if you will. The first of these, chapter 2, "Babies Blood, Phenylketonurea and the Rise of Public Health Genetics," documents the first breakthrough, or moment of truth, in which improper phenylalanine metabolism is identified as the cause of mental retardation in about "one in fifteen thousand neonates in the United States" (p. 28). The third chapter, "Provenance and the Pedigree, Victor McKusick's Field Work with the Pennsylvania Amish," explores the efforts of one researcher to connect genetic findings in a carefully tended social network in the early 1960s.

In chapter 4, "Squashed Spiders, Standardizing the Human Chromosome and other Unruly Things," Lindee tracks the development of the field of human cytogenetics. "The subjects of this interest were twenty-four X-shaped objects, visible in the nucleus of the cell only during certain phases of cell division: the twenty-two pairs of autosomes and the two sex chromosomes, X and Y. These were accurately counted only in 1956 [due to improved lab equipment] and not conclusively distinguished from each other until the 1970s" (p. 92), when standardization of nomenclature occurred due to the monumental efforts of scientists. In chapter 5, "Two Peas in a Pod, Twin Science and the Rise of Human Behavior Genetics," twins are presented as the golden opportunity to see genetics in action, so to speak; to identify the line between nature and nurture, especially among twins separated at birth. In chapter 6, "Jewish Genes, History, Emotion, and Familial Dysautonomia," the author discusses familial dysautonomia as a classic genetic disease among Ashkenazi Jews that has inspired significant parental and social support group activity.

In her concluding chapter, Lindee uses cancer to make a central point: "What does it mean to say cancer is a genetic disease? . . . It can mean that cancer cells have disordered chromosomes . . . [and/or] it can mean that there is a higher risk of cancer in some individuals because they are genetically vulnerable" (pp. 190–191). She goes on to point out that "all disease is not any one thing" (p. 192). But seeing disease as genetic enables the marketplace to identify "small pieces of nature that can be patented, hoarded, distributed, mass-produced and isolated. . . . They are the right disease vectors for the early twenty-first century in the developed world" (p. 192).

Each chapter exemplifies Lindee's social history argument that breakthroughs occur due to the combined and happenstance efforts of parents, physicians, social advocates, laboratory advances, community resources, legislators, researchers, and many others; at some point, when enough information collects around a topic, a "moment of truth" occurs. In some sense, it reminds me of the current popular notion of "a tipping point" but at a much higher intellectual level. The book is beautifully written, thoroughly researched, and logically constructed. Although it covers a topic of dense content, it reads easily and entertainingly. I highly recommend it as fascinating reading for anyone with an interest in the field of genetics and for anyone wanting to see how history should be done.

Ellen D. Baer, PhD, FAAN
Professor Emerita of Nursing
University of Pennsylvania
732 Village Rd.
North Palm Beach, FL 33408

Observing Bioethics

By Renée C. Fox and Judith P. Swazey
(New York: Oxford University Press, 2008) (388 pages, $45.00 cloth)

In *Observing Bioethics*, two world-renowned social scientists, Renée C. Fox (sociologist) and Judith P. Swazey (historian), join forces to present their ethnographic views on the evolutionary field of bioethics. Commonly known as the "team of two," the authors quickly point out that they are not, in fact, bioethicists, nor are they engaged in bioethical research or clinical practice related to bioethics. They are, however, genuinely concerned with the field's ability to address the salient values, beliefs, and norms central to its professional domain and the influence that bioethics has had on what philosopher-bioethicist Daniel Callahan called the larger moral struggles of our society. Fox and Swazey received funding from the National Science Foundation in the late 1990s to interview forty-four first- and second-generation figures—the majority of whom were involved in the development of American bioethics—to ascertain their diverse accounts on the origins of the field. They also rely heavily on their own participant observations, including national and international involvement in bioethics-related conferences and working groups, as well as a comprehensive collection of media accounts, court decisions, and other substantive materials. Indeed, they have done their homework, and leave no doubt of their thoroughness and dedication to their cause.

The authors conducted face-to-face semi-structured interviews with iconic leaders in bioethics ranging from moral theologians to analytical philosophers and, in particular, the likes of Ruth Macklin and Ruth Faden. There are very few women bioethicists in the country who have significantly advanced the field as much as these two women. Both are impressive in their own right on topics of informed consent, social justice, and global health. Although the valued contributions of Macklin and Faden were discussed, the authors missed a unique opportunity to shed more light on their feminist perspective, including their professional advancement within the nascent field of bioethics and how their voices have shaped the intellectual, social, and cultural bioethics agenda. That being said, the author masterfully articulate the sentinel events that permeated the *discourse* of bioethics in its formative years, including events such as the Nazi Doctor's Trial; Henry K. Beecher's revelations on human subject abuses in research and his landmark publication in the *New England Journal of*

Medicine in 1966;[1] Willowbrook; Principalism; the Belmont Report; the promulgation of the Hastings Center Report; and the creation of Dolly, the cloned sheep.

The "Inauguration of the Kennedy Institute of Ethics" chapter was especially poignant because of the recent loss of both Senator Edward Kennedy and Eunice Kennedy Shriver. Fox and Swazey remind us of the political savoir faire so often needed to champion socially conscience issues and address them within the public domain. At the Kennedy Symposium in 1971, the Kennedys set the stage for a broader interdisciplinary forum on ethical issues of procreation, disabilities, genetics and disease, and the caring needs required for the most vulnerable among us. To this day, these issues remain a central focus of bioethical scholarship, and in some part, a true testament to their ability to give voice to the voiceless, raise considerable awareness about ethical issues important to various stakeholders, and address the value of ethics education.

A scholarly field of inquiry cannot grow or sustain itself without critical self-reflection or introspection of its core values and beliefs. At the very least, it must accommodate diversity of thought and argumentative discourse. Every student and scholar of bioethics knows the ethical principles outlined in The Belmont Report, and the classic book, *Principles of Biomedical Ethics*, now it its sixth edition, by Tom L. Beauchamp and James Childress.[2] This work has guided clinical and research ethics for over 25 years. As such, Fox and Swazey question why American bioethics has not done more to reflect on its own principles and modify them accordingly.

The last chapter of the book, "The Coming of the Culture Wars to American Bioethics," is particularly relevant as the polarization of the field of bioethics—conservative versus liberal—reflects the national dialogue on complex moral questions regarding stem cell research, cloning, human reproduction, and more recently, health care reform. The authors seek to understand if bioethicists can disentangle themselves from the polarization and politicization surrounding bioethical questions of importance to society and whether they can clearly separate scholarship from politics. The discussion begs one to reflect on the purpose of bioethics: is it a field meant solely for academic scholarship or is political advocacy a role it cannot escape?

Fox and Swazey's book is truly about "Celebrating the 'Birth of Bioethics' and Its 'Pioneers.'" It is well constructed, informative, and a fine contribution to bioethics.

CONNIE M. ULRICH, PhD, RN
Associate Professor of Bioethics and Nursing
University of Pennsylvania School of Nursing
418 Curie Blvd.
Philadelphia, PA 19104

Notes

1. Henry K. Beecher, "Ethics and Clinical Research," *The New England Journal of Medicine* 274 (1966): 1354–60.

2. Tom L. Beauchamp and James Childress, *Principles of Biomedical Ethics*, 6th ed. (Oxford: Oxford University Press, 2009).

The Adelaide Hospital School of Nursing 1859–2009: A Commemorative History

By Gerard M. Fealy
(Dublin, Ireland: The Columba Press, 2009) (148 pages, 29.99€, cloth)

What is the nature of "commemorative" history? What are the politics involved in its production, and what are the conventions of such commemoratives? Should such a history be critiqued differently than any other? These are questions of concern when reading *The Adelaide Hospital School of Nursing 1859–2009: A Commemorative History*, by Gerard Fealy.

Fealy is an associate professor of nursing at University College Dublin School of Nursing, Midwifery and Health Systems. His previously published A *History of Apprenticeship Nurse Training in Ireland* is a helpful companion piece to this work as a source to clarify the nature of apprentice-style nurse training.[1] The Adelaide Hospital School of Nursing is historically important in that it "was the first nurse training school for lay women in Ireland" (p. 129). Fealy lays out the school's trajectory in a well-written, accessible manner, starting with its conception and tracking ups and downs through the present day culminating in a partnership with Trinity College Dublin School of Nursing and Midwifery. The book's chapters, with the exception of the last, address the school's history in blocks of time from ten to thirty years. Sometimes the book reads more like a history of nursing at the Adelaide Hospital rather than the development of the nursing school, perhaps because the school and hospital were so intimately intertwined, with limited "education" in the early days of the school when tuition was directly tied to providing patient care.

A number of questions arise as one reads the text. How was this "peculiar" school with its "Protestant students only" (p. 9) rule perceived in a national context? With little support for his claim, Fealy states that the "school developed a national reputation as a place for training nurses who excelled in their standards of nursing" (p. 129). The commentary would be enhanced by sources outside of the school, such as, contemporaneous newspaper reports. Were the comments in these sources positive and supportive or otherwise? Who owned these newspapers? What was it like to be an institution dedicated to educating a particular religious minority when that minority had political power, and then what was the experience when that power source was no longer in place? How was the school viewed by the Catholic majority? The political issues confronting Ireland and its institutions in the last 150 years are a very limited and carefully couched part of this presentation. Knowing the political context is important to understanding of the impact of the school.

What exactly was the "Adelaide ethos" (p. 112)? Fealy seems to skirt this idea until well into the book. And then it is all implied with distancing language. What is meant by "preservation of the Protestant ethic" and "different ethical approaches" (p. 113)? Was the disharmony that occurred with the Adelaide's merge to form Tallaght Hospital based on more than whether the institution provided abortions? For non-Irish readers, it would help to provide the context. What are/were the ethical impositions placed on other hospitals by the Catholic Church? What is meant by "liberal tradition" (p. 115)? Is privacy between patient and physician not available in Catholic institutions in Ireland? And how did these issues affect the students at the school? Fealy makes the assumption that the reader can provide these answers.

Since this is a history of a school, a discussion of the evolving curriculum would be helpful. What was important to teach? When were topics introduced? This kind of information would say something about the era, about the institution, and about its philosophy. While a list is given for curricular topics proscribed by the state in 1920, what did the topics look like when they were translated by Adelaide tutors into an educational experience? A deeper analysis of the rules and regulations for probationers would help illuminate the culture of the organization. The discussion does get richer when Fealy addresses training in the 1950s to 1980s, where prime student educational experience based on oral history is presented.

And who were the students at this school? We know that they were Protestant, but were diaries available to get perspective from probationers' points of view? It would be interesting to know what the earlier students thought of the training, and what they thought of their school. Did those affiliated with the school have a sense of superiority because of they were Protestant? Did the charitable nature of the hospital motivate students to attend the school? Were they actually from the middle classes as was the aim of the school?

The oddities in the book include the date range given in the title (*The Adelaide Hospital School of Nursing 1859–2009*). In the body of the text it appears the school was conceptualized in 1858 but never came to fruition until 1861. The start date of 1859 is never clearly explained. In addition, the last chapter appears to have been written for another purpose, giving a brief overview of the school's history, a view of the Adelaide nurse focusing on graduates from the 1970s and 1980s, and current-day goals of the Adelaide Hospital Society.

Although there is a tradition of nursing school histories in the United States, not many are written by nurse historians. This book makes a contribution in that it is the first published work focusing on the history of a school of nursing in Ireland. What is presented is carefully documented with primary sources of evidence drawn from the Adelaide Hospital Archives housed at Trinity College Dublin, the Adelaide Nurses' League Archives, oral histories provide by the Meath Foundation, and documentary materials from Sunbeam House Services.

Ann Marie Walsh Brennan, RN, PhD
Practice Assistant Professor
University of Pennsylvania
School of Nursing
418 Curie Boulevard
Philadelphia, PA 19104–4217

Note

1. Gerard Fealy, A *History of Apprenticeship Nurse Training in Ireland* (London: Routledge, 2006).

NEW DISSERTATIONS

Compiled for the *Nursing History Review* by Jonathon Erlen, PhD, History of Medicine Librarian, Health Sciences Library System, and Assistant Professor, Graduate School of Public Health at the University of Pittsburgh, Pittsburgh, Pennsylvania. These dissertations can be obtained through Proquest Dissertations.

Carol Silverberg, "IQ Testing and Tracking: The History of Scientific Racism in the American Public Schools: 1890–1924," 2008 PhD dissertation, University of Nevada, Reno (Publication Number: AAT 3311920).

Hilary A. Smith, "Foot Qi: History of a Chinese Medical Disorder," 2008 PhD dissertation, University of Pennsylvania (Publication Number: AAT 3309509).

Mary Glennon Okin, "'Madwomen' in Quebec: An Analysis of the Recurring Themes in the Reasons for Women's Committal to Beauport, 1894–1940," 2008 PhD dissertation, The University of Maine (Publication Number: AAT 3309231).

Christi Keating Sumich, "Soul-sick Stomachs, Distempered Bodies, and Divine Physicians: Morality and the Growth of the English Medical Profession," 2008 PhD dissertation, Tulane University (Publication Number: AAT 3310077).

Kathleen L. Wessels-Cruz, "A History of Drug Regulation in the United States 1902–2008: Effects on Women's Health," 2008 EdD dissertation, Dowling College (Publication Number: AAT 3313053).

Christina Kathryn Fradelos, "The Last Desperate Cure: Electrical Brain Stimulation and its Controversial Beginnings," 2008 PhD dissertation, The University of Chicago (Publication Number: AAT 3309034).

Deborah I. Levine, "Managing American Bodies: Diet, Nutrition, and Obesity in America, 1840–1920," 2008 PhD dissertation, Harvard University (Publication Number: AAT 3312441).

Louis Paul (Gus) Hill, "Understanding Indigenous Canadian Traditional Health and Healing," 2008 PhD dissertation, Wilfrid Laurier University, Canada (Publication Number: AAT NR38005).

Jeannine Uribe, "Nurses, Philanthropies, and Governments: The Public Mission of Chilean Nursing 1900–1945," 2008 PhD dissertation, University of Pennsylvania (Publication Number: AAT 3309517).

Michael Stobbe, "The Surgeon General and the Bully Pulpit," 2008 DrPH dissertation, The University of North Carolina at Chapel Hill (Publication Number: AAT 3304293).

Jacqueline Doreen Wright, "Understanding the Decline in Prevalence of Hypertension in U.S. Adults between 1976–1980 and 1999–2002," 2008 DrPH dissertation, The University of North Carolina at Chapel Hill (Publication Number: AAT 3304306).

Cristina Hanganu-Bresch, "Faces of Depression: A Study of Antidepressant Advertisements in the American and British Journals of Psychiatry, 1960–2004," 2008 PhD dissertation, University of Minnesota (Publication Number: AAT 3313444).

Diane M. O'Heron, "Renunciation and Resistance: Confessions of the Alcoholic and Addicted Experience in the 19th and 20th centuries," 2008 PhD dissertation, State University of New York at Binghamton (Publication Number: AAT 3310690).

Ellen R. Boucher, "'An Imperial Investment': British State-Assisted Child Emigration to Australia and Southern Rhodesia, 1869–1967," 2008 PhD dissertation, Columbia University (Publication Number: AAT 3317532).

Mary C, Miles, "Democracy Within: Religious Outsiders and the Americanization of Psychoanalysis during and after World War II," 2008 PhD dissertation, Cornell University (Publication Number: AAT 3317448).

David Joseph Caruso, "War and Knowledge Production: American Military Medicine, 1898 to 1918," 2008 PhD dissertation, Cornell University (Publication Number: AAT 3317472).

David L. Ferro, "Selling Science in the Colonial American Newspaper: How the Middle Colonial American General Periodical Represented Nature, Philosophy, Medicine, and Technology, 1728–1765," 2001 PhD dissertation, Virginia Polytechnic Institute and State University (Publication Number: AAT 3313206).

Matthew Lavine, "A Cultural History of Radiation and Radioactivity in the United States, 1895–1945," 2008 PhD dissertation, The University of Wisconsin–Madison (Publication Number: AAT 3314335).

Stephen E. Wald, "Minds Divided: Science, Spirituality, and the Split Brain in American Thought," 2008 PhD dissertation, The University of Wisconsin–Madison (Publication Number: AAT 3314264).

Marian Moser Jones, "Confronting Calamity: The American Red Cross and the Politics of Disaster Relief, 1881–1939," 2008 PhD dissertation, Columbia University (Publication Number: AAT 3317567).

Thomas P. Jundt, "The Origins of the Environmental Movement," 2008 PhD dissertation, Brown University (Publication Number: AAT 3318335).

Crispin Robert Claude Barker, "From Atom Bomb to the 'Genetic Time Bomb': Telomeres, Aging, and Cancer in the Era of Molecular Biology," 2008 PhD dissertation, Yale University (Publication Number: AAT 3317061).

Manuella Meyer, "Enlightened Reason in the Tropics: Madness, Society and the State in Rio de Janeiro, Brazil, 1808–1930," 2008 PhD dissertation, Yale University (Publication Number: AAT 3317176).

Todd Michael Olszewski, "Cholesterol: A Scientific, Medical, and Social History, 1908–1962," 2008 PhD dissertation, Yale University (Publication Number: AAT 3317192).

Deborah Ann Davidson, "The Emergence of Hospital Protocols for Perinatal Loss, 1950–2000," 2007 PhD dissertation, York University (Canada) (Publication Number: AAT NR39000).

Christopher R. Freed, "Doctors and Drunks: Addiction Medicine and Addiction Psychiatry in America," 2008 PhD dissertation, City University of New York (Publication Number: AAT 3311204).

Hui Liu, "The Times They Are a Changin': Marital Status and Health Differentials from the 1970s to the 2000s," 2008 PhD dissertation, The University of Texas at Austin (Publication Number: AAT 3315246).

Linda K. Walline, "The Life of Patricia Morin: A Nursing Dean," 2008 PhD dissertation, The University of Nebraska–Lincoln (Publication Number: AAT 3311305).

Marlene Frances Cimons, "The Medicalization of Menopause: Framing Media Messages in the Twentieth Century," 2008 PhD dissertation, University of Maryland, College Park (Publication Number: AAT 3315435).

Joseph A. Provenzano, Jr., "Federal Nurse Training Legislation: A Study in Legislative Opportunity," 2008 PhD dissertation, The American University (Publication Number: AAT 3323600).

Stephen Wills Murphy, "'It Is a Sacred Duty to Abstain': The Organizational, Biblical, Theological, and Practical Roots of the American Temperance Society, 1814–1830," 2008 PhD dissertation, University of Virginia (Publication Number: AAT 3322517).

Jessica Lynn Grogan, "A Cultural History of the Humanistic Psychology Movement in America," 2008 PhD dissertation, The University of Texas at Austin (Publication Number: AAT 3311487).

Mie Nakachi, "Replacing the Dead: The Politics of Reproduction in the Postwar Soviet Union, 1944–1955," 2008 PhD dissertation, The University of Chicago (Publication Number: AAT 3322619).

Stephen Inrig, "In a Place So Ordinary: North Carolina and the Problem of AIDS, 1981–1997," 2007 PhD dissertation, Duke University (Publication Number: AAT 3321835).

Rob Wilson, "The Disease of Fear and the Fear of Disease: Cholera and Yellow Fever in the Mississippi Valley," 2008 PhD dissertation, Saint Louis University (Publication Number: AAT 3324235).

Sara Maria Sliter-Hays, "Narratives and Rhetoric: Persuasion in Doctors' Writings about the Summer Complaint, 1883–1939," 2008 PhD dissertation, The University of Texas at Austin (Publication Number: AAT 3329869).

Sarah L. Russo, "Women's Self-writing and Medical Science: Harriet Martineau, Charlotte Brontë, Harriet Jacobs, and Elizabeth Stoddard," 2008 PhD dissertation, Syracuse University (Publication Number: AAT 3323081).

Sarah Jo Lock, "The People in the Neighborhood: Samaritans and Saviors in Middle-Class Women's Social Settlement Writings, 1895–1914," 2008 PhD dissertation, Texas Christian University (Publication Number: AAT 3324871).

Donna A. Patterson, "Expanding Professional Horizons: Female Pharmacists in Twentieth-Century Dakar, Senegal," 2008 PhD dissertation, Indiana University (Publication Number: AAT 3319926).

Jonathan C, Bergman, "The Shape of Disaster and the Universe of Relief: A Social History of Disaster Relief and the 'Hurricane of '38,' Suffolk County, Long Island, New York, 1938–1941," 2008 PhD dissertation, State University of New York at Buffalo (Publication Number: AAT 3320427).

Audra R. Jennings, "With Minds Fixed on the Horrors of War: Liberalism and Disability Activism, 1940–1960," 2008 PhD dissertation, Ohio State University (Publication Number: AAT 3325734).

Kazuhiro Oharazek, "Japanese Prostitutes in the Pacific Northwest, 1887–1920," 2008 PhD dissertation, State University of New York at Binghamton (Publication Number: AAT 3320155).

Diana T. Reinhard, "Bodies on Display: Gender, Sexuality, and the Visual Culture of American Medicine, 1870–1920," 2008 PhD dissertation, Temple University (Publication Number: AAT 3326372).

Tuba Inci Agartan, "Turkish Health System in Transition: Historical Background and Reform Experience," 2008 PhD dissertation, State University of New York at Binghamton (Publication Number: AAT 3320170).

Laura S. Taylor, "The National Smallpox Vaccination Program: Opinion Leaders Perceptions of State Health Department Roles and Responsibilities during the

Vaccination Initiative," 2008 PhD dissertation, Temple University (Publication Number: AAT 3326604).

Sujani Reddy, "Women on the Move: A History of Indian Nurse Migration to the United States," 2008 PhD dissertation, New York University (Publication Number: AAT 3330167).

Patricia Dockman Anderson, "'By Legal or Moral Suasion Let Us Put It Away': Temperance in Baltimore, 1829–1870," 2008 PhD dissertation, University of Delaware (Publication Number: AAT 3329783).

Megan Elizabeth Birk, "Alone in the Country: Rural Social Welfare for Dependent Children, 1865–1920," 2008 PhD dissertation, Purdue University (Publication Number: AAT 3330230).

Suzanne Elizabeth Evans, "Parental Eugenics: Congenitally Anomalous Newborns and the Continuing Debate Over Selective Non-treatment and Neonatal Euthanasia in the United States, 1915–2008," 2008 PhD dissertation, University of California (Publication Number: AAT 3331590).

Sarah Frances Rose, "No Right to Be Idle: The Invention of Disability, 1850–1930," 2008 PhD dissertation, University of Illinois at Chicago (Publication Number: AAT 3327434).

Katherine Leonard Turner, "Good Food for Little Money: Food and Cooking among Urban Working-Class Americans, 1875–1930," 2008 PhD dissertation, University of Delaware (Publication Number: AAT 3324472).

EunJeong Ma, "Medicine in the Making in Post-Colonial Korea (1948–2006)," 2008 PhD dissertation, Cornell University (Publication Number: AAT 3329982).

Dominique Avril Tobbell, "Pharmaceutical Networks: The Political Economy of Drug Development in the United States, 1945–1980," 2008 PhD dissertation, University of Pennsylvania (Publication Number: AAT 3328664).

Brian Rostron, "Convergence and Discontinuities: Trends in Mortality by Cause in Developed Countries, 1950–2000," 2008 PhD dissertation, University of California, Berkeley (Publication Number: AAT 3331771).

Neel Ahuja, "Cultures of Quarantine: Race, U.S. Empire, and the Biomedical Discourse of National Security, 1893–1960," 2008 PhD dissertation, University of California, San Diego (Publication Number: AAT 3330845).

Meredith B. Linn, "From Typhus to Tuberculosis and Fractures In Between: A Visceral Historical Archaeology of Irish Immigrant Life in New York City 1845–1870," 2008 PhD dissertation, Columbia University (Publication Number: AAT 3333487).

Howard Philip Padw, "Narcotics vs. the Nation: The Culture and Politics of Opiate Control in Britain and France, 1821–1926," 2008 PhD dissertation, University of California, Los Angeles (Publication Number: AAT 3332550).

Assefa B. Negwo, "Church-based Healing and the State in Ethiopia, 1900–1980," 2008 PhD dissertation, Emory University (Publication Number: AAT 3332333).

Michael K. Heaney, "Uncounted Costs: The Civil War's Impact on an Infantry Company's Men and Their Families," 2008 PhD dissertation, Rutgers University (Publication Number: AAT 3335534).

Melissa Norelle Stein, "Embodying Race: Gender, Sex, and the Sciences of Difference, 1830–1934," 2008 PhD dissertation, Rutgers University (Publication Number: AAT 3335559).

Michael Yudell, "Making Race: Biology and the Evolution of the Race Concept in 20th-century American Thought," 2008 PhD dissertation, Columbia University (Publication Number: AAT 3333492).

Concha German Bes, "History of the Institutionalisation of the University Degree in Nursing: An Analysis under a Gender Perspective," 2006 Dr dissertation, Universidad Complutense de Madrid, Spain (Publication Number: AAT 3333983).

Kathy Hille, "Veblen on Medicine: A Sociological Analysis of the Cultural and Organizational Development of Medicine as a Social Institution, "2008 PhD dissertation, Texas A&M University (Publication Number: AAT 3333686).

Susan Parry, "Power Shifts: How Patient Activism Shapes the Practice of Medicine," 2008 PhD dissertation, University of Minnesota (Publication Number: AAT 3336424).

Carlina de la Cova, "Silent Voices of the Destitute: An Analysis of African American and Euro-American Health during the Nineteenth Century," 2008 PhD dissertation, Indiana University (Publication Number: AAT 3331240).

Emily A. Berry, "From Criminals to Caretakers: The Salvation Army in India, 1882–1914," 2008 PhD dissertation, Northeastern University (Publication Number: AAT 3336477).

Deirdre Benia Cooper Owens, "'Courageous Negro servitor' and Laboring Irish bodies: An Examination of Antebellum-Era Modern American Gynecology," 2008 PhD dissertation, University of California, Los Angeles (Publication Number: AAT 3335952).

David Hood, "The Homeless and Reformers: Negotiating Progress in the Upper Streets of Halifax, 1890–1914," 2008 PhD dissertation, Carleton University, Canada (Publication Number: AAT NR43896).

Jonathan David Hagood, "Cells in the Body Politic: Physicians, Social Medicine, and Public Health in Peronist Argentina," 2008 PhD dissertation, University of California, Davis (Publication Number: AAT 3336263).

Michael K. Rosenow, "Injuries to All: The Rituals of Dying and the Politics of Death among United States Workers, 1877–1910," 2008 PhD dissertation, University of Illinois at Urbana-Champaign (Publication Number: AAT 3337899).

Michael B. Guenther, "Enlightened Pursuits: Science and Civic Culture in Anglo-America, 1730–1760," 2008 PhD dissertation, Northwestern University (Publication Number: AAT 3336448).

Heather L. Moran, "Stretcher Bearers and Surgeons: Canadian Front-Line Medicine during the First World War, 1914–1918," 2008 PhD dissertation, The University of Western Ontario, Canada (Publication Number: AAT NR43077).

Eduardo J. Gomez, "Responding to Contested Epidemics: Democracy, International Pressures, and the Civic Sources of Institutional Change in the United States and Brazil," 2008 PhD dissertation, Brown University (Publication Number: AAT 3335657).

Robyn Olson, "The Politics of Water Fluoridation from a Problem Definition Perspective," 2008 PhD dissertation, Northeastern University (Publication Number: AAT 3331233).

Margaret Regensburg, "The Religious Sisters of the Good Shepherd and the Professionalization of Social Work," 2007 PhD dissertation, State University of New York at Stony Brook (Publication Number: AAT 3337604).

Rebecca J. Culyba, "Classification and the Social Construction of Disease in Medical Systems: A Historical Comparison of Syphilis and HIV/AIDS in the United States," 2008 PhD dissertation, Northwestern University (Publication Number: AAT 3336513).

Jin-Kyung Park, "Corporeal Colonialism: Medicine, Reproduction, and Race in Colonial Korea," 2008 PhD dissertation, University of Illinois at Urbana-Champaign (Publication Number: AAT 3337881).

John M. Nemecek, "The Vaccines for Children Program: A Decade Later," 2008 PhD dissertation, Walden University (Publication Number: AAT 3336675).

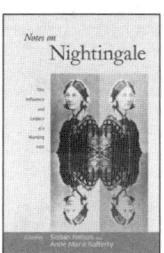

NOTES ON NIGHTINGALE
The Influence and Legacy of a Nursing Icon
EDITED BY SIOBAN NELSON AND ANNE MARIE RAFFERTY

"*Notes on Nightingale* is an extraordinary achievement, bringing together some of the world's most eminent Nightingale scholars. It explodes myths, develops sophisticated lines of analysis, and reveals the full range of achievement of one of the world's most iconic figures."
—CHRISTINE HALLETT, DIRECTOR, THE UK CENTRE FOR THE HISTORY OF NURSING AND MIDWIFERY
$18.95 paper | AN ILR PRESS BOOK | THE CULTURE AND POLITICS OF HEALTH CARE WORK

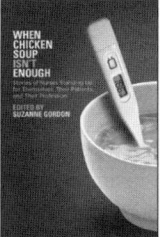

WHEN CHICKEN SOUP ISN'T ENOUGH
Stories of Nurses Standing Up for Themselves, Their Patients, and Their Profession
SUZANNE GORDON

"*When Chicken Soup Isn't Enough* is an excellent collection capturing the real work done by nurses. It demonstrates that the triumphs and struggles of nurses are universal."
—KATHLEEN BURKE, RN-BC, BSN, UCSF MEDICAL CENTER
$24.95 cloth | AN ILR PRESS BOOK | THE CULTURE AND POLITICS OF HEALTH CARE WORK

CORNELL UNIVERSITY PRESS
www.cornellpress.cornell.edu

American Nursing
A History of Knowledge, Authority, and the Meaning of Work

Patricia D'Antonio

Narrating the experiences of nurses, Patricia D'Antonio captures the possibilities, power, and problems inherent in the different ways women defined their work and lived their lives.

"D'Antonio's argument will upend many of the standard beliefs about nursing and its history. She stays sensitive to the psychological and cultural tropes and debates while demonstrating a wildly sophisticated historical imagination and scholarly apparatus. This will become *the* book on the history of nursing."
—Susan M. Reverby, Wellesley College
$30.00 paperback

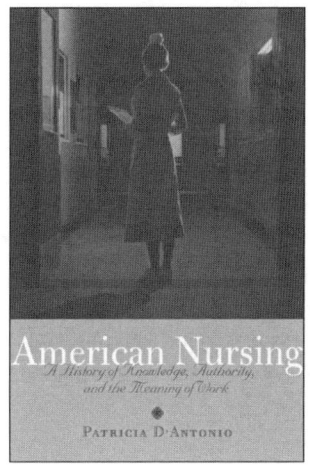

The Johns Hopkins University Press
1-800-537-5487 • press.jhu.edu

Teaching Cultural Competence in Nursing and Health Care
Second Edition

Marianne Jeffreys, EdD, RN

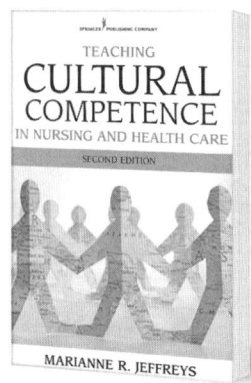

Newly updated and revised, this book presents ready-to-use materials for planning, implementing, and evaluating cultural competence strategies and programs. Users will learn to identify the needs of diverse constituents, evaluate outcomes, prevent multicultural-related workplace conflict, and much more. Complete with vignettes, case exemplars, illustrations, and assessment tools, this book is required reading for those working in academic settings, health care institutions, employee education, and nursing and health care organizations and associations.

Key Features:

- Offers a wide selection of educational activities and techniques for diverse learners
- Presents guidelines for helping educators, students, and professionals to maximize strengths, minimize weaknesses, and facilitate success
- Describes toolkit questionnaires for measuring and evaluating cultural learning and performance
- Provides guidelines for employee orientation programs to achieve cultural competence in the workplace

The Digital Cultural Competence Education Resource Toolkit:

Offering a wealth of hands-on, user-friendly tools, this kit provides specialized resources to measure cultural competence for all levels and settings-both academic and professional. This toolkit incorporates the 7 essential steps toward achieving cultural competence, and contains numerous evaluation and assessment tools, data sheets, and much more!

June 2010 · 424 pp · Paperback · 978-0-8261-1787-8

---

11 West 42nd Street, New York, NY 10036-8002 • Fax: 212-941-7842
Order Toll-Free: 877-687-7476 • Order Online: www.springerpub.com

SPRINGER PUBLISHING COMPANY

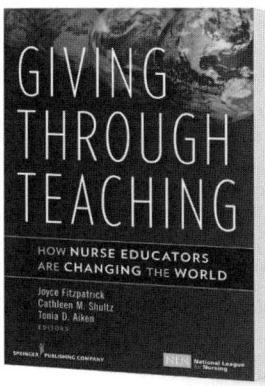

Giving Through Teaching
How Nurse Educators Are Changing the World

Joyce Fitzpatrick, PhD, RN, FAAN
Cathleen Shultz, PhD, RN, CNE, FAAN
Tonia Aiken, JD, RN

This book celebrates the remarkable stories of nurse educators from around the globe. The volume editors have gathered an extensive and compelling body of stories from more than 70 nurse educators, detailing their professional and personal experiences-their goals, challenges, and tremendous breakthroughs in the field.

A major component of the book is to profile the international work of US educators. In doing so, the volume showcases the exciting diversity of the nursing profession itself. This collection of stories will quickly become an inspiration for nurse educators everywhere.

Key topics include:

- Disaster nursing, including stories by nurses working during Hurricane Katrina, in Iraq, and other disaster-stricken areas
- Global- and US-based education partnerships, with stories of nurses working to improve schools, hospitals, and communities around the world
- Nurse philanthropy and the stories of nurses' personal philanthropic and fundraising initiatives
- And much more!

June 2010 · 262 pp · Paperback · 978-0-8261-1862-2

---

11 West 42nd Street, New York, NY 10036-8002 • Fax: 212-941-7842
Order Toll-Free: 877-687-7476 • Order Online: www.springerpub.com

Subscription Order Form

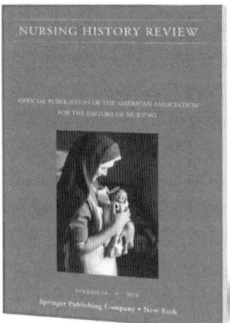

Official Journal of the American Association for the History of Nursing

Editor:
Patricia D'Antonio

❏ **Yes! Start my subscription to *Nursing History Review* with the current issue.**

	Individuals	Institutions
Print	❏ $90	❏ $90
Online	❏ $300	❏ $300
Print and Online	❏ $300	❏ $300

Outside the United States please add $40.

Nursing History Review, an annual peer-reviewed publication, is a showcase for the most significant current research on nursing and the health care history. Contributors include national and international scholars who represent many different disciplinary backgrounds.

Subscribe to the online edition and receive access to all back issues!

International subscriptions are also available. Please visit www.springerpub.com/nhr for more information.

4 Easy Ways to Order
- Web: www.springerpub.com
- Toll Free Phone: 1-877-687-7476
- Fax This Form: 212-941-7842
- Mail this form to address below

❏ Start my subscription to **Nursing History Review**

Checks or International Money Orders must be in U.S. dollars drawn on a U.S. bank made payable to Springer Publishing Company. All prices are subject to change, and are slightly higher outside the U.S.

Check or money order enclosed: $ _____ payable to Springer Publishing Company

Charge to: ❏ Visa ❏ MasterCard ❏ American Express ❏ Discover

Card No. _____ Exp. date _____

Signature _____

Name _____

Institution _____

Address _____

City _____ State _____ Zip _____

Telephone _____ E-mail _____

By providing us with your e-mail address, you agree to receive occasional book and journal announcements. You may unsubscribe at any time.

SPRINGER PUBLISHING COMPANY
11 West 42nd Street, 15th floor, New York, NY 10036